# The Sorcerer's Apprentice

# The Sorcerer's Apprentice

## How Medical Imaging Is Changing Health Care

Bruce J. Hillman, MD

*Editor-in-Chief*
*Journal of the American College of Radiology*
*Theodore E. Keats Professor of Radiology*
*Professor of Public Health Sciences*
*University of Virginia*
*Charlottesville, Virginia*

Jeff C. Goldsmith, PhD

*President, Health Futures, Inc.*
*Associate Professor of Public Health Sciences*
*University of Virginia*
*Charlottesville, Virginia*

OXFORD
UNIVERSITY PRESS

2011

## OXFORD
UNIVERSITY PRESS

Oxford University Press, Inc., publishes works that further
Oxford University's objective of excellence
in research, scholarship, and education.

Oxford  New York
Auckland   Cape Town   Dar es Salaam   Hong Kong   Karachi
Kuala Lumpur   Madrid   Melbourne   Mexico City   Nairobi
New Delhi   Shanghai   Taipei   Toronto

With offices in
Argentina   Austria   Brazil   Chile   Czech Republic   France   Greece
Guatemala   Hungary   Italy   Japan   Poland   Portugal   Singapore
South Korea   Switzerland   Thailand   Turkey   Ukraine   Vietnam

Copyright © 2011 by Oxford University Press, Inc.

Published by Oxford University Press, Inc.
198 Madison Avenue, New York, New York 10016
www.oup.com

Oxford is a registered trademark of Oxford University Press.

Library of Congress Cataloging-in-Publication Data

Hillman, Bruce J.
The sorcerer's apprentice : how medical imaging is changing health care / Bruce J. Hillman, Jeff C. Goldsmith.
p. ; cm.
Includes bibliographical references.
ISBN 978-0-19-538696-7
1. Diagnostic imaging—Social aspects.   I. Goldsmith, Jeff Charles.   II. Title.
[DNLM:   1. Diagnostic Imaging—trends.   2. Diagnostic Imaging—economics.   3. Diagnostic Imaging—
utilization.   4. Radiography, Interventional—trends. WN 180 H654s 2011]
RC78.7.D53H55 2011
616.07'54—dc22
2010013328

9 8 7 6 5 4 3 2 1

Printed in the United States of America
on acid-free paper

*For Aaron Hillman and Karen Walker*

# *Acknowledgments*

The authors are greatly indebted to the following individuals who provided information during our research, helped review the manuscript, or contributed images. Their efforts are a testament to the fact that sometimes "it takes a village."

Dr. Nadeem Ishaque and numerous colleagues at the GE Global Research Center spent an entire day giving us insight into the miraculous new technologies that might comprise medical imaging in the future. Jack Taggart and Steve Haberlein of Fuji Medical Systems discussed with us how the business of imaging is likely to change over the next five years. Steven Seltzer, Ramin Khorasani, Ferenc Jolesz, and Ron Kikinis of the Brigham and Women's Hospital described their vision of the "electronic radiology round trip" imaging information technology of the future and demonstrated their concepts of advanced neurovisualization and MRI-guided focused ultrasound treatment. At the Massachusetts General Hospital, James Thrall and Giles Boland provided insights into the business of radiology; Ralph Weissleder regaled us with accounts of how molecular imaging will be adopted into clinical practice.

Numerous actors in the imaging business also played a role. Dr. Michael Brant-Zawadzki described his entrepreneurial experiences in establishing a CT screening center chain. Curtis Kauffman-Pickelle, of the *Radiology Business Journal,* provided useful guidance on sources of industry intelligence and history. Steve Duvoisin, CEO of Inland Imaging, Paul Berger, founder of NightHawk Radiology, and Paul Viviano, CEO of Alliance Healthcare, gave us extended interviews on their businesses and their perspectives on the broader industry. David Lee and Nick Caffentzis of GE Healthcare provided access to industry analysis that made its way into our figures.

Steven Horii of the University of Pennsylvania provided extensive historical background based on his participation in the working groups that produced the DICOM standard. Jean Mitchell of George Washington University and Rebecca Smith-Bindman of the University of California at San Francisco both found time to talk about their work on imaging utilization and its drivers. Jonathan Sunshine of the American College of Radiology generously provided both research access to and special analysis of the size of the imaging business and radiology profession. We thank Gail Prochaska of IMV Medical Information Division for analysis of the installed base of high technology imaging in the United States. We thank Jenna Kappel at the Society of Interventional Radiology for materials concerning the practice and economics of interventional radiology.

We thank the following persons who reviewed individual chapters to help make certain that we were not writing egregious untruths: Spencer Gay, Chapter 1 on radiological practice; Jane Morley on the historical aspects and Mark Williams on the physics aspects of Chapter 2 on the development of modern imaging technologies; Jeffrey Weinreb, Chapter 4 on the risks of imaging; John Patti, Barry Pressman, Bob Berenson, Greg Raab, and Nathan Kaufman, Chapter 5 on economics; Paul Berger and David Levin, Chapter 6 on digital imaging and business structures; David Levin, Chapter 7 on moral hazard; Bill Black, Chapter 8 on screening. Their efforts saved us many a misstep. Any remaining factual errors are entirely our own.

We are especially grateful to Frank Lexa, Gregg Raab, Jonathan Sunshine, and Jack Wickens for reading and commenting on a late draft of the entire manuscript. Their insights encouraged us to rethink some of our conclusions.

The images are a critical aspect of this book, particularly to help lay readers understand our descriptions of the great power of medical imaging. The following individuals were kind enough to contribute images: Mehdi Adineh, Tally Altes, Fritz Angle, Michelle Barr, Mathew Bassignani, Bill Brant, Michael Cohen, Ed DeLange, Fred Epstein, Cree Gaskin, Spencer Gay, Klaus Hagspiel, Chris Hiss, Jeff Hoffmeister, Lee Jenson, Ferenc Jolesz, Ron Kikinis, Chris Kramer, Drew Lambert, Alan Matsumoto, Nathan McDonald, Patrick Norton, Bob Older, Marc Sarti, Clare Tempany, Ralph Weissleder, and Brian Williamson.

Peggy Brown, Marion Dewalt, Susan Guerrant, Linn Harrison, Sharon Hostler, and Gerry Krueger, as patient a reading group as ever existed, provided grammatical instruction and invaluable advice on how to make the book more approachable for lay readers.

# Contents

# Introduction: The Sorcerer's Apprentice

Any sufficiently advanced technology is indistinguishable from magic.
—*Sir Arthur C. Clarke*

Four decades ago, radiologists were cave dwellers, living in the damp and dingy basements of hospitals amid yellowed linoleum flooring and flickering fluorescent lights. The primary job of these physician specialists was interpreting backlit anatomical images on film exposed to X-rays. Their work spaces stank of chemical developer and overflowed with dusty celluloid images archived in manila files. While useful, radiological images were only occasionally definitive enough to resolve diagnostic uncertainty, and many patients subsequently underwent exploratory surgery to define and treat their illnesses.

How remarkably things have changed! Radiology has become the archetypical medical specialty of the digital age. Thanks to ubiquitous broadband Internet and their embrace of digital technology, diagnostic radiologists can practice their specialty from anywhere they choose to be—their private offices, imaging centers across the street from the hospital, their dens at home, or their hotel rooms while away at conferences anywhere in the world. They can consult with colleagues on images sent to Barcelona, Bangalore, or Sydney and sleep soundly at night while radiologists in these and other cities interpret their off-hour examinations. During the past decade, radiology has become the first truly global medical discipline.

Just as remarkably, radiologists no longer only interpret images. They use medical imaging to guide lifesaving interventions of critical illness—implanting coils in brain aneurysms, threading stents into the carotid arteries of stroke patients, alleviating blood clots in patients' legs. Radiologists have become pivotal actors in critical care medicine, expanding their scope of practice into areas formerly the exclusive preserve of neuro-vascular and general surgery.

Imaging advances also threaten some of the traditional practices of other medical specialties, such as cardiology and gastroenterology, by replacing invasive diagnostic procedures with more benign, image-guided techniques that are less expensive, reduce patients' discomfort, and speed recovery. New, even less invasive technologies, like image-guided focused ultrasound, are poised to broaden further radiology's advance into curative medicine. In a very short period of time, radiologists have vaulted over many of their clinical colleagues in medicine's food chain. Other specialists have responded by acquiring sophisticated medical imaging technologies for their offices and centers, setting off a "turf war" for control of imaging as intense as that fought by the cattlemen and sodbusters of the old West.

The modalities radiologists have exploited—primarily computed tomography (CT) scanning, magnetic resonance imaging (MRI), positron emission tomography (PET) scanning, and ultrasonography—are now mature technologies. However, as the mathematical algorithms and the computing engines that facilitate them have grown more powerful, these modalities have markedly improved, allowing more precise anatomical definition, better differentiation between normal and abnormal tissues, and insight into the mechanisms of disease. With the contemporary advent of molecular medicine, radiology is poised to invade the traditional preserve of laboratory medicine, detailing the functioning of human cells—portraying the products of gene expression, tracing molecular pathways of disease inside the cell, and identifying threatening pathology at an earlier, more treatable stage. Advances in miniaturization, image enhancement, computer-aided diagnosis, and molecular imaging appear likely to broaden further the scope and power of medical imaging specialists.

The rise of radiology over the past three decades is an extraordinary story of accomplishment, even in the context of the great strides that have been made across all aspects of medicine. However, all this achievement has come at an economic cost. Imaging expenditures have increased dramatically in the past decade, becoming the fastest-growing component of all physician-directed services and altering the economic shape of national medical expenditures. There is a broadly held belief that not all of the increase in imaging utilization is clinically necessary. As a result, imaging has become a proverbial "tall poppy" to both governmental and private insurance payers—a prominent target for cost reduction. The success of medical imaging has thrust it and the practitioners who use it into the center of the nation's health care cost debate.

Many will remember the "Sorcerer's Apprentice" segment of the Disney film *Fantasia*—a perfect metaphor for medical imaging as it stands today.[1] The apprentice magician, played by Mickey Mouse, tests his nascent skills at sorcery by bringing common household items to life and putting them to work. At first, things go well, but eventually Mickey loses control, and chaos ensues.

Medical imaging, too, could spin out of control. Some policymakers believe it already has. While the benefits of imaging are undeniable, there exists significant potential for human and economic harm through inappropriate use. Where is imaging technology and its partnership with clinical practice headed? Can the patient care benefits produced by imaging be enhanced by further technological advances? What is the potential for harm that accrues along with these benefits? How will the health

---

[1] Actually, Disney brought to animated life a poem called *Der Zauberlehrling* by Johann Wolfgang von Goethe, published in 1797. *Fantasia*'s "Sorcerer's Apprentice" eerily presaged the Manhattan Project, which was launched while *Fantasia* was under development and gave rise to nuclear fission and atomic weapons.

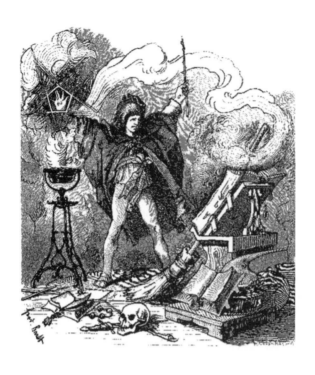

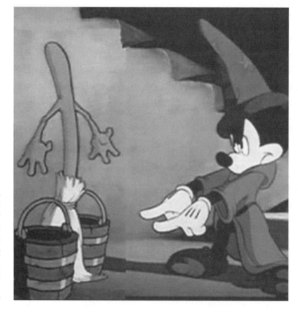

*Two contrasting renderings of the sorcerer's apprentice: Goethe's and Disney's Mickey. © Disney Enterprises, Inc. Reprinted with permission.*

care system adopt future emerging technologies, and how will it pay for them? How can society learn to make more intelligent use of these powerful tools?

These are the central questions we address in this book for our intended audiences of lay readers, radiologists and their medical colleagues, industry analysts, health reform advocates, health insurers, and those interested in health services research and policy. Chapter 1 introduces the reader to the radiologist, the physician specialist of medical imaging who, in many ways, sits at the center of the storm. This chapter discusses who the radiologist is, what he or she does, how he or she does it, and why many people are unfamiliar with the radiologist's contributions to their care.

The next two chapters acquaint readers with the key imaging technologies and their applications, how they developed into clinical use and how they work. Chapter 2 addresses diagnostic modalities like plain X-ray, CT, and MRI. Chapter 3 details how these primarily diagnostic techniques gave rise to and guide new, less invasive treatment methods that created the radiological subspecialty of interventional radiology. Chapter 4 focuses on common risks associated with medical imaging, including those associated with inappropriate use, the health effects of ionizing radiation (like X-rays), and contrast media (also known as *dyes*).

The remainder of the book builds on what the reader has learned about imaging in the early chapters to address key policy issues affecting medical imaging currently and in the future. Chapter 5 addresses the principal economic issues—how imaging is paid for, who are the principal players in the imaging industry, and what incentives exist in the current payment system that encourage the abuse of imaging procedures. Chapter 6 focuses on how the advent of digital imaging and advanced information technology has made radiology the first global medical specialty. This chapter explains how the capacity to transmit images over the Web has opened the door for corporate enterprises to disrupt traditional radiology practice models. Chapter 7 expands on a theme first introduced in Chapter 5: how the acquisition of advanced imaging technologies by practitioners who can refer their patients to imaging facilities they own presents an opportunity for financially motivated abuse. Chapter 7 frames this possibility in the context of physicians' moral hazard[2] and presents policy options for dealing with the problem.

Chapter 8 details issues related to imaging screening—using imaging methods to detect important disease early in healthy-seeming individuals. This topic merits a separate chapter because it is a popular topic in the lay media and because the use of imaging methods in healthy individuals differs in some important respects from its use in the diagnosis of symptomatic disease. Chapter 9 describes a vision of the future of radiology. There are extraordinary possibilities for imaging to contribute to improved health, influenced by the transition of medical diagnosis and treatment to the molecular level, where much complex disease originates. This chapter provides readers with examples of how imaging could make care more convenient, safer, and more personalized than it is presently. It also discusses the economic, regulatory, and cultural influences that will strongly influence whether the great potential of imaging will become reality.

---

[2] The concept of moral hazard will be explained at length in the chapter. For now, consider moral hazard to be financially motivated, rather than clinically justified, treatment by physicians who stand to increase their incomes by doing potentially unnecessary work.

The final chapter pulls everything together and considers how society should manage the benefits of medical imaging, its risks, and its costs. It addresses where health policy has failed with respect to imaging and what alternative approaches might maximize the value society receives from advanced medical imaging examinations.

Radiology is on the move. Where it is going and what the medical care system will look like when it gets there are concerns to be addressed in the following pages.

Bruce Hillman and Jeff Goldsmith
February 2010

# The Sorcerer's Apprentice

# The Most Important Doctor You've Never Met

*Susan Whiting was having trouble concentrating on the Vogue in her lap. It wasn't just that the magazine was an older issue she had already seen or that the table lamp beside her was a bit dimmer than necessary to read comfortably. Susan was anxious about undergoing a computed tomography (CT) scan, which her physician had recommended to evaluate what might be causing the sharp abdominal pains she'd been having off and on for over a month. She'd arrived well before the scheduled time of her exam to undergo tests to ensure that she was not pregnant and that her kidney function was normal.[1] She'd had plenty of time to stew over her concerns about what the impending examination might show.*

*Susan took another couple of gulps of the thinly flavored liquid in the quart cup. The drink had a bitter aftertaste, and she had to force herself to swallow the last bit. The woman at the reception desk had emphasized how important it was that the drink completely fill her intestines[2] and improve her chances of having an accurate diagnostic study. Feeling bloated after drinking what seemed like gallons of fluid, Susan tried again to focus on the elegantly dressed woman striding across the page of the magazine.*

*"Ms. Whiting?" said a short young woman in bright blue scrub pants and a vividly floral short-sleeved top. The woman wore tennis shoes and had seemed to materialize from nowhere.*

[1]  Both are important considerations before a CT exam. The dose of X-radiation a patient receives during the scan is potentially dangerous to a fetus, especially during the first trimester. As we'll discuss later, normal kidney function is important for excreting the intravenous contrast material Susan will receive as part of her scan.

[2]  Oral contrast material is commonly given before a CT scan. Although clear to the eye, the fluid is radiodense, appearing white on a CT scan and helping the radiologist to differentiate the intestines from adjacent anatomical structures or abnormal masses.

*Susan rose, sensing the stares of several other patients who believed that they had been waiting longer than she. She followed the woman down a hallway to a cramped room containing little more than some shoulder-height cabinets and a couple of bare plastic chairs. The woman introduced herself as Robin, the X-ray technologist who would be performing Susan's CT scan. She told Susan to make herself comfortable in one of the chairs.*

*Robin explained that for the type of scan her doctor had ordered, an X-ray dye, also known as contrast material, needed to be injected into a vein in her arm. The dye might make her feel a little odd, but it was not dangerous. Did she have any allergies? It seemed that a very small number of patients reacted badly to the dye, developing hives, shortness of breath, or, very rarely, a life-threatening lowering of blood pressure. The technologist wondered if she had experienced any of these reactions in the past. Assured that she had not, Robin inserted a needle connected to a thin, short tube (i.e., a catheter) into a vein in Susan's arm. Noting the free return of blood into the tubing, Robin advanced the catheter, removed the needle, released the tourniquet, and taped the catheter firmly in place. She then walked Susan across the hall and helped her onto a table that protruded from the hole of what looked like a giant, thick-walled, white plastic donut. Another technologist joined Robin and, together, they slid Susan under the red laser cross-hairs that positioned her for her CT exam.*

*It had all happened so quickly that Susan had little time to be frightened. But now, lying on the scanner table, her view obscured by the walls of the machine, listening to Robin's electronically processed voice, she quickly reviewed everything Robin had said could go wrong. She was moving toward panic when she heard Robin telling her that they were about to inject the dye. Susan was not to move.*

*"Take a deep breath"—Robin hesitated for an instant—"and hold it," she said with an upward lilt.*

*Susan felt a deep, slightly unpleasant warmth creep throughout her body, but the sensation passed quickly. She held her breath, not wanting to have to repeat this experience if it could be avoided by her cooperation. She could feel the table sliding her smoothly through the donut. Although the whole procedure took only about 20 seconds, Susan exhaled with enormous relief when told by Robin that she could once again breathe normally. The technologist emerged from behind the glass wall of an adjacent room and pulled out the table from the scanner so that Susan would feel less constrained.*

*"I'll be right back," said Robin. "We just need to check the images to be sure that they look okay and that we've completely covered the area your doctor requested."*

*Robin was back in just over a minute to help Susan off the table and assure her that the scan was fine.*

*"When will my doctor get the pictures to look at?" asked Susan.*

*"Well, the radiologist needs to interpret them first. Your doctor will get a report as soon as the radiologist finishes looking at the images," Robin responded.*

*The radiologist? What radiologist? I thought my doctor was going to read my scan.*

Given the ubiquity of medical imaging nowadays, you may have experienced something quite similar to Susan's CT scan. The high-technology nature of medical imaging and, most often, the invisibility of the physician responsible for interpreting the exam can make the experience feel very impersonal. It's as though you walked in on the middle of a movie and then had to leave early. You missed everything that went on before you arrived, and something important will happen after you leave. There's an absence of context to many radiological exams that, if understood, would give broader meaning to the experience.

In fact, Susan's exam was preceded by several visits to her physician over a few weeks. On the first occasion, her doctor observed, listened, palpated, and completed a history documenting Susan's symptoms. On the second visit, the doctor asked about any changes in the frequency or character of the pains, repeated the physical exam, and ran a panel of *blood chemistries*.[3] The doctor's assistant passed a handheld portable ultrasound machine over Susan's stomach, an increasingly common event nowadays. But when all of these tests proved unenlightening and the pains continued, her doctor decided to go further, pursuing his diagnostic concerns with high-technology medical imaging.

Doctors make the choice to image their patients based on a number of factors — the expectations of the patient, their belief that the patient might have a serious illness, whether the physician's group owns its own imaging equipment, the habits and norms of practice in the group or the geographic region, and, sadly, their assessment of the risk of a malpractice suit if something were missed, to name a few of the considerations.

In Susan Whiting's case, the doctor asked his office manager to fax a requisition (more formally, a request for a radiologist's consultation) to his nearby hospital outpatient radiology department for an abdominal and pelvic CT scan with intravenous contrast material.

What happened from that point on is the subject of this chapter. Specifically, this chapter will introduce the physician specialist in imaging: the radiologist. It will discuss the supervision and interpretation of imaging examinations, the applications of medical imaging to patient care, and the unseen infrastructure and processes that underlie the performance of medical imaging examinations. It will also consider some of the challenges facing the clinical practice of imaging in the twenty-first century.

## "Pay No Attention to the Man Behind the Curtain"[4]

Like Susan, many patients don't realize that their imaging examination may be interpreted by a radiologist rather than by their own physician. In a 2007 survey conducted by the American College of Radiology (ACR) of people living in Burlington Vermont, Miami, Florida, and Washington, D.C., only 55% of respondents knew that radiologists were physicians. Forty-four percent had had an imaging exam during the six months prior to the survey, but only 39% of these individuals could assert that the procedure had been conducted by a radiologist.[5]

In fact, radiologists are physicians who uniquely receive comprehensive, specialized training in and exclusively practice medical imaging and/or image-guided

---

3  Blood chemistries usually consist of a number of automated tests that can be run on a single tube of blood. The panel provides insight into abnormalities of electrolytes, proteins, and enzymes that can potentially lead a doctor to the source of the patient's complaints.

4  From the *Wizard of Oz*.

5  Unpublished ACR survey results; Shawn Farley, personal communication, September 2009.

treatment. If your imaging study is performed in a hospital or in a hospital outpatient imaging department, a radiologist will almost certainly interpret your images. Radiologists also perform imaging in their own private offices and in imaging centers. Increasingly, nonradiologists are acquiring high-technology imaging devices and performing scans in their offices. If your doctor is among these physicians, he or she may interpret your exam personally or, more frequently, consult a radiologist with whom he or she has contracted to interpret the examinations. To simplify things, and because radiologists practice imaging more comprehensively than other physicians, this chapter will focus on the work of radiologists. There will be more to say about nonradiologists who practice medical imaging in Chapter 7.

There are two main reasons why patients often are unaware of the involvement of radiologists in their care. First, with few exceptions, radiologists receive patients only by referral from another physician. Even in the rare circumstance in which a patient calls to request an imaging examination, most radiologists refuse to accept such patient-initiated referrals.[6] The second reason many patients don't know about the involvement of radiologists is that, for the great majority of imaging studies, the only person they actually see is the radiological technologist who performs the imaging [often called *X-ray technologists*, although they also perform studies that don't use X-rays, like ultrasonography and magnetic resonance imaging (MRI)]. The radiologist interprets the exams later and out of the patient's view.

There are exceptions to these generalizations. For instance, many women refer themselves to radiologists for screening mammography. Interventional radiologists directly evaluate patients and perform image-guided interventional procedures like angioplasties, catheter drainages of abscesses, and needle-guided biopsies. However, such exceptions account for only a small fraction of imaging care. Most patients never meet the radiologist and may be unaware that he or she has reviewed and interpreted their images, then sent their doctor a report of the findings and diagnostic conclusions, until they receive the radiologist's bill.

*The Making of a Radiologist*    So, who is this shadowy figure—this radiologist—and how does he or she come by this special expertise in medical imaging? To qualify to take the American Board of Radiology (ABR) certification examinations to become a radiologist, a physician, having graduated from medical school, must serve a one-year internship in a field of medical practice (like general medicine or surgery) other than radiology and then train for four years in a dedicated radiology residency program. Over 90% of radiology trainees choose to add one to three years of fellowship training in a subspecialty area like breast imaging, interventional radiology, or MRI (Smith et al. 2009). Thus, a radiologist spends two to four years longer in medical training than does a general internist or family practitioner.

---

[6]  Radiologists refuse patient-initiated referrals for a number of reasons, including not wishing to alienate their referring physicians, the legal implications of assuming responsibility for the care of patients beyond the interpretation of the imaging examination, and because, with few exceptions, insurers require a referral from a physician with primary responsibility for medical care as a prerequisite for payment.

Radiology residency training is comprehensive with regard to medical imaging. Training addresses such topics as the underlying physical basis for imaging exams, the interactions of radiation with human tissues, the risks and benefits of medical imaging, selecting the most appropriate imaging studies for a given clinical presentation, managing the performance of imaging studies, techniques for image-guided invasive procedures, and the interpretation of imaging examinations, to name just a few. By far the largest segment of diagnostic radiological training focuses on the last of these: learning to recognize and synthesize the imaging findings that signal the presence of important disease. This is a complex task, learned during what amounts to a multiyear apprenticeship under experienced radiologists.

Radiologists-in-training progress through a series of rotations focused on individual imaging modalities, organ systems, and procedures. The principal method of learning involves residents interpreting cases on their own, making the critical decisions about the presence of imaging findings. They decide for themselves what diagnoses should be considered and, if pertinent, what follow-on imaging examinations they should recommend. Faculty radiologists "overread" each case with the resident beside them before it is reported out to the referring physician, discussing with the resident the important features and correcting any misapprehensions. The overread is not purely pedagogical; insurers require that a licensed staff physician be the ultimate interpreter of any examination for which payment is requested.

National and hospital requirements for the supervision of radiology residents mandate that residency training programs set forth the curriculum that constitutes the program and that there be regular and frequent evaluation of all trainees to ensure that they are progressing at an acceptable rate. An ABR written examination during training tests trainees' medical and imaging knowledge, as well as their understanding of the physics underlying imaging examinations, their risks and hazards, and the biological effects of imaging. At the end of training, the ABR tests residents' interpretive capabilities via one-on-one oral examinations covering each of the major organ systems and imaging technologies.

Radiology residents spend most of a year studying in their spare time to prepare for the ABR examinations. Since 2004, the percentage of those passing the written examinations has ranged from the high 80s to the low 90s. From 83% to 90% have passed the oral examination on their first attempt during the same period.[7] Failed candidates may retake the entire examination or repeat failed portions of it. However, ultimately, a trainee must pass all parts of the written and oral tests to be certified as a diagnostic radiologist.

**The Organization of Radiological Practice**   Nearly all radiologists practice in groups. Approximately 55% of them are engaged in private practice (also know as *community practice*). Nearly all of the remainder practice in academic medical centers (19%) and multispecialty groups (16%) (Smith et al. 2009).[8] Given the increasing use of imaging, the responsibility of 24-hour coverage, and the need to cover the unpaid responsibilities listed below, the size of both academic and community radiology

---

7  http://theabr.org/ic/ic_dr/ic_dr_score.html#result.
8  The remainder comprise a diverse group. Many work in government or for large corporations.

groups is increasing to spread the financial and manpower burdens and achieve effi-ciencies of scale (Bhargavan and Sunshine 2008).

Academic radiologists practice in university medical centers. Most academic radiologists are subspecialists, meaning that they typically focus their clinical prac-tice, and related teaching and research, on a single organ system or imaging technol-ogy. The advantage of subspecialization (for example, in gastrointestinal or cardiac radiology) is greater depth of knowledge in the area of interest but at the expense of losing much of what was learned in other fields of imaging during radiology training.

In contrast, historically, the dominant community practice model for radiology has been generalism. General radiologists practice across the entire breadth of the specialty. In the basic general practice model, all the radiologists in the group do similar types and amounts of work. In a purely generalist practice, everyone inter-prets all types of examinations for all body systems. This tends to be more efficient than subspecialization in handling the peaks and valleys that inevitably occur for any type of examination during the day. When the "stack" of brain MRI studies is temporarily depleted, the radiologist moves on to ultrasound of the abdomen; while waiting for a patient to be prepped by a nurse for an image-guided catheter drainage of a pelvic abscess, he or she reads a few thoracic CT scans. As described later in this book, external forces are compelling a reconsideration of this model of practice. Nowadays, many general radiologists spend a large fraction of their time in a particular subspecialty while still covering other areas during the remainder of their working hours.

In virtually all settings, radiologists underpin and, in many cases, manage the imaging process, providing services to their hospitals or imaging facilities well beyond image interpretation. Radiologists advise on equipment purchases, ensure adherence to federal and state regulations, manage imaging-related information technology, maintain and upgrade equipment, and interface with referring physi-cians and hospital administrators, to name just a few of their roles. Because imaging has become central to the provision of emergency and hospital inpatient care, radi-ologists must either provide their services around the clock or make arrangements with other radiologists to do so.[9]

## The Processes and Resources Underlying the Delivery of Imaging Care

Returning to our story of Susan Whiting, there is a great deal of unseen structure and process that underlies a successful radiological examination. This section provides some insight into what goes on behind the scenes between the request for an exam and the transmission of the radiologist's report to the referring physician promised by Susan's technologist.

Earlier, it was stated that Susan's doctor's office faxed a request for referral to the radiology department. The fax was received by a radiology scheduler, who looked for the first slot available on an outpatient CT scanner. She then phoned Susan to confirm that she would be able to come to the hospital's outpatient radiology

---

[9] Chapter 6 will discuss how radiologists are outsourcing their night and weekend call responsibilities to other radiologists—often on the other side of the world.

department two days later to be scanned at 11:30 in the morning.[10] She took pains to explain to Susan that she had to come in 90 minutes before her scheduled scan time to drink the fluid that would outline her intestines and have the procedure properly explained.

Entering Susan's name into the schedule prompted the hospital's electronic information system to search for her history of previous radiological examinations. Knowing about Susan's imaging history is critical because the accuracy of radiologists' interpretations is improved by comparing the findings of the current exam with those of any previous studies. The search revealed that Susan had had a CT scan of the abdomen in the same department but in the distant past. The images were in remote computerized storage. The system brought the images forward into short-term storage for rapid accessibility on the day of Susan's scan.[11]

The day of the exam, Susan appeared on time at the radiology department's registration desk. A receptionist logged her into the system and then led her to the waiting area. As detailed at the beginning of this chapter, shortly before her exam, the technologist greeted her, explained the procedure, and prepared her for the study.

After Susan's scan was completed, while Susan was still resting on the CT scanner table, the technologist returned to her seat behind the glass wall and scrolled image by image through the entire series. She checked to see that the first view, or slice,[12] was above the diaphragm and the last view was below the symphysis pubis, where the bones of the pelvis come together in the front of the body (anteriorly), as required for an abdominal and pelvic scan. The technologist made sure that there was no blurring of the images because Susan had moved or breathed when the images were being exposed and that there were no artifacts caused by metal objects like coins or an underwire bra inadvertently left on Susan's person. In some departments, experienced technologists may consult the radiologist before allowing the patient to leave, either because there is a particular clinical question that needs to be answered or because they see something that might require further imaging for clarification.

Even before Susan left the department, her examination had been sent to the radiologist's electronic queue. Computed tomography scanners produce images much faster than a radiologist can interpret them, so Susan's exam had to await interpretation after the two other exams that had preceded hers. The radiologist reviewed the clinical history provided by Susan's physician. He also drew up her electronic medical record through the hospital's information system in case the imaging findings raised questions that could be explained by her medical history, blood chemistries, or other tests. Finally, the radiologist interpreted Susan's exam, noting only some minor and unimportant findings that were unchanged since her prior CT scan.

---

[10] The most modern departments have computerized this step, so it can be handled by the doctor's receptionist, in real time, before the patient leaves the doctor's office.

[11] Radiology departments used to maintain vast file rooms and large numbers of employees to accomplish these functions. Some still do. However, most modern departments have digitized their past exams. Digital storage has greatly improved the speed and reliability of finding previous examinations (see Chapter 6).

[12] CT images look as though someone has used a band saw to cut across the body, exposing a gray scale (like a black-and-white photograph) view of the organs, fat, bones, and superficial soft tissues at the level at which the cut was made. CT scan slices are sometimes referred to as cuts.

The traditional picture of a radiologist at work is that of a lone figure in a dark cave-like room, laboriously inspecting an overly blackened image on a light box. This view is so twentieth century. While the old-fashioned radiology practice still exists in some places, X-ray films are increasingly a thing of the past. Susan's radiologist viewed her images on a computer workstation, which brought the images up on several high-resolution monitors in the configuration chosen by the radiologist. The workstation offered him a series of options that make image interpretation easier, faster, and more accurate. The radiologist's review of Susan's exam included his inspection of nearly 1000 images, scrolling through them as though he were watching a movie.

As the radiologist reviewed the images, he dictated his report into a microphone connected to a voice recognition system. The system printed the report in real time on a computer screen as he spoke, allowing the radiologist to make corrections as he dictated and edited the final report. He signed the document electronically with his attestation that he had personally reviewed the images (required for insurer payment) and transmitted the report to the referring clinician. The images and the interpretation report were filed in Susan's electronic folder along with her other imaging exams, available for review in the future.

It took quite a while for Susan to exit the hospital parking lot. So, by the time she arrived in her physician's office, about 45 minutes later, her physician had already reviewed the radiologist's report and looked at a few selected images via his secure connection to the hospital information system. The source of Susan's abdominal symptoms remained a puzzle, but her pains slowly abated over the following week and did not return. The imaging examination had played an important role in ruling out the possibility that Susan had a serious condition.

## What Radiologists Do and How They Do It

In considering what distinguishes radiological practice from that of other medical specialties, noted radiologist Harry Mellins, once said, "The radiologist perceives a shadow, sees a lesion, and imagines the man. The bedside physician sees the man, perceives the signs, and imagines the lesion. They practice from the outside in and we from the inside out."[13]

It's no small task. Given the permutations of imaging technologies, body parts, and clinical presentations, there are literally thousands of different medical imaging examinations currently employed in medical practice. In order for the reader to understand how imaging examinations have improved medical care, we will focus on the four major imaging applications: screening and early disease detection; directing image-guided treatment; disease diagnosis and staging; and using imaging to evaluate the effectiveness of treatment. In the future, medical imaging may also play important roles in predicting the outcomes of disease and determining in advance which treatments might be most effective for a given patient. In the jargon of our times, advanced imaging will serve as *prognostic* and *predictive* biomarkers (see Chapter 9).

---

[13]  Personal communication, Stuart Silverman, MD, August 2009.

The remainder of this section summarizes how medical imaging is used in each major clinical application.

*Screening and Early Detection*    Using modern imaging to detect important diseases, like cancer and cardiovascular disease, before they become symptomatic (what is called *screening*) is, in important ways, different enough from the other applications that we devote an entire chapter to the subject (see Chapter 8). To provide an overview of the applications of imaging here, Chapter 8 will only review the basic principles and provide an example of successful screening.

The rationale for imaging screening is intellectually compelling: that detecting life-threatening diseases earlier in disease development allows more effective, less harmful, and less costly treatment than when an abnormality is discovered later, after symptoms have developed. The hoped-for outcome of screening large populations is that fewer people will suffer serious illness and early death from the condition targeted by the screening.

For this to occur, screening must fulfill a number of crucial preconditions. There must be an accurate and acceptable screening test that can be uniformly performed and interpreted over broad geographic areas and long periods of time. For example, a mammogram in Miami must be essentially the same test as a mammogram in Omaha. Even allowing for improvements in technology and interpretation, a mammogram performed in 2004 should be similar to one performed in 2008. For screening to be effective in improving health, there must also be more effective treatment for earlier disease than for more advanced disease. Finally and crucially, the benefits of screening must be cost-effective for society.

Various authors have proposed many combinations of medical conditions and imaging screening examinations [including using whole body CT, MRI, and positron emission tomography (PET)] to find disease (Hillman et al. 2005). Most of them have not yet been sufficiently validated by clinical research to be broadly accepted in medical practice. However, at least one imaging screening examination—mammography to detect asymptomatic breast cancer—has become accepted internationally as standard medical practice because it has been shown repeatedly to reduce breast cancer–related deaths (Smith et al. 2003). The ACR and the American Cancer Society (ACS) have established screening guidelines for the optimal frequency of screening and which, if any, additional technologies (such as MRI and ultrasound) are best suited to a woman's risk of developing breast cancer. These recommendations are based on such criteria as age, breast density (i.e., amount of glandular versus fatty tissue), family history, ethnicity, and genetic makeup. However, as discussed further in Chapter 8, there is still controversy over the costs and benefits associated with these recommendations, particularly with regard to whether less frequent screenings, begun later than recommended by ACR and ACS, might be equally effective.[14]

*Image-Guided Intervention*    Some of the greatest advances in the contribution of imaging to patient care during the last decades of the twentieth century occurred in the field of image-guided intervention (also known as *interventional radiology*). Indeed, image-guided intervention is such an important topic that an entire

---

[14] http://www.ahrq.gov/clinic/uspstf/uspsbrca.htm.

chapter (Chapter 3) is devoted to the emergence of the field and an exploration of its applications. This topic is addressed here only briefly as part of our overview of the applications of medical imaging.

The goal of image-guided intervention is to provide health outcomes similar to those of traditional surgical treatment but less invasively—with less pain, fewer complications, shortened convalescence, and, ideally, lower overall costs.[15] A variety of imaging methods can be employed to perform various image-guided interventional procedures. Advanced imaging technologies like CT and MRI are increasingly used to guide interventional procedures. Examples of open surgical procedures partly or completely replaced by image-guided interventions are legion; a few prominent examples include ultrasonic lithotripsy[16] versus surgical removal of kidney stones; uterine artery embolization[17] of benign uterine fibroids versus hysterectomy; dilatation and/or stenting[18] of vascular narrowings and occlusions versus operative vascular surgery;[19] embolization of vascular abnormalities like brain aneurysms,[20] tumors, and bleeding varices[21] versus open surgical treatment; and catheter drainage of postoperative abscesses obviating the need for a second surgery.

General radiologists often perform interventional procedures. However, many of the more exacting procedures are performed by subspecialists who have received an added year or more of training in interventional radiology beyond radiology residency and have passed a specialized ABR certifying examination to receive a Certificate of Added Qualifications.

*Diagnosis and Staging*    Susan Whiting's encounter with CT imaging is representative of diagnosis and staging. By far the greatest number of applications of and encounters with imaging fall into this category. So, it is no surprise that most people identify diagnosis and staging as the principal use of medical imaging. To provide a practical understanding of what we mean by diagnosis and staging, here are a few examples of this use of medical imaging:

- A patient goes to his physician with a three-month history of occasional, intermittent mid-abdominal pain and nausea. He reports an 8-pound weight loss since the symptoms began but attributes it to a reduction of appetite. The doctor detects no specific physical findings, with the exception of very mild yellowing of the whites of the eyes (she suspects jaundice). Concerned about a disease process affecting

---

[15] The calculation of costs is a complicated issue. For image-guided intervention to provide lower overall costs, there are several possible targets: reducing the cost of the procedure itself, reducing the costs associated with hospitalization, reducing the patient's costs in travel to see health care providers and reducing time away from work.

[16] High-powered sound waves shatter kidney stones; the fragments flow down the ureter to the bladder and are passed during urination.

[17] Various materials are used to block off the arterial branches to a fibroid (a benign but sometimes symptomatic tumor) via a catheter placed in the artery by the Seldinger technique.

[18] A stent is a tube left in a vessel or another lumen to hold it open.

[19] Numerous surgical methods have been used to bypass a blocked artery.

[20] An outpouching of a blood vessel in the brain that has the potential to rupture, causing a stroke and sometimes death.

[21] Patients with a cirrhotic liver can have increased pressure in the veins of the digestive system. The veins dilate and can bleed, causing serious complications and even death.

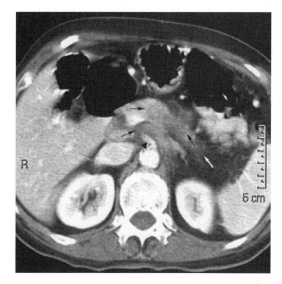

FIGURE 1-1

*CT scan reveals inoperable cancer of the pancreas. A pancreatic mass (black arrows) infiltrates a considerable portion of the pancreas and extends posteriorly (downward) to surround the superior mesenteric artery (arrowhead). The cancer infiltrates the fat in the left midabdomen (white arrow). (Courtesy of Spencer Gay, MD, the University of Virginia.)*

the biliary system[22] or adjacent organs, she refers the patient for a CT scan of the abdomen and pelvis with intravenous contrast material. The scan reveals a vague change in the normal density (the *grayness*, from pure white to pure black, depicted on the image) of the head of the pancreas[23] with some filamentous *dirtying*, or graying, of the fat in the region around the organ, which includes major blood vessels (Fig. 1-1). The bile ducts are slightly larger than normal. A subsequent endoscopic ultrasound[24]-guided needle biopsy of the abnormal focus in the pancreas reveals pancreatic cancer.

- A muscular young man is playing touch football for his fraternity team when another player accidentally is pushed into the back of his knees. His lower leg twists awkwardly to the side. He is unable to continue playing without pain. The student health service doctor refers him to an orthopedist. On examination, the knee is found to be tender and swollen. The knee joint moves more loosely than it should. The orthopedist refers the patient for an MRI scan of the knee to determine if there is damage to the ligaments. A musculoskeletal radiologist interprets the scan as showing completely torn anterior and posterior cruciate ligaments (Fig. 1-2).[25]
- An unconscious woman arrives in the emergency room. Her husband says that they were having dinner in a downtown restaurant when she began to drool out

---

[22] The gallbladder and ducts that channel the products of liver metabolism into the intestines.

[23] The head of the pancreas resides to the right of the midline and behind (i.e., posterior to) the stomach.

[24] A scope is placed through the mouth or nose into the small bowel adjacent to the pancreas. The tip of the scope is both an ultrasound transducer (which sends and receives sound waves) and a passage for a biopsy instrument. The operator uses the ultrasound image to locate the abnormal focus and to guide the biopsy.

[25] These and other ligaments are crucial in holding together the knee joint and ensuring correct joint motion.

of the left side of her mouth and her speech became slurred. Soon afterward, she became unconscious and slumped in her chair. The emergency physician requests a CT scan of the brain. A white rim surrounding brain tissue on the scan signals an intracranial (within the skull) hemorrhage. The neuroradiologist performs arteriography,[26] which shows a leaking basilar artery aneurysm (Fig. 1-3).[27] The neuroradiologist immediately repairs the leak by injecting material through the arteriography catheter to seal off the aneurysm (an example of image-guided treatment).

Radiological diagnosis and staging is a three-step process that involves recognizing signs on the image when an abnormality is present (detection), synthesizing what is seen into a coherent hypothesis about the condition the findings might represent (characterization), and determining how severe or extensive the disease is.

*Disease detection* means differentiating an abnormal finding from normal anatomy and/or physiology. This sounds simple enough, and in some circumstances it is. Many laypersons with only a faint notion of human anatomy could, for example, point to a slice of a CT scan with a large lung cancer surrounded by inflated lung and say, "This doesn't look right to me." However, most abnormal findings are more subtle—small and concealed within an organ with a density and texture similar to those of the normal tissue that surrounds it. Such abnormalities are detected only by the disciplined application of learned patterns of eye movement that reliably review all parts of each image, image after image for hundreds (or even thousands) of images, until the entire sequence of images that make up an examination is exhaustively evaluated. By such patterns of examination, the radiologist's years of training and experience are brought to bear in extracting the *signal* (the abnormality) from the *noise* (the normal structures). The task is further complicated by the

FIGURE 1-2

*Sagittal (a) and coronal (b) MRI images of a young man with a traumatic tear of the anterior cruciate ligament. (a) The anterior cruciate ligament is normally seen as a thin black line near its insertion on the tibia (small arrow); here the ligament becomes edematous (swollen with fluid), hence white (higher signal), as it nears (but never is seen to attach to) its usual origin on the posterior femur (arrowhead). The posterior cruciate ligament is normal (large arrow). An effusion (fluid) (e) is present in the joint space. (b) Coronal view of the knee joint. The edematous anterior cruciate ligament (small arrow) is separated from its origin on the femur by a slip of joint fluid (arrowhead). The speckled white region of the tibia represents a bone contusion (large arrow)—a common occurrence with cruciate ligament injuries. (Courtesy of Cree Gaskin, MD, the University of Virginia.)*

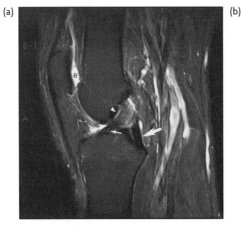
(a)

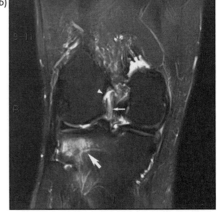
(b)

[26] This procedure involves inserting a catheter into an artery of the leg or arm and, watching the movement of the catheter under fluoroscopy and placing the catheter tip into the artery leading to the abnormality. When contrast material is injected, the artery can be imaged on X-ray along with any arterial abnormality.

[27] The basilar artery and its branches supply blood to the back of (posterior aspect) the brain.

(a) 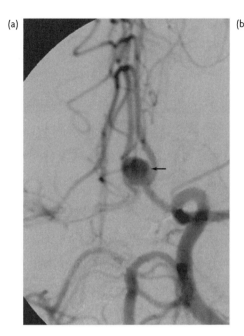   (b)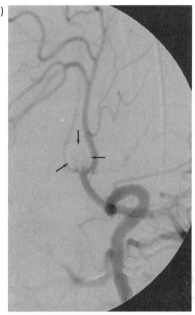

FIGURE 1-3

*Digital subtraction angiography (DSA) images pre- and postembolotherapy for an aneurysm of the posterior brain circulation. (a) Initial diagnostic angiogram demonstrating a sizable posterior circulation aneurysm (arrow). (b)Following the placement of platinum coils into the aneurysm (seen as a faint gray area in the image—arrows) via a catheter selectively placed in the aneurysm, the aneurysm is blocked off. (Courtesy of Mary Lee Jensen, MD, the University of Virginia.)*

considerable variability of normal human anatomy. Nearly every organ has a large variety of acceptable sizes and shapes, as well as lumps and bumps that can simulate the appearance of disease.

Once the radiologist has thoroughly reviewed the images for possible abnormalities, his or her cognitive faculties take over. This is the *characterization* phase, wherein the radiologist must mentally discard the irrelevant findings and extract from all he or she has seen the salient features that will allow him or her to make an accurate diagnosis. To do so effectively, the radiologist must cull from memory or from readily available sources—like books, journal articles, and Web sites—the pertinent facts about anatomy, disease processes, and radiological signs. In essence, the radiologist tests what he or she sees in each new case against patterns and information that form his or her past experiences to establish a likely set of diagnostic possibilities. Innate and learned talent for integrating information, depth and breadth of experience, and a penchant for keeping up with rapidly advancing knowledge all improve the likelihood of making an accurate diagnosis.

Occasionally, what the radiologist observes on the images is an *Aunt Minnie*. He or she has seen the findings before, and they always have turned out to represent a single diagnosis that is as familiar as an old relative (hence the term). Much more often, he or she is only able to narrow the diagnostic possibilities to a small number and assign to each a relative likelihood to guide the referring physician's considerations of diagnosis and how to proceed with further diagnostic testing, if necessary. In such an instance, the radiologist is said to have provided a *differential diagnosis*.

As an example, consider the hypothetical case described earlier in this section of the patient with three months of abdominal pain and weight loss. From the information provided by the referring physician on the request for the imaging examination, the radiologist knows that the symptoms have had a slow onset and the patient is jaundiced. The imaging signs are suggestive of an infiltrating process that involves the organ itself rather than pushing on it from a nearby location. The bile ducts are dilated, suggesting that they are partially blocked. The radiologist's *impression*—involving the radiologist's conclusions and a listing of possible explanations for the findings (i.e., the differential diagnosis)—would be:

> Radiological findings most consistent with pancreatic carcinoma extending posteriorly to involve the superior mesenteric artery and vein. Much less likely considerations include pancreatitis[28] and the recent passage of a gallstone with resultant inflammation and edema (swelling).

The final step in diagnosis and staging is to ascertain the extent or severity of disease. This is essential in helping referring physicians determine the appropriate therapy for a given patient. The task is highly variable, depending on the disease process involved. For instance, in the previously described case of pancreatic cancer, the radiologist commented in his impression importantly that the malignancy extended beyond the pancreas itself to involve the adjacent major blood vessels. Such involvement usually precludes an attempt at a surgical cure for the patient's pancreatic cancer. Other considerations for cancer care include determining if the disease has spread to lymph nodes or involves other organs (i.e., *metastases*).

There are entirely different considerations for the most common cardiovascular disease, atherosclerosis, wherein *plaques* of fat, fibrosis, inflammation, and calcification invest the wall of the large and medium-sized arteries. The important determinations of the extent of disease for atherosclerosis include which arteries are involved in the process and to what extent the arteries are narrowed. A narrowing of more than 50% in cross-sectional diameter is usually considered *hemodynamically significant*, meaning that the lesion has the potential to affect blood flow and cause symptoms or affect organ function.

From the foregoing discussion, it should be evident that radiologists must not only be cognizant of the imaging signs but must also have a thorough grasp of disease anatomy and pathological processes in order to comprehensively discharge their responsibilities to both the referring physician and the patient.

*Imaging to Evaluate the Effectiveness of Treatment*    For many conditions, medical imaging is a one-shot deal. Either nothing is found and the patient's symptoms eventually disappear or the findings are dealt with definitively and no further imaging investigation is necessary. Very often, however, treatment is either incremental and must be monitored or there are potential unintended aftereffects of the treatment that demand additional evaluation. To appreciate the role of imaging in monitoring patients' response to treatment, consider the following commonly encountered circumstances:

• A 62-year old woman is found on her first screening CT colonography examination[29] to have an invasive colon cancer. A subsequent CT scan of her chest,

---

[28] An inflammatory condition of the pancreas, usually presenting with acute pain.

[29] ACS recommendations are to begin regular colon screening at age 50. CT colonography is a new colon screening technique recently recommended by the ACS.

abdomen, and pelvis with intravenous contrast material, prior to surgery, shows no distant tumors that could represent metastases. However, a routine follow-up CT scan performed a year later reveals two new 1-centimeter nodules in her right lung and a 3-centimeter mass in her liver (Fig. 1-4).[30] When an ultrasonography-guided needle biopsy of the liver lesion reveals metastatic colon carcinoma, the patient is placed on a chemotherapeutic regimen. The patient begins a regimen of CT scanning every three months to determine whether the chemotherapy is effective or if different or additional agents should be considered. The radiologist employs an option on his workstation to measure electronically the cross-sectional diameters of each lung and liver mass, reporting on changes from scan to scan, as well as noting the appearance of any new metastases.

- A 13-year-old boy has increasingly severe pain in the right lower quadrant of his belly. The doctor in the emergency room notes the patient's discomfort when he presses on the area, particularly when he applies pressure and releases it suddenly (known as *rebound tenderness*). He suspects appendicitis, and the patient is taken to surgery, where the diagnosis is confirmed and the appendix removed laparoscopically.[31] Despite the surgery, the patient continues to feel bad and has a low-grade fever. An ultrasound examination performed at the patient's bedside three days after the surgery reveals a 4-centimeter, complicated-appearing fluid collection in the region of the surgery (Fig. 1-5). The radiologist uses the ultrasound imaging to guide a needle through the patient's skin into the fluid collection. Pus returns through the needle hub, confirming the diagnosis of a post-surgical abscess. The radiologist guides a flexible sterile wire through the needle into the fluid collection to hold the position and then threads a catheter over the

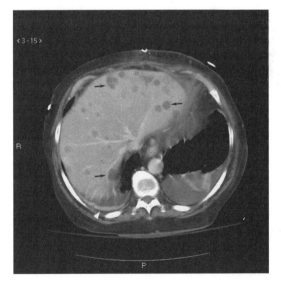

FIGURE 1-4

*The multiple lucencies in the liver (examples indicated by arrows) shown on CT scan represent metastatic tumors from colon cancer. There is fluid (ascites—arrowhead) in the peritoneal space of the abdomen related to metastatic spread to the peritoneum. (Courtesy of Mathew Bassignani, MD, the University of Virginia.)*

---

[30] The measurements traditionally are made in the longest diameter.
[31] A scope is placed through a small skin incision into the peritoneum (a space in the abdomen containing, among other organs, the appendix); through the scope, the surgeon closes off the connection of the appendix with the colon and takes out the diseased organ.

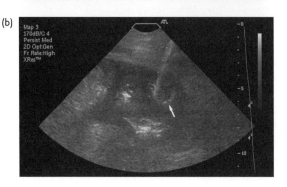

wire (another example of image-guided intervention). He sutures and tapes the catheter to the boy's abdomen to allow for continuous drainage of the abscess over the next several days. The combination of catheter drainage and intravenous antibiotics obviates the need for further surgery.

Modern medical imaging allows for more accurate, less invasive monitoring of the effectiveness and complications of treatment than existed prior to the advent of computerized cross-sectional imaging methods like ultrasonography, CT, and MRI. As with these cases, the use of imaging to recognize changes in patients with serious conditions allows for improved treatment. The job of the radiologist is similar to his or her responsibilities for the diagnosis and staging function. The radiologist must differentiate what is normal from what is not, determine what the abnormality represents in the context of the known underlying condition and any previous or ongoing treatment, and delineate its extent. These tasks can be complicated by the changes wrought by the therapy, particularly in surgical cases, wherein the normal anatomy may be considerably distorted.

## Summary

The goal of this chapter was to describe who interprets medical imaging examinations and how they do it, as well as how imaging is organized and practiced. Readers were introduced to the radiologist, gained an understanding of why his or her work is under-recognized (or unrecognized) by patients, and now understand that having a qualified radiologist interpret their images has important implications for quality of care.

This chapter also described the different clinical applications of medical imaging—screening and early detection, diagnosis and staging, gauging the response to treatment, and image-guided therapy—and explained the radiologist's role in each of these circumstances. Each imaging application represents a unique role for the radiologist as a consultant to two clients: the physicians who refer patients and the patients themselves.

The practice of radiology is changing. The traditional model of small, independent group practice is giving way to an assortment of business structures designed to provide enhanced efficiency, greater geographic breadth, subspecialized expertise, and financial leverage. These changes are being enforced by the economic pressures of our times. Several later chapters will explore the economics of medical imaging.

## References

Bhargavan M, Sunshine JH. The growing size of radiology practices. *J Am Coll Radiol.* 2008;5:801–805.

Hillman BJ, Amis ES, Weinreb JC, et al. The future of imaging screening—Proceedings of the Fourth Annual ACR Forum. *J Am Coll Radiol.* 2005;2:43–50.

Smith GS, Thrall JH, Pentecost MJ, et al. Subspecialization in radiology and radiation oncology. *JACR.* 2009;6:147–159.

Smith RA, Saslow D, Sawyer KA, et al. American Cancer Society Guidelines for breast cancer screening: update 2003. *CA: A Cancer Journal for Clinicians.* 2003;53:141–169.

# 2

# The Rise of Medical Imaging

*"I have seen my death," said Berta.*[1]

    *It was 1895. Berta's physicist husband, Wilhelm Conrad Roentgen (Fig. 2-1), had just shown her an image revealing the skeleton of her hand, her wedding band encircling the fourth finger (Fig. 2-2). This iconic "first medical image"—requiring immobilization and a 15-minute exposure—had been produced by X-rays, a previously unknown type of radiation.*

    *The actual discovery of X-rays had occurred several evenings before. Roentgen, like many of his contemporaries, was interested in defining the properties of the emanations of various high-energy vacuum tubes. One evening, he completely darkened the workroom below his living quarters at the University of Wurzburg to experiment with a Crookes/Lenard cathode ray tube.*[2] *The tube was completely covered by blackened cardboard, so Roentgen was surprised to see a glow emanating from a fluorescent screen*[3] *he had unintentionally left leaning against a nearby wall.*

    *Others had almost certainly seen this phenomenon before, since experimenting with cathode ray tubes was extremely popular with physicists and amateur scientists of this era. Most notable among them was Philipp Lenard, a close friend of Roentgen and the modifier of the Crookes tube that Roentgen employed that historic night. Roentgen's genius, however, was that he was the first to recognize the importance of what he saw—a new kind of radiation that would ultimately prove extraordinarily useful to the practice of medicine. Indeed, while Roentgen never personally*

---

[1] This statement is widely quoted, but we have been unable to determine its source.

[2] These tubes are the predecessors of modern tubes used for television and computer screens.

[3] The screen was coated with barium platinocyanide salts, which, like some other salts, have the capacity to translate high-radiofrequency energies like X-rays into light.

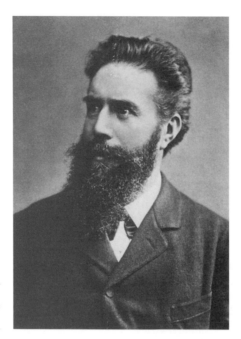

FIGURE 2-1

*Portrait of Wilhelm
Conrad Roentgen.*

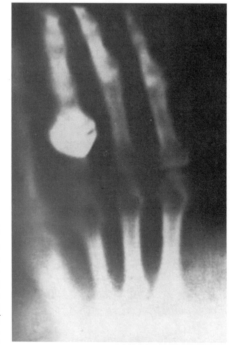

FIGURE 2-2

*The first human
radiograph—Berta
Roentgen's ghostly skel-
etal hand—exposed by
her husband, Wilhelm
Conrad Roentgen, within
weeks of his discovery of
X-rays.*

*investigated the practical applications of the Roentgen rays (as his physicist colleagues dubbed them), he presaged their eventual medical use. On this first evening of recognition, he moved his hand between the Crookes tube and the fluorescent screen and saw the vague, wavering outline of the bones of his hand.*[4]

Roentgen's epiphany was the first in a lengthening chain of discoveries that has brought us an array of modern computerized imaging modalities. The imaging innovations of the past 115 years have fundamentally altered nearly every aspect of medical practice. The amplification and refinement of medical images through digital technology brought into being powerful clinical tools like CT, MRI, ultrasonography, and PET scanning. A *fin de siecle* survey of physicians identified medical imaging as among the most important medical innovations of the last three decades, with CT and MRI achieving the highest ranking (Fuchs and Sox 2001).

A comprehensive history of medical imaging is beyond the scope of this book. Indeed, some have argued that imaging began with Anton von Leeuwenhoek's seventeenth-century use of lenses and light to observe microbes (what he called "wee beasties"). It would be hard to disagree. However, in this chapter, we have chosen to focus on the development of selected contemporary medical imaging technologies that employ penetrating radiant energies (for example, both X-rays and ultrasound waves are radiant energies) to depict disease in humans.

Rather than provide a strict chronological history, this chapter highlights a number of recurring themes in the development and adoption of the major medical imaging innovations in use today. Dominant themes of the history of medical imaging include:

- The role of serendipity;
- How developments in fields other than medicine have contributed to advances in imaging;
- The impact of wartime research and development on civilian use of imaging;
- The role of multidisciplinary collaboration;
- The transition from the depiction of anatomy to the depiction of physiology.

The ascent of imaging technologies to their current eminence is, in fact, an anthology of compelling narratives. From the discovery of the X-ray to the invention of today's cross-sectional imaging technologies, these stories illustrate the convergence of happy accidents with the receptivity of the prepared mind, competition and collaboration among investigators, the exhilaration of discovery, and the disappointment of near misses. This chapter will detail the life work of men and women whose ingenuity and perseverance led to the clinical uses of imaging we enjoy today and provide brief, hopefully lucid, descriptions for the lay reader of how the various modalities work to produce medical images.

These highly selective and abbreviated histories draw heavily on two major sources: the remarkable compendium celebrating the centennial of the discovery of the X-ray, *A History of the Radiological Sciences—Diagnosis*, edited by Bruce McClennan (Gagliardi and McClennan 1996), and Kevles' illuminating cultural

---

[4] http://wilhelmconradroentgen.com/wilhelm-conrad-roentgen-relevant-facts.

history, *Naked to the Bone* (Kevles 1997). Factual assertions are referable to these works unless otherwise indicated.

## A Shot in the Dark

On the evening of November 8, 1895, when Roentgen first observed, then deduced, the existence of what he called *X-rays*,[5] he was little known beyond the small enclave of European physicists. What he did in the months immediately following was to change that status. Roentgen worked with a fury to verify and expand upon what he knew about the mysterious rays. "I didn't think. I investigated," he later wrote to a colleague. And he did so in utter secrecy:

> I had spoken to no one about my work. To my wife I merely mentioned that I was working on something about which people would say, when they found out about it, "Roentgen has surely gone crazy." (Zehnder 1935)

Within six weeks, Roentgen detailed most of the physical properties of X-rays. Roentgen's original paper, "On a New Kind of Rays" ("Eine Neue Art von Strahlen"), was published on December 28, 1895. Among the properties he described were these:

- "…the density of the bodies is the property whose variation mainly affects their [X-ray] permeability."
- "Increasing thickness increases the hindrance offered to the rays by all bodies."[6]
- "…other bodies [than barium platinocyanide] exhibit fluorescence [to X-rays], e.g. calcium sulfide, uranium glass, Iceland spar, rock-salt, etc."
- "…we cannot conclude any regular reflection or refraction of the X-rays."
- "I have not succeeded in observing any deviation of the X-rays even in very strong magnetic fields."
- "The retina of the eye is quite insensitive to these rays; the eye placed close to the apparatus sees nothing (i.e. X-rays are invisible). It is clear from the experiments that this is not due to want of permeability on the part of the structures of the eye."[7]

The report was picked up by newspapers around the world and republished in English in *Nature, Science,* and *Scientific American*. Its appearance in the press caused a sensation among a lay public just emerging from the Victorian era and enamored of science, but there remained considerable skepticism among Roentgen's physicist colleagues. On January 23, 1896, Roentgen put an end to their doubts. He presented his findings to a gathering of prominent European physicists in Wurzburg, concluding with a demonstration that astounded his audience. Watched by the doubting crowd, he produced an image of the hand of one of the attendees, a famous professor of anatomy named Geheimrat von Kolliker.

---

[5] Roentgen preferred the term *X-rays* to signify their unknown properties, perhaps analogous to a mathematician solving for *X*.

[6] For materials of the same density, the thicker the material, the greater the absorption of the X-rays and the more radiodense, or whiter, the image.

[7] http://web.lemoyne.edu/~giunta/roentgen.html.

Roentgen became an instant celebrity—a rock star of his era. He was made rector of the university, the highest honor the institution could bestow. He received medals and other honorifics around the world. In 1901, the newly formed Swedish Nobel Academy awarded Roentgen the first Nobel Prize for physics.

The recognition Roentgen received sparked controversy. Lenard insisted that he had been the first to see the effects of the mysterious rays.[8] In fact, in Roentgen's original paper (he published two more articles in 1896 and 1897), he acknowledged Lenard and others whose work underlay his observations. But in the end, he was the one who had made the critical connection.

Medical applications of the X-ray followed with remarkable speed. Dr. John Macintyre established a medical imaging service at the Glasgow Royal Infirmary in 1896 and produced a number of radiographic firsts, such as demonstrating a kidney stone and a coin swallowed and lodged in the throat of a child. In the United States, also in 1896, Dartmouth surgeon Edwin Frost showed the potential of the X-ray for orthopedic diagnosis, depicting the broken wrist of a patient brought to him by his brother, also a physician. Harvard physiologist Walter Cannon fed a barium-coated meal to a cat and revealed fluoroscopically[9] how food was propelled by peristalsis through the gastrointestinal tract. The first U.S. textbook of medical imaging, *The Roentgen Rays in Medicine and Surgery*, was published by Dartmouth's Dr. Francis Williams in 1901.

The use of X-ray examinations expanded greatly with the advent of the Boer War and World War I. The new technology showed its mettle on the battlefield in locating bullets and shrapnel for surgical guidance and elucidating the causes of cryptic injuries. When the soldiers returned home, they brought with them expectations of continued access to this marvelous new technology. The use of X-ray diagnosis in wartime promoted the broader dissemination of medical applications during the ensuing peace.

The frenzy over the discovery of X-rays was not limited to medicine. Thomas Edison, among others, patented a number of X-ray-generating products for use as popular entertainment. Sideshow barkers and pitchmen hawked products that had been exposed to X-rays as curatives for everything from headaches to hemorrhoids. Indeed, the X-ray has remained part of popular culture up to recent times. As one example, older baby boomers may remember playing with the foot fluoroscope at their local shoe store.

In time, the enthusiasm for uncontrolled X-radiation was tempered by the evidence first emerging within months of Roentgen's discovery that excessive exposure could be harmful—even deadly. Many of the early experimenters experienced acute burns. Some died of tumors produced by massive X-ray exposures over time and are frequently referred to as "martyrs of radiology" (Brown 1936). As one example of how

---

[8] The Nobel advisory committee actually voted to give the prize to both Roentgen and Lenard, but the full Nobel assembly determined that Nobel's bequest was for a single prize. The practice has since been changed, and a shared prize is more the rule nowadays. This is more in keeping with the way science operates—a convergence of various contributions that, combined, produce something of importance. Lenard received the Nobel Prize in 1905 for his work on cathode ray tubes.

[9] Fluoroscopy replaces film with a fluorescent plate, allowing the visualization of motion as it is happening.

extreme X-ray injury could be, the early pioneer Emil Grubbe—who began building his own X-ray tubes and experimenting with X-rays in 1896—was said to have had over 100 surgeries and amputations related to X-radiation before his death.[10]

The concerns about the dangers of chronic radiation exposure were buttressed by a growing body of scientific evidence in biophysics that coincided with the birth of atomic power in the 1940s. These discoveries only enhanced the public's fascination with X-rays. Numerous popular films exploited the plot device of an accidental exposure to X-radiation leading to dire consequences. X-rays have mutated harmless creatures into well-meaning fictional crusaders like Spiderman (bitten by an irradiated spider); tragic victims of science (like the character in *The Fly*); and monsters like Godzilla (whose strontium-laden footprints evidenced his exposure to the fallout of a nuclear blast).

Advances in film technology, methods for reducing scatter radiation that clouds the sharpness of the image, and the replacement of film by digital receptor technology to allow the display of medical images on computer monitors have all contributed to the improvement of X-ray diagnosis over the past 115 years. However, most crucial to the development of X-ray diagnosis was the emergence of the new medical specialty, radiology. It is doubtful whether without the focused interest of these specialized physicians and their collaboration with their colleagues in physics and engineering we would today enjoy the benefits of modern medical imaging.

Even today, with all of our complex cross-sectional imaging methods, the humble radiograph remains by far the most frequently performed imaging procedure in the United States and around the world. Its principal applications are in orthopedic, abdominal, and chest diagnosis, mammography, and emergency room trauma (Figs. 2-3 and 2-4). Frequently, X-ray examination is used as a first test to help determine if additional, more sophisticated imaging is warranted.

FIGURE 2-3

*Radiograph of a premature infant with severe necrotizing enterocolitis due to poor blood flow from a congenital coarctation (narrowing) of the aorta. The infection has cause infarction (tissue death from lack of oxygen) of the intestinal wall, allowing air into the branching portal venous system (veins draining the gastrointestinal tract—arrow). The gas indicates the diagnosis of bowel wall infarction. (Courtesy of Marc Sarti, MD, the University of Virginia.)*

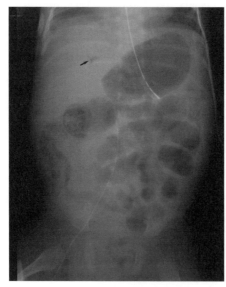

[10] Personal communication, Otha Linton, May 2009.

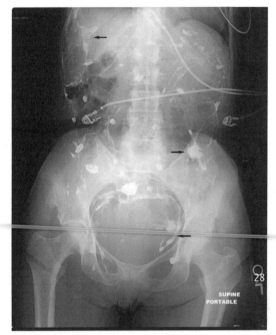

FIGURE 2-4

*Radiograph of the abdomen of an 88-year-old patient with barium peritonitis (inflammation of the space surrounding the intestines). The patient had previously undergone a barium enema examination. The barium leaked through a rupture in the colon into the peritoneum and is seen as dense material surrounding the intestines (arrows). (Courtesy of Marc Sarti, MD, the University of Virginia.)*

## Box 2-1  Radiography

Electric energy boils off electrons from the negatively charged cathode of an X-ray tube, and the electrons are accelerated to high speed toward the anode. Striking the anode causes rapid deceleration and the emission of X-rays. Alignment of the patient in the proper position relative to the X-ray beam causes the X-rays to enter the intended body part of the patient. Some of the X-rays are absorbed by tissues, others pass directly through the body onto the X-ray receptor, and still others are scattered by physical interactions with the molecules in the tissue. How many X-rays pass through to the receptor depends on the energy of the X-rays and the thickness and density of the tissues they traverse. Different thicknesses and densities of tissues cause different anatomical structures to appear darker or whiter on the X-ray image (called the *radiograph*). Dense tissues like bone absorb more of the radiation and appear whiter (radiologists say *denser*) than soft tissues like liver or kidney, which are shades of gray (more *lucent*). Fat is more lucent than other soft tissues. Gas, normally contained within the intestines, is the most lucent and appears nearly black.

### From Warfare in the North Atlantic to TomKat's Baby

Another widely applied imaging technology is ultrasonography. Ultrasonography uses high-frequency sound waves to interrogate a broad range of organ systems.

The development of medical ultrasonography owes much to World War II naval research and development. However, that's not how ultrasonography initially began. Sonographic imaging is based on the physical principle of piezoelectricity, first described by the Curie brothers, Jacques and Pierre, in 1877.[11] They found that electricity has the power to deform crystals, which then emit sound waves at frequencies far beyond the range of human (or even canine) hearing—hence the term *ultrasound*.[12] And there the discovery sat, with no practical application, for roughly 40 years.

The 1912 sinking of the *Titanic* revived scientific interest in the piezoelectric effect. The tragedy gave physicists the idea of employing high-frequency sound to provide earlier warning of an impending collision than simple sighting of an obstacle. Carl and Friedreich Dussik first reported a medical application in 1937. They placed the ultrasound transducer (the instrument emitting the ultrasound) and the receptor (the instrument detecting the transmission of sound waves) on opposite sides of a patient's head and produced a crude image of the brain. The brain, as it turns out, was a tough place to start, and a number of early medical ultrasound researchers foundered on the shoals of the human skull. This is because bone is highly reflective of ultrasound waves, complicating adequate representational imaging of the brain. Ultimately, ultrasonography did find an application in detecting intracranial abnormalities in the form of A-mode ultrasonography, which produces a waveform rather than a pictorial representation of anatomy, and aided the diagnosis of abnormalities like blood clots and tumors shifting the midline of the brain.

The definitive boost toward practical application was provided by antisubmarine warfare in the north Atlantic during World War II. Beginning in the late 1930s, German submarines savaged Allied shipping, threatening the supply lines between the United States and Europe and even menaced commercial shipping along the U.S. Eastern seaboard within sight of land. High frequency sound waves travel nearly unimpeded through a homogeneous substance like water. Its reflections off a solid object can travel great distances and provide information about the location of the detected object relative to the source. The resultant technology was called *SONAR* for "sound navigation and ranging." Ultrasound technology also found uses in the burgeoning industrial war effort, where it was used to look for non-uniformities in the metallic armor plating of tanks.

In the immediate postwar era, researchers who had participated in the science that promoted the Allied victory sought new civilian applications for wartime discoveries. Four major medical ultrasound laboratories developed in the United States—at the Massachusetts Institute of Technology (led by Richard Bolt), the University of Illinois (William Fry), the University of Minnesota (John Wild), and the University of Colorado (Douglas Howry). By the mid-1950s, the efforts of these research groups led to the invention of the pulse-echo technique, which allowed the consolidation of the transducer and receptor into the same unit, as well as B-mode scanning,

[11] Pierre is better known as the husband of Marie Curie, although his work earned a Nobel Prize too.
[12] Humans hear sounds in the low tens of thousands of Hertz range, while medical ultrasound employs frequencies in the megaHertz range—two orders of magnitude higher.

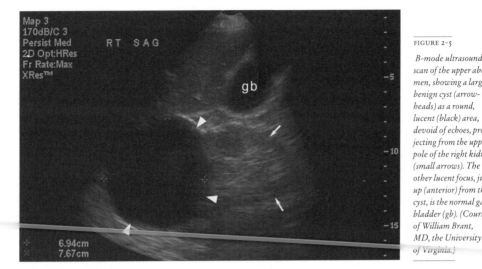

FIGURE 2-5

*B-mode ultrasound
scan of the upper abdo-
men, showing a large,
benign cyst (arrow-
heads) as a round,
lucent (black) area,
devoid of echoes, pro-
jecting from the upper
pole of the right kidney
(small arrows). The
other lucent focus, just
up (anterior) from the
cyst, is the normal gall-
bladder (gb). (Courtesy
of William Brant,
MD, the University
of Virginia.)*

which generated the now familiar black-and-white, fan-shaped image of a segment
of the body (Fig. 2-5).

John Wild was among the prime innovators responsible for the discoveries that
underlie modern ultrasonography. Using equipment derived from military SONAR,
he was able to use A-mode scanning to show characteristic differences among normal
intestine, inflamed bowel wall, and cancer in tissue specimens. Wild was a talented
but controversial scientist, whose colleagues looked askance at the testing he did on
himself and the informal way he dealt with human subjects. Even so, the National
Cancer Institute (NCI) continued to fund his research program well into the 1950s.
At that point, NCI's ultrasound imaging project managers decided to focus their
funding on what they considered the more promising Colorado techniques and
asked Wild to adopt Howry's methods. Wild refused to alter his approach. He sued
the federal government over the withdrawal of his federal funding and continued
his work well into the 1990s with private money as director of his own research
institute.[13]

The ultrasound devices of these early researchers were unwieldy and impractical.
As an example, one of Howry's early scanners—depicted in *Life* magazine in 1954—
required that subjects be immersed in a water bath to be scanned.[14] More important
was the fact that, there was no compelling clinical need for the technology to drive
commercial interest. What changed that situation was the work of Dr. Ian Donald
of Scotland and his obstetrician colleagues. Donald had worked with SONAR during the war. Using an A-mode scanner based on a military metal flaw detector, he
experimented with ultrasonography as a way of measuring fetuses less invasively
in situations where he was concerned that a large fetal head might endanger the
mother's health. Other obstetricians adopted sonography for this purpose, as well
as for a growing list of other gynecological and fetal indications. The development
of so-called B-mode scanning (*B* for "brightness") made possible representational

[13] http://www.ob-ultrasound.net/jjwildbio.html.
[14] http://www.ob-ultrasound.net/howry.html.

FIGURE 2-6

(a) M-mode ultra-
sound scans showing a.
a living fetus (arrow)
with normal cardiac
motion represented
by the waveform
(arrowheads) beneath
the image. Compare the
cardiac waveform of the
normal fetus shown in
image (a) with the flat
waveform associated
with fetal demise in
image (b). (Courtesy of
William Brant, MD, the
University of Virginia.)

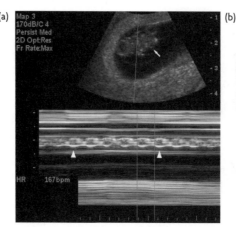
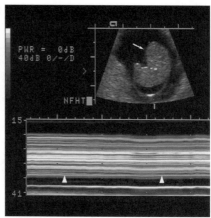

scanning that produced an image of a section of the body. In Sweden, cardiologist Inge Edler and physicist Helmuth Hertz developed M-mode scanning (*M* for "motion"), another graphic technique that proved useful in cardiac diagnosis (Fig. 2-6). By the mid- to late 1960s, the major imaging equipment manufacturers had become interested in the commercial possibilities of medical ultrasound imaging.

Early commercial B-mode systems produced images that were strictly black and white and low resolution. The images revealed only major interfaces between organs or between normal and abnormal tissues. It took great expertise to produce the scans and interpret them. The clinical ultrasound pioneer Dr. Barry Goldberg of Thomas Jefferson University recalled a common perspective of established radiologists when he trained in ultrasonography during its early years of clinical use:

> In radiology, the established hierarchy was skeptical, particularly because tissue representation in the ultrasound image was different from that of conventional radiologic images, so physicians with considerable skill and experience in interpreting X-ray images could not readily interpret sonograms. The relatively poor resolution and the difficulty in imaging tissue such as lung, bowel, and bone also proved barriers to acceptance even though different tissue properties were evident on sonograms as compared with radiographs. As a result, radiologists striving to make their mark in ultrasound often received less than optimal departmental support. (Goldberg et al. 1993, p. 193)

One of the authors of this book (BJH) experienced much the same attitude when, during his residency, he took several months of training with the renowned early Danish practitioner Hans Hendrick Holm. Holm, a urologist, was among the first to use ultrasound to guide therapeutic procedures. The snide comments by colleagues may have had more to do with the fact that the fellowship was in Copenhagen than that it focused on ultrasonography.

What changed physicians' perceptions were several key developments enabled by the computerization of ultrasound technology. These innovations have resulted in a modality that is perhaps the most versatile in all of imaging and is second only to X-radiography in worldwide use. The development of gray-scale ultrasonography (images portrayed as shades of gray, rather than the black and white of B-scale) revealed the internal features of organs and masses (Fig. 2-7) and greatly expanded the indications for the use of ultrasound throughout the body. Real-time technology allowed operators to see what they were pointing at as they moved the transducer, allowing them to make subtle adjustments in the positioning of the transducer for improved diagnosis.

Doppler sonography is another advance that has extended the capabilities of ultrasonography to the evaluation of the cardiovascular system. Based on the discovery of the Austrian Johann Doppler, who first described the changing frequency of sound as a moving object (like a train) approaches, then departs from, a stationary listener, this technique has been applied to medical diagnosis. Doppler sonography depicts the extent, direction, and velocity of blood flow, enabling the diagnosis of vascular conditions like stenoses (narrowings) of key arteries, malfunctioning heart valves, and the obstruction of dialysis access shunts, and in some cases, the differentiation of benign from malignant masses (Fig. 2-8).[15] With Doppler interrogation of blood vessels, ultrasonography progressed from the purely anatomical to the physiological, or functional, realm.

The current principal uses of ultrasound are for prenatal examination of the fetus; the evaluation of premature infant brains; the evaluation of flow through blood vessels; diagnosing abnormalities of the abdomen, eye, and heart; the further evaluation of breast masses seen on screening mammography; and guidance of nonvascular interventional procedures like directing needle biopsies of tumors and catheter drainages of fluid collections. In performing image-guided interventions,

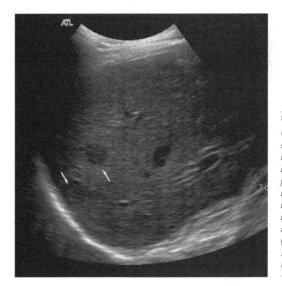

FIGURE 2-7

*Contemporary gray scale sonogram angled through the liver. The image reveals abnormal foci of mixed echoes that are less dense than liver representing fungal* (Candida albicans) *abscesses (arrows). (Courtesy of Marc Sarti, MD, the University of Virginia.)*

[15] A dialysis access shunt is surgically created in the arm of a patient with kidney failure to make feasible the periodic cleaning of the blood by a dialysis machine, which acts as an artificial kidney.

FIGURE 2-8

*Modern gray scale
breast sonogram
depicting a solid mass
(arrows) (a cyst would
have no echoes within
it). The scan is in
Doppler mode, showing
moderately high blood
flow (boxed region)
typical of breast cancer.
(Courtesy of Michael
Cohen, MD, Emory
University.)*

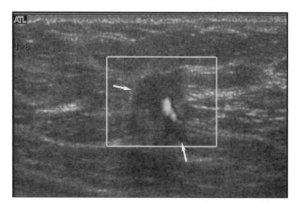

the capacity to visualize structures in real time[16] is a particular advantage. The radiologist watches the target organ move with respiration as the biopsy needle approaches and enters a suspicious mass. Real-time ultrasound guidance reduces the time required for the procedure, makes it safer, and affords the patient a less painful and risky intervention.

Modern ultrasonography has captured the professional and lay public imagination. Fetal ultrasound has become a rite of pregnancy (some would say "a right!"). It has become routine to have at least one sonography examination during the course of fetal development, if only to obtain the baby's first picture for the family scrapbook. Actors Tom Cruise and Katie Holmes famously bought their own machine to keep track of their baby's maturation. Modern three-dimensional ultrasound imaging has become sophisticated enough that medical practices, hospitals, and suburban mall stores have been able to develop successful businesses purely for ultrasonic fetal photography.[17] All of them tout the capacity of these devices to produce life-like featuring of the baby's face, fingers, and toes. In doing so, they have molded patients' expectations. Ultrasound images have become so life-like that the technology has become a legislative and public relations tool in the anti-abortion movement's fight against fetal termination (Sack 2010).

The virtues of ultrasonography are that the technology does not rely on potentially harmful ionizing radiation like X-rays and is portable enough to be taken to the patient's bedside (a real advantage for evaluating very sick patients). Ultrasound is more flexible and tends to be faster for guiding interventional procedures than other modalities when the target is superficial and/or large. Contributing to the global adoption of the technology is that ultrasonography devices are far less expensive to buy and operate than other cross-sectional imaging methods, like CT and MRI. In recent years, manufacturers have emphasized this distinction by making units smaller, and hence more portable, and inexpensive enough ($20,000–$30,000) for even solo practicing nonradiologist physicians to acquire them. The attraction is that physicians can use these "modern-day stethoscopes," as companies market them, to diagnose conditions that might not be detected by the traditional tools of physical

---

[16] Seeing what the transducer is "seeing" at the same time that it is seeing it.
[17] Commercial stores selling ultrasound photography have been banned in some states where ultrasonography is restricted to purely medical use.

examination—observation, palpation, percussion, and auscultation.[18] If the miniaturization trend continues, the ultrasound machine will soon rival the cell phone for
portability, and its use (and perhaps misuse) will become ubiquitous.

---

**Box 2-2**  Ultrasonography

---

Ultrasonography depends on the piezoelectric effect, which is generated by
passing an alternating electric current through bipolar (think of north/south, as
with a magnet) crystals. The electric current deforms the crystal. When the burst
of electricity is shut off, the crystal seeks to return to its more stable, original
configuration. The repeated process of deformation and reconfiguration causes
the emission of a high-frequency sound wave. The frequency of the sound is
dependent on both the nature of the crystal and the electric field. The frequency
of ultrasound used for medical imaging ranges from 1 to greater than 10 MHz.[*]
Ultrasound travels poorly through air, so the abrupt difference in sound transmission between air and the surface of the body requires that the ultrasound
transducer be "coupled" to the body by a thick gel. As the ultrasound waves enter
the body, they encounter heterogeneous tissues. Some of the sound waves are
reflected back to the transducer by major interfaces, as where two body organs
abut. Ultrasound also bounces off of smaller interfaces, such as at the junction of
different tissue components within an organ. The ultrasound device uses a computer to localize these *echoes* spatially on the image by calculating the elapsed
time between their transmission and reception.

[*]Ultrasound frequencies are 1,000 or more times higher than the 15 kHz limit of human
hearing.

---

### CT Scanning and the Foundations of Modern Cross-Sectional Imaging

The CT scanner is the workhorse of modern diagnostic imaging. Contemporary CT
scanning depends on multiple X-ray sources and multiple detectors (up to 320 of
them) surrounding the patient to produce *tomograms*—images appearing as horizontal slices through the body. Powerful microprocessors translate the numerous
resultant electronic signals into a stream of coherent horizontal (called *axial*) slice-
like images through the human body and also enable image reconstruction into life-
like three-dimensional representations of anatomy. Hundreds to more than 1000 of
these slices—each as thin as 1 millimeter for some clinical applications—plus recon-
structions of the data into complementary vertical and depthwise (sagittal and coronal, respectively) planes comprise the complete CT examination.

Unlike the situation with radiography, no single event marks the seminal moment
in the invention of the CT scanner. However, it is fair to say that neither CT nor any
of the other major cross-sectional technologies we employ today would exist without the work of several foundational investigators. All cross-sectional technologies

---

[18] Looking, feeling, tapping, and listening, respectively.

require a complex mathematical algorithm that permits the "reconstruction" of the image from its various component signals. Development of the initial algorithm originated as a part-time job for mathematician Alan Cormack, who was asked by Capetown, South Africa's Groote Schuur Hospital to develop a means of gauging the effects of the differences in the way radiation passes through the tissues of patients undergoing radiation therapy. The eventual use of this work in the algorithm for reconstructing CT slices of the body from multiple X-ray signals was critical to the actualization of the technology.

However, it was Godfrey Hounsfield who, while working for the British electronics firm EMI (Electrical and Musical Industries, Ltd.), was principally responsible for the invention of the CT scanner. His background would not have predicted it. Hounsfield was raised in rural England and did not pursue an advanced education. Rather, he was an autodidact who, after serving as a radar mechanic during World War II, became intrigued by the potential applications of postwar electronics, including primitive computers.

EMI was Hounsfield's sole employer for his entire career. He became EMI's resident genius. A seemingly unrelated development was critical to Hounsefield's great accomplishment. A sidelight for EMI was its participation in the recording industry. In the early 1960s, EMI signed on a little known mop-headed music quartet from the rougher part of Liverpool. The Beatles eventually sold more than 200 million records, more than doubling EMI's revenues. Suddenly EMI had the financial wherewithal to pursue longer-range projects. The Beatles' explosive success made CT imaging possible.

One of the new projects was assigned to Godfrey Hounsfield. EMI wanted to pursue investigations in pattern recognition, which had been popularized during the war to address the problem of identifying camouflaged targets from other geographic features. Hounsfield was thinking about his work as he took one of his frequent strolls in the English countryside. He had an epiphany. Combining measurements of X-ray transmissions derived from multiple different angles would allow him to reconstruct a new type of medical image. Hounsfield's country idyll led directly to his group's development of a primitive version of CT. A 1968 prototype featured a rotating table and took nine days using gamma rays to produce an image of a *phantom* (an inanimate model used in testing imaging equipment). Interestingly, David Kuhl at the University of Pennsylvania, one of the founders of clinical PET scanning, had earlier tried, and dismissed as impractical, using gamma rays to produce cross-sectional images. Using X-radiation instead was the critical advance of the EMI research group that made CT scanning more time-efficient. Even so, given the level of available computing power, early CT image generation still took an impractical length of time.

Despite its robust financial state, EMI was averse to assuming the risk of fully funding the CT project on its own. The company found a partner in the British Department of Health and Social Security and a clinical collaborator in neurosurgeon James Ambrose at the Atkinson Morley Hospital. Typical of most proprietary research, the work proceeded in absolute secrecy for fear of corporate espionage.[19]

---

[19] The incentive for most academic researchers is recognition, so they tend to publish results as rapidly as possible. The principal motivation for companies is financial profit, so such niceties as publication and public presentation rarely occur before a product is patented and clears regulatory hurdles for fear of another company's copying the idea.

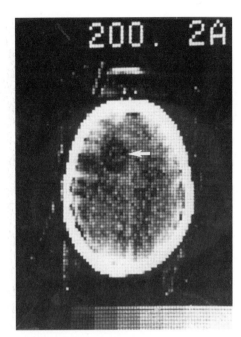

FIGURE 2-9

*First human CT scan, performed by the EMI Corporation at the Atkinson Morley Hospital, Wimbledon, England, in 1972 on a woman thought to have a brain tumor. The pixels comprising the image are quite large, meaning that the scan can resolve only larger abnormalities. The scan shows a cyst in the left frontal lobe (arrow). Following the woman's operation, the surgeon said, "It looks exactly like the picture." Reprinted with permission from Beckmann EC. CT scanning the early days.* British Journal of Radiology 2006;79(937):5–8.

The first CT image (Fig. 2-9) was presented at the British Institute of Medicine in April 1972. The first commercial scanner emerged later the same year. Initially, EMI's CT device was designed strictly for brain scanning. It featured a sealed plastic water bag that fitted over the top of the patient's head. With only a single radiation source and a single detector, the gantry slowly clicked its way around the patient, discharging a pencil-thick X-ray beam. A computer took an hour or more to reconstruct the separate images into a picture of the brain.

The presentation of the first human scan at British and American medical meetings caused a sensation among radiologists and other providers interested in brain imaging. Prior to CT scanning, the brain and its diseases could only be viewed by open brain surgery or, indirectly by invasive, severely discomforting procedures like catheter angiography, The initial CT images were grainy, but a knowledgeable and experienced radiologist could diagnose major abnormalities like tumors, hemorrhages, and strokes. As CT disseminated into practice, patients were spared the anguish of pneumoencephalography, which became obsolete overnight and ceased to be performed within several years.

Modifications to the technology soon allowed scanning of other parts of the body. EMI sold its CT business to the Picker Corporation, and a host of other companies entered the CT market. There were naysayers who said that the technology was too expensive and that its actual contributions wouldn't live up to the hype. In response to these concerns, during a 1976 department of radiology grand rounds at Harvard's Peter Bent Brigham Hospital, radiologist Herbert Abrams predicted that CT would not only dominate diagnosis, but that a still-to-be-invented modification he named the *computerized axial tomography (CAT)-cutter* would one day obviate the need for surgery (author BJH attended the session). What Abrams intended as a humorous prod of his surgical colleagues was remarkably prescient.

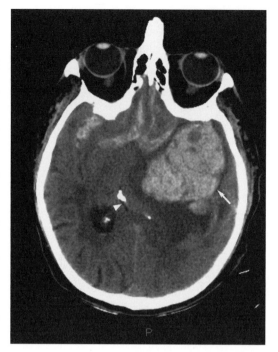

FIGURE 2-10

*Compare the much
better visualization of
structure in this modern
CT scan with that in
Figure 2-9. The patient
has had a massive
stroke. The large, lobu-
lar, dense focus (arrow)
at the base of the skull
represents a hemor-
rhage, which is displac-
ing normally midline
structures, like the third
ventricle (arrowhead),
to the right. The very
dense foci are calcified
choroid plexus (a
frequent finding of no
importance). (Courtesy
of Mary Lee Jensen,
MD, the University of
Virginia.)*

Over the years, the allied efforts of academic radiology departments and their corporate partners have resulted in the continuous evolution of CT technology. Enormous leaps in computing power have greatly improved the quality of the images (Fig. 2-10) and expanded the diagnostic reach of the technology. The combination of ever more powerful microprocessors, increasing numbers of sources and detectors,[20] as well as novel scanning and reconstruction approaches, have resulted in higher spatial resolution and more speed (known in the trade as *temporal resolution*). These technical advances have led to a continuous stream of new applications, which have incorporated into radiologists' practices. Today, CT is used to investigate innumerable conditions in every part of the body. New applications like CT angiography and CT colonography[21] threaten to disrupt the order of medicine by replacing existing invasive procedures like catheter evaluation of blood vessels and traditional colonoscopy.

The ongoing increase in the use of CT scanning continues to generate controversy. On the one hand, it is incontrovertible that CT has been revolutionary in expanding the diagnostic reach of health care, in eliminating the morbidity associated with pre-CT diagnosis, and in saving many a patient from a more invasive procedure. On the other hand, CT has been held up (for more than 30 years!) as the poster child for high-technology medicine run amuck—too often used in situations where it is

---

[20] The sources are the components emitting the X-rays; the detectors pick up the X-rays as they pass through the other side of the patient.

[21] CT colonography and CT angiography are new ways to visualize abnormalities of the colon and blood vessels, respectively. We discuss both of these procedures in several other chapters.

unnecessary, thereby adding unnecessary cost. Emblematic of how the rapid rise in CT utilization has been viewed by its detractors is a statement in the *New England Journal of Medicine* during the early euphoric years of clinical use:

> CAT fever has reached epidemic proportions and continues to spread among physicians, manufacturers, entrepreneurs, and regulatory agencies. A cursory review of any radiologic or neuroscience journal attests to the virulence of this new disease. Within the United States, alone, the costs of this epidemic are staggering. (Shapiro and Wyman 1976, p. 954)

The Nobel Assembly awarded the 1979 Nobel Prize to Alan Cormack and Godfrey Hounsfield, noting that "ordinary X-ray examinations of the head had shown the skull bones, but the brain had remained a gray, undifferentiated fog. Now, suddenly, the fog had lifted." (Goetz 2010) Upon hearing the news, Hounsfield denied having ever heard of his fellow laureate, nor, he said, did he know of Cormack's contributions. The prize conferred recognition of the value of CT but did not end the debate over its costs. Concerns over the marginal and inappropriate use of CT have increased in parallel with its use. The usage of CT is characteristic of a problem inherent in much of medical innovation. Dissemination and use outpace scientific consensus on the utility and appropriate use of the technology. The dearth of reliable evidence for when imaging is best employed and when imaging improves the balance between benefit and harm is a major and recurring theme of this book.

## Box 2-3  Computed Tomography

Computed tomography scanners use X-rays as the radiant energy to interrogate the body's structure. However, rather than irradiating the body from a single direction, as with X-radiography (also known as *plain X-ray*), irradiation is performed from many directions around the body. Each of the many measurements of transmitted X-rays contributes a fragment of the cross-sectional image. The computational power of modern computers combines the X-ray images from many different directions into a composite that depicts a complete *slice* through the body. Moving the patient's body through the ring of surrounding detectors allows for the reconstruction of numerous adjacent slices. The resultant images can be viewed sequentially to mentally build a comprehensive view of a body part or the computer can reconstruct them into a three-dimensional representation.

### Magnetism and Spinning the Atom

Magnetic resonance imaging is based on physical phenomena quite different from .those thus far described. As a result, the technology provides quite different information about anatomy and function than X-radiation or ultrasonography.

That atomic nuclei with an odd number of protons or neutrons can be induced to display a characteristic spin has been known since the 1920s. This spin was first measured in the 1930s by the American physicist I.I. Rabi, who termed the phenomenon *nuclear magnetic resonance* (NMR).[22] A decade later, chemists Felix Bloch, working at Stanford, and Edward Purcell, working at Harvard, independently measured the NMR effect in bulk materials by placing them in an alternating magnetic field of increasing and decreasing strengths and published their results simultaneously.[23] In doing so, they established what ultimately would become the physical basis for medical MRI.

Decades later, laboratories headed by Paul Lauterbur and Raymond Damadian made practical use of Bloch and Purcell's discovery. From the start, Lauterbur concentrated on producing cross-sectional images. Damadian initially focused his efforts on producing chemical spectra that would differentiate the metabolism of normal from cancerous tissues. Indeed, Damadian's early experiments showed the potential to do exactly that in test tube specimens. With a small grant from the National Institutes of Health (NIH) and private funding, he built the first magnetic NMR machine for interrogating the human body. He called his machine "Indomitable."

During the early 1970s, Lauterbur headed a small NMR company. The struggling company needed help, and he had an idea. He could produce a coherent NMR image of the human body from numerous contributing signals by interrogating the body with magnetic fields oriented in different directions, much the same as the concept for CT scanning. The application of this idea allowed Lauterbur to plot the signals coming from specific points in the body, which he could assign to an image. This was an advance over the early system developed by Damadian, which provided no spatial information.

Lauterbur's insight came in 1971, a year before the introduction of commercial CT. The mathematics he employed were similar to those of Cormack and Hounsfield, but he was unaware that he was reinventing earlier work. He predicted in his notebooks that his new technique might eventually replace X-rays for medical diagnosis. Overcoming initial rejections of his work by scientific journals, Lauterbur finally published his description of the new method of making medical images in *Nature* in 1973. The short article included the first known NMR images of water-filled test tubes. The choice of water by Lauterbur and other early NMR researchers was telling. Water is by far the most common substance in the human body, and its hydrogen atoms, having a single proton, are particularly susceptible to NMR imaging. The imaging of the body's water is what lies at the root of MRI's superior definition of soft tissue structures.

In England, physicist Peter Mansfield independently came up with the same imaging solution as Lauterbur, but his work was primarily with nonorganic substances. As he became aware of the works of Damadian and Lauterbur, Mansfield switched his focus to biological imaging.

By this time, there was bad blood between Damadian and Lauterbur. They had had an unhappy first meeting, and Damadian blamed Lauterbur for some of the impediments he perceived to have been placed in his path. The differences between the two men were considerable. From his early involvement in MRI development, Damadian had been an aggressive self-promoter who, to the present, has proclaimed

[22] The discovery earned Rabi the Nobel Prize in 1944.
[23] Bloch and Purcell shared the 1952 Nobel Prize. Imagine the disappointment if one lab had come in with its results just a little later.

his primacy in NMR research. In sharp contrast, Lauterbur was a self-effacing academic type. Mansfield's growing eminence in the field unwittingly placed him in competition with two men engaged in an acrimonious race to see who could first develop a viable imaging device.

By the early 1980s, a number of small companies were springing up to manufacture and sell MRI devices. The companies variously developed scanners based on three magnet technologies: permanent, resistive, and superconducting. A discussion of the differences among these types of systems is beyond the scope of this book, but suffice it to say that they were significant enough to cause uncertainty among potential customers.

The acceptance of CT as an important advance in medical care during the 1970s both helped and hindered the introduction of MRI in the early 1980s. The development of CT largely overcame the technical problems of reconstructing usable medical images from multiple cross-sectional signals, but there were intense debates over the incremental value of MRI beyond what CT offered. From the start, MRI was (and remains today) a more expensive technology, and it was not immediately clear to its many detractors what advantages MRI offered over CT.

Despite the voices contending that MRI was simply an expensive add-on to CT, which would add little to clinical care, a number of leading academic radiology departments—at the University of California San Francisco, Washington University, and the Cleveland Clinic, to name a few—vied for leadership in exploring the clinical uses of the new modality.

However, the early leaders in the field perceived a potential marketing problem: the name *nuclear magnetic resonance*. Advocates of the technology posited that people might be frightened of NMR because of the strong association between the word *nuclear* and weaponry. The name NMR also incorrectly implied that dangerous ionizing radiation was involved.

As NMR was developing, the Cold War was heating up. It was rumored that India was working on a bomb. The antinuclear movement was coalescing and becoming more vocal about the threat of global annihilation. The Three-Mile Island nuclear power plant meltdown had occurred just a few years earlier, in 1979. Perhaps more to the point, there was the issue of who would control the clinical applications. Radiologists, who were among the first to install NMR imaging devices, were concerned that the word *nuclear* might embolden nuclear medicine physicians, and even other specialists, to compete with radiologists for MRI ownership. Alexander Margulis, then chair of the Department of Radiology at the University of California, San Francisco, described his epiphany about the name NMR:

> I was visiting the Cleveland Clinic in the early 1980s. The Clinic was looking for a new chair of radiology, and they asked me to advise them. They were very proud of their two MRI units, which they had put in an outpatient building and labeled it with a sign: "World's Best NMR Center." The building was located in an African-American neighborhood, and the residents were very vocal about how the Clinic wouldn't have placed a nuclear facility in a white neighborhood. I recall thinking—magnetic resonance imaging ... MRI.[24]

[24] Personal communication, Alexander Margulis, August 2009.

Despite the technical, competitive, and economic concerns, corporations began to sense that there might be big money in MRI. Driven both by the uniqueness of the diagnostic information MRI conveys and by competition among imaging providers, the technology quickly diffused into clinical practice.

But what became of the angry competition between Damadian and Lauterbur? As MRI gained the same level of acceptance as CT, backers of each of these men increasingly agitated behind the scenes for their man to receive the Nobel Prize. The chairman of the Nobel Committee for Medicine or Physiology in 2005 was Hans Ringertz, professor and chairman of radiology at Stockholm's Karolinska Institute. The time and leadership were right for a Nobel Prize for MRI, and those who believed they had a claim pursued it. Damadian was particularly aggressive, to the point of visiting Ringertz in Stockholm in 2005 and offering him, gratis, a scanner for his department.[25]

The proceedings of the Nobel Assembly are locked for 50 years, so what exactly happened will not be known until 2055. After an unusual wait beyond the expected time of the announcement, the Nobel Assembly announced that Lauterbur and Mansfield would share the Nobel Prize. Damadian was left out. Neither the subsequent full-page ads his supporters placed in *The New York Times* nor the letter-writing campaign they coordinated decrying the unfairness of his exclusion would change the outcome.

Over time, MRI has earned its way into broad worldwide use for its better soft tissue resolution, its lack of ionizing radiation, and its value in situations where the use of CT might be dangerous to the patient.[26] Magnetic resonance technology has the potential to provide important molecular information about disease processes at both the organismal and cellular levels. As a result, MRI has found applications in every organ system (Figs. 2-11 and 2-12), with particular utility in the anatomical

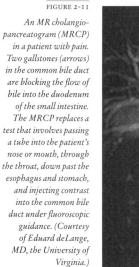

FIGURE 2-11

*An MR cholangio-pancreatogram (MRCP) in a patient with pain. Two gallstones (arrows) in the common bile duct are blocking the flow of bile into the duodenum of the small intestine. The MRCP replaces a test that involves passing a tube into the patient's nose or mouth, through the throat, down past the esophagus and stomach, and injecting contrast into the common bile duct under fluoroscopic guidance. (Courtesy of Eduard deLange, MD, the University of Virginia.)*

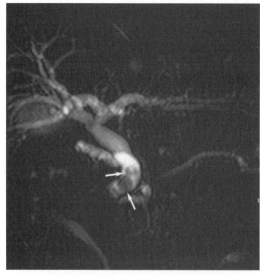

[25] Personal communication, Hans Ringertz, March 2007.
[26] We'll discuss the risks of imaging in Chapter 5, but briefly, some patients can be allergic to the CT contrast material (also called *X-ray dye*), and there are growing concerns about the radiation dose of CT.

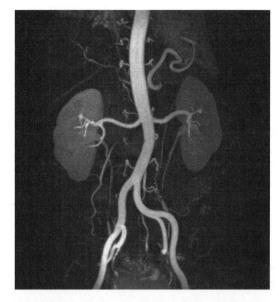

FIGURE 2-12

*Normal MR angio-
gram (MRA) of the
aorta and branch arter-
ies. (Courtesy of Klaus
Hagspiel, MD, the
University of Virginia.)*

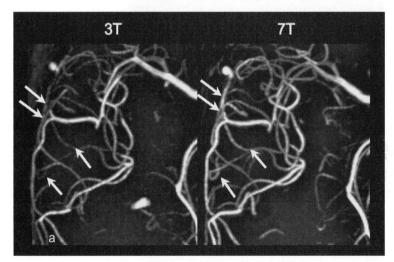

FIGURE 2-13

*Normal research vol-
unteer comparing the
same midsized branches
of the cerebral blood
vessels at (a) 3 Tesla and
(b) 7 Tesla. The higher
magnetic field creates
images with a better sig-
nal (the vessels) to noise
(background) ratio so
that observers perceive
improved vessel contrast
and better anatomical
detail (arrows point to
examples). (Courtesy of
Cornelius von Morze,
PhD, the University
of California, San
Francisco.)*

depiction of diseases of the brain, spine, and joints, the female reproductive tract, the prostate, and the breasts. Fast scans depict the cardiovascular system. Functional MRI (fMRI) is a fertile area of investigation for its clinical potential to provide insight into brain dysfunction. A number of companies are touting using fMRI as a lie detector technology, but there is little supporting evidence of its value.

Continuing technological innovations have advanced the role of MRI both in surgical planning and in the intraoperative guidance of therapeutic procedures. Increasing field strength has become a principal theme of MRI development. More powerful 3 Tesla machines are becoming commonplace because they offer better signal-to-noise ratios (producing cleaner images of smaller abnormalities) than the 1.5 Tesla units. Some academic centers are experimenting with 4 and 7 Tesla units (Figs. 2-13 and 2-14). The hope is that higher magnetic field strengths will advance

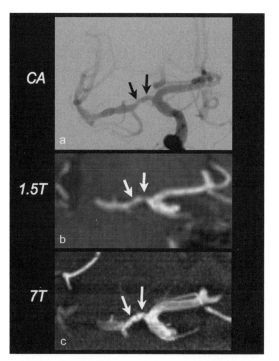

## Box 2-4  Magnetic Resonance Imaging

Magnetic resonance imaging is based on the principle of NMR. Some elements—ones that have an odd number of protons or neutrons—are *paramagnetic*. They resonate and produce a signal in strong magnetic fields. One such element is hydrogen, which has only a single proton and is the most common element in the body. Placing a patient in an MRI scanner exposes the patient to a strong magnetic field (most modern scanners use a 1.5–3.0 Tesla field). The magnet aligns most of the paramagnetic hydrogen nuclei along the axis of the scanner. A transducer (also called a *coil*) emits a radiofrequency signal that both flips the nuclei out of alignment with the magnetic field and sets them spinning around an axis oriented in the direction of the field. When the radiofrequency pulse ends, the nuclei return to alignment while the spinning weakens. Both processes emit radiofrequency signals that are received by the coil and transmitted to the computer for construction into a cross-sectional image similar to that seen with CT scans. The operator can change the strength and timing of the radiofrequency signals to generate a range of images that emphasize different details about the organs and their abnormalities.

the applications of MRI beyond detailing gross anatomical abnormalities to the evaluation of physiological processes and its use in the diagnosis of the molecular abnormalities underlying human disease.

## From Gross Anatomy to Cellular Metabolism—Nuclear Medicine and PET

The imaging modalities described to this point are transmission technologies. The formation of an image depends on some form of penetrating radiant energy transmitted from outside the patient and detected by a receptor that is also outside of the body. Nuclear medicine, in contrast, employs injected agents that emit radiation from inside the body to a detector that is outside of the patient.

The history of nuclear medicine parallels that of transmission imaging, coursing from the initial discovery of naturally occurring radioactivity (in the year after Roentgen's reporting of X-rays) through the ongoing development of modern PET imaging. Perhaps more than any other field of imaging, progress in nuclear imaging has been dependent on advances in physics.

The relationship between physics and nuclear medicine began in 1896. Henri Becquerel, a third-generation French physicist, was interested in natural phosphorescence—the glow certain materials give off after being exposed to sunlight. Once again, it was a happy accident meeting the prepared mind that produced an important discovery. Becquerel had planned an experiment using uranium salts, but he put it off because of dreary weather. He placed the pitchblend (uranium ore) in a drawer, wrapped in black paper and, serendipitously, in close proximity to a photographic plate. Developing the plate several days later, he noted:

> ... one recognizes that the phosphorescent substance appears black on the negative. If one places between the phosphorescent substance and the paper [wrapping the substance] a piece of money or a metal screen pierced with a cutout design, one sees the image of these objects ... the phosphorescent substance in question emits rays which pass through the opaque paper and reduces silver salts.[27]

Becquerel won a Nobel Prize for his discovery, sharing it with Marie and Pierre Curie in 1903. Why the Curies? Marie was a student of Becquerel who, working with her professor husband, isolated the new radioactive elements polonium—named for Marie's homeland, Poland—and radium.[28]

Naturally occurring radioactivity was further characterized by Becquerel, Ernest Rutherford, Marie Curie, and others. Investigators described three types of radiation—alpha and beta particles and gamma rays—their emission depending on the specific radioactive element.[29] They found that radioactivity could produce heat and light and could redden the skin. Each radioactive element decayed with a defined

---

[27] Translated into English and available at http://web/lemoyne.edu/~giunta/becquerel.html.

[28] Her continued work in the field also made her the sole recipient of the 1911 Nobel Prize.

[29] Because of their penetrating power, gamma emissions have proven to be most useful for diagnostic purposes.

half-life distinct to the specific radioactive element. The half-life is the amount of time required for half of the remaining radioactivity to decay. Thus, if a hypothetical half-life were 24 hours, it would take a day for 1000 emissions to decay to 500, another day to diminish to 250, another day to decline to 125, and so on.

The first biological application of radioactivity was an unusually practical one. Around 1910, George von Hevesy, a student of Rutherford and the Dane, Niels Bohr, suspected his landlady of reusing the leftovers of meals she prepared at her boarding house. He added a small amount of radium to the meat pie served on Sunday and then assayed Wednesday's soufflé for radioactivity. Despite his landlady's protestations, he had caught her "red-handed." It was a Pyrrhic victory. She threw him out of her house.

Hevesy's experiment is an example of using a radioactive substance as a *tracer*, wherein a radioactive substance is used to track a process over time. The use of radionuclide tracers allows researchers or clinicians to track not just meat pies, but also physiological processes within the body. An important quality of a tracer is that only a small amount of the radioactive substance is needed. This means that the study will not interfere with the physiological process under evaluation.

Hevesy famously experimented on himself (as did many others until institutional ethics committees became commonplace), showing that he could use radioactive deuterium ($H_2$) to evaluate water turnover in his own body. Hevesy's tracer experiments with bone metabolism, intestinal mucosa, and blood volume earned him the 1943 Nobel Prize and began a new field of medical endeavor, which has evolved into the specialty of nuclear medicine. Injecting trace amounts of gamma-emitting elements is the basis for a host of nuclear medicine procedures like bone scanning (used to find bone infections and cancerous metastases), lung scanning (for pulmonary emboli),[30] and the evaluation of kidney function.

Ultimately, though, the slow decay rate of naturally occurring radioactive elements proved limiting, given the rapidity of biological processes. What were needed were short-lived, rapidly decaying radioactive elements. Scientists surmised that faster-decaying elements could be artificially produced. The first proof of the concept occurred in 1933, when Irene and Frederic Joliot-Curie bombarded boron and aluminum with alpha particles and demonstrated positron emissions derived from new, artificial radioactive elements. The pride was evident on the face of Marie Curie, Irene's mother, when she was called to witness the evidence of the first artificially produced radionuclide. Now there were elements with half-lives in minutes, rather than days, months, or years.

The production of medically useful artificial isotopes[31] requires powerful equipment such as a cyclotron to generate enormous energies to cleave nuclei. Most of the medically useful artificially generated radionuclides are produced by high-energy bombardment of naturally occurring substances. The catalog of such elements was greatly expanded by the efforts to develop an atomic bomb during World War II. At the conclusion of the war, the federal government released many new radionuclides for civilian use, shipping them mostly from the Oak Ridge, Tennessee, nuclear facility. The gamma emitter iodine-131, from this period, and later technetium-

---

[30] Blood clots traveling through the venous circulation from the legs or pelvis to the lungs.
[31] Variants of the same element with different numbers of protons and neutrons.

99m, along with others, became widely-used artificially produced radionuclides for evaluating medical conditions.

The instrumentation used to detect nuclear emissions has progressed over time, more or less in synchrony with the demands of imaging the radionuclide substrates. The Geiger counter was replaced by the rectilinear scanner, first constructed by Benedict Cassen in 1951. In 1956, Hal Anger introduced the Anger camera, which used a more efficient sodium iodide crystal as the receptor substance. Later iterations of the Anger camera used photomultiplier tubes to convert the detected nuclear emissions into light and then into electrical signals, which the device constructed into nuclear medical images. The progress in technology allowed for faster, higher-resolution examinations. In 1976, David Kuhl, at UCLA, invented computerized cross-sectional emission imaging known as *single-photon emission computed tomography* (SPECT). This technology allows for cross-sectional imaging and has a better signal-to-noise ratio. These advances permit improved visualization of abnormal focuses.

The World War II nuclear research effort also led to techniques for producing positron-emitting radionuclides. Certain of these very rapidly decaying elements—isotopes of fluorine, oxygen, and carbon,[32] to name a few—can be tagged onto essential molecules that are components of human metabolism. As such, they have the capability to portray fast-moving biological processes central both to the depiction of disease and the patient's response to treatment. However, because positron emitters decay so rapidly, they must be generated in a cyclotron and quickly transported to the patient so that they can be injected and the images obtained before too much of the decay occurs. A number of major medical centers purchased cyclotrons for the purpose of generating their own positron emitters.

Over the last decade, commercial operations have sprung up across the country specifically to manufacture the most commonly used positron-emitting substrate, fluorine-18-desoxyglucose (18-FDG),[33] a glucose look-alike. It is taken into cells like regular glucose, but it is not metabolized, allowing the locations where it accumulates to be imaged. Certain disease states, like cancer and inflammatory processes, have higher rates of metabolism than in surrounding normal tissues. Deposits of cancer take up and burn sugar more rapidly and, as a result, show up as increased densities on PET images. FDG-PET imaging is employed to characterize abnormalities seen on anatomical imaging studies, stage the extent of disease (e.g., to evaluate whether cancer, for example, has metastasized), and assess whether the treatment is working effectively to improve the condition.

Depending on the proximity of the manufacturer to the provider, this workhorse imaging agent is either driven or flown to the exam site immediately after it is produced. Commercial fluorine-18-FDG manufacturing has allowed PET to disseminate to smaller community hospitals, as well as imaging centers and physician practices, providing broad patient access to PET imaging that would otherwise be impossible.

---

[32] Fluorine-18 is produced in a cyclotron by bombarding oxygen with protons; oxygen-15 by deuteron (deuterium) bombardment of nitrogen; carbon-11 by proton bombardment of nitrogen.

[33] Fluoro-desoxyglucose.

The basic instrumentation of PET imaging dates from 1953, when Gordon Brownell, a physicist working at the Massachusetts General Hospital, used dual positron detectors to capture the two simultaneously emitted positrons[34] of artificially produced, positron-emitting radionuclides. Michael Ter Pogossian and colleagues at Washington University improved imaging by computerizing PET to portray cross sections of the body similarly to what is done for CT and MRI. Modern PET involves arrays of detectors and microprocessors that have improved both the speed of imaging and the spatial resolution.

Over the last decade, PET has become the vehicle for the progression of medical imaging into the realm of cellular metabolism. Many believe that PET is the harbinger of new imaging technologies that will make enormous contributions to the early detection, characterization, and treatment of serious diseases. Whole-body PET imaging can detect subcentimeter metabolic abnormalities like metastases from cancer or small inflammatory foci. Specialized imaging contrast agents that target receptors for specific applications in brain or breast imaging are capable of portraying even smaller deposits of disease.

While PET imaging is very sensitive to variations in cellular and tissue metabolism occurring with disease, the images appear fuzzy and vague compared to the exquisite anatomical detail of CT or MRI scans (Fig. 2-15). It can be difficult to localize the area of greater uptake of the tracer to a specific anatomical locale. For this reason, nearly all new PET scanners sold today are combined CT-PET scanners, which allow for *fusion* imaging—superimposing PET's metabolic information on the detailed CT anatomy (Fig. 2-16). Manufacturers are developing and beginning

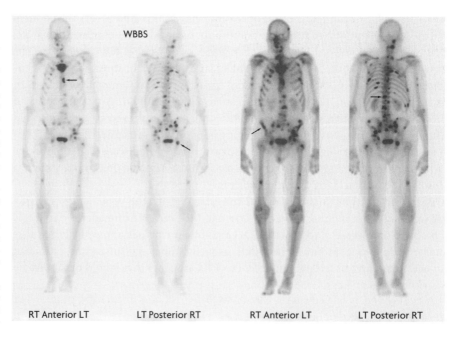

FIGURE 2-15

*Whole body 18-FDG PET scan in a patient with diffuse metastases from prostate cancer. The four images represent different projections to best show the metastases on different sides of the body (see notations at the bottom of the figure). The metastases appear as numerous dense foci (arrows point to a few examples) because they have a higher metabolic rate than normal bone and, hence, take up more of the 18-FDG. (Courtesy of Brian Williamson, MD, the University of Virginia.)*

WBBS

RT Anterior LT          LT Posterior RT          RT Anterior LT          LT Posterior RT

34 Positrons can be thought of as positively charged electrons.

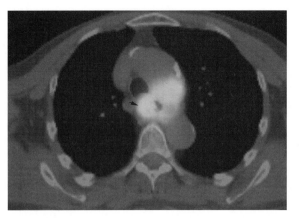

FIGURE 2-16

*Coronal cross-sectional image from an 18-FDG PET/CT scan through the upper thorax showing a large esophageal cancer (bright white area with arrow) in a patient who had difficulty swallowing. The CT scan provides anatomical context for the physiological findings of the PET scan. (Courtesy of Brian Williamson, MD, the University of Virginia) (See Color Figure 2-16 in the insert.)*

## Box 2-5  Nuclear Medicine/Positron Emission Tomography

Nuclear medicine relies on the inhalation, ingestion, or injection of a radioactive substance (*radionuclide*) into the body. The radionuclide is *tagged* to a molecule designed to be taken up by normal and/or abnormal tissues. Most diagnostic uses of nuclear medicine employ gamma ray–emitting radionuclides. Gamma rays are emitted through radioactive decay. They pass through the body to strike a crystalline receptor external to the patient. The gamma rays generate light. Light particles, called *photons*, are translated into an electrical signal that retains the spatial information of the receptors to allow the construction of an image.

Positron emission tomography is a form of diagnostic nuclear medicine that employs an administered radioisotope that decays by the emission of positrons. Positrons can be thought of as positively charged electrons. Positron-emitting radionuclides decay rapidly. The positrons collide with electrons in the body, producing an *annihilation*. Positron-electron annihilation generates two high-energy gamma rays (511 keV), which are emitted in diametrically opposite directions, permitting localization of the line along which the point of annihilation occurred in the body by the PET system. Linking the positron-emitting radionuclide to a biological substance allows PET to interrogate specific metabolic processes. Positron emission tomography is a computerized imaging technology that produces cross-sectional slices of the body or target organ.

to sell MRI-PET scanners to take advantage of the unique imaging information MRI provides.

Until very recently, Medicare coverage of PET for clinical care has progressed slowly with few covered indications. Around 2005, in response to growing single-site research on the effectiveness of PET in cancer diagnosis, staging, and evaluation of response to treatment, the Academy of Molecular Imaging joined with the clinical trials cooperative group, the American College of Radiology Imaging Network, the

ACR, and others to develop a registry for clinical PET sites to submit data indicating the effect of PET interpretations on physicians' treatment of cancer patients. In response to data accrued by the National Oncologic PET Registry,[35] the Centers for Medicare and Medicaid Services (CMS) have recently approved new PET coverage for a number of cancers and cancer-related indications.[36] Anecdotally, the coverage decision has had the expected effect of greatly increasing PET utilization.

## Summary

This chapter presents brief vignettes about the origins of the major contemporary imaging technologies and the basics of how they work, emphasizing the personalities and cultural and environmental influences that played such important roles in their development. There are several recurring themes that influenced the progress of medical imaging—serendipity, discoveries borrowed from scientific and technical fields outside medicine, and multidisciplinary collaboration.

The last of these has been the most critical. Applications in physics, engineering, mathematics, and software have played a synergistic role in this emerging story—a synergy that has benefited both individual patients and society. Time and again, intellectually curious and venturesome clinical investigators found medical applications for knowledge and technology developed in other fields. A great deal has been left out due to space constraints. Many individuals not mentioned in these pages have made important contributions without which patients would not benefit from modern medical imaging as they do today.

The developments in imaging of the past century have indelibly changed the practice of medicine. Medical imaging has become pivotal to both diagnosis and treatment for nearly every organ system and medical specialty. Imaging has both influenced and been pulled along by the advances in the rest of medicine. Almost certainly, a similar pattern will hold in the future.

Indeed, the gains of the past century may pale in comparison to the benefits medical imaging may offer to patients 20 years from now. Our understanding of how to apply imaging to improve human health is expanding very rapidly. Imaging researchers stand on the brink of another revolution—taking imaging inside the human cell and characterizing disease at a personal level. What is unknown is whether the economic and political environments will be favorable to continuing the advances in medical imaging. How society can create the economic, financial, regulatory, and cultural conditions to continue the remarkable development of this technology is a principal focus of this book and one that will be discussed in much greater detail in the concluding chapter.

## References

Brown P. *American Martyrs to Science Through the Roentgen Rays*. Springfield, IL: Charles C. Thomas, 1936.
Fuch VR, Sox HC. Physicians' views of the relative importance of thirty medical innovations. *Health Aff*. 2001;20:30–42.

[35] http://www.cancerpetregistry.org/what.htm.
[36] http://www.cancerpetregistry.org/news.htm.

Gagliardi RA, McClennan BL. *A History of the Radiological Sciences—Diagnosis.* Reston, VA: 1996 Radiology Centennial, Inc., 1996.

Goetz T. Good day, CT scan: the Beatles' legacy compounds health costs. *The Washington Post*, Feb. 21, 2010, G4.

Goldberg BB, Gramiak R, Freimanis AK. Early history of diagnostic ultrasound. The role of American radiologists. *Am J Roentgenol.* 1993;160:189–194.

Kevles BH. *Naked to the Bone.* New Brunswick, NJ: Rutgers University Press, 1997.

Sack K. In ultrasound, abortion fight has new front. *The New York Times*, May 27, 2010. Available at http://www.nytimes.com/2010/05/28/health/policy/28ultrasound.html?emc= etal. Accessed on May 28, 2010.

Shapiro SH, Wyman SM. CAT fever. *N Engl J Med.* 1976;294:954–956.

Zehnder LA. *WC Roentgen: Briefe an L. Zehnder.* Zurich: Rascher, 1935.

# 3

# Imaging's Leap to Curative Medicine

*Sven-Ivar Seldinger, a radiology resident at the Karolinska Institute in Stockholm, faced a difficult problem. Seldinger was working on a new technique to improve percutaneous angiography—a procedure for imaging the arterial circulation by placing a needle through the skin and into a blood vessel, then injecting X-ray dye and viewing the result by fluoroscopy. Portuguese neurologist Egas Moniz[1] had initially described percutaneous angiography a quarter century earlier, in 1927. Despite refinements over time, Moniz's procedure of direct needle puncture and X-ray dye injection through the needle into the aorta or the carotid artery remained an uncomfortable and potentially dangerous procedure for patients. Seldinger needed a breakthrough to write his PhD thesis, a virtual requirement in Europe (though not in the United States) to become a successful academic physician.*

*Seldinger's first thought was to use a very long needle that had a cutting edge. The half-meter-long needle could be placed inside a flexible catheter, with the tip of the needle protruding just beyond the edge of the catheter. Seldinger's plan was to feel for the pulsations of a major branch artery of the aorta near the skin surface—like the femoral artery in the groin or the brachial artery in the armpit—and take aim with the needle. Once the needle had penetrated the skin and the fat layer and entered the artery, he would retract the needle while advancing the catheter to the desired location under the guidance of a fluoroscope.[2] Because the catheter was so flexible, a wire*

---

[1]  Moniz won a Nobel Prize but not for percutaneous angiography. Moniz developed techniques for performing prefrontal lobotomy, a procedure that has fallen into disrepute.

[2]  Fluoroscopy uses X-rays, but the imaging receptor is a fluorescent plate rather than film. The plate allows the radiologist to track the movement of the catheter as it happens. Modern fluoroscopy systems add an electronic means of getting more light energy from the X-rays reaching the plate to improve image quality.

*had to be inserted into the catheter once the needle was removed so that the catheter
could be directed to the desired location.*

*Working with a phantom, Seldinger realized that his approach was still too unreli-
able. He described what happened next:*

> *Now! After an unsuccessful attempt to use this technique I found myself dis-
> appointed and sad, with three objects in my hand—a needle, a wire and a
> catheter—and ... in a split second I realized in what sequence I should use
> them: Needle in[3]—wire in—needle off—catheter on wire—catheter in—
> catheter advance—wire off.*

*What Seldinger meant by this shorthand describes the essence of his method:*

1. *With a needle, penetrate the skin and vessel wall until there is free flow of pul-
   sating arterial blood through the needle hub (i.e., the widened part that can
   connect to a syringe).*
2. *Pass the guidewire through the needle hub into the vessel to hold the position in
   the artery.*
3. *Remove the needle by retracting it over the wire.*
4. *Slide the catheter over the wire into the blood vessel and, under fluoroscopic
   guidance, direct the catheter to the aorta or branch artery of interest.*
5. *Remove the wire from the catheter. Inject contrast material and film the
   appearance of the blood vessel.*

*Seldinger continued:*

> *I have been asked how this idea turned up, and I quote Phokion, the Greek.
> "I had a severe attack of common sense." With the "beginners luck," the first
> angiography performed with this technique was successful. A subclavian
> arteriography,[4] with one single exposure, the catheter introduced through
> the brachial artery after puncture at the cubital level[5] revealed a mediastinal
> parathyroid adenoma,[6] unsuccessfully searched for by the surgeon at a former
> operative exploration.[7]*

The import of Seldinger's advance was not immediately recognized. His own department considered Seldinger's new method to be too trivial to warrant granting him his
PhD until he later applied the same technique to visualizing the biliary ducts within
the liver. However, time has proven Seldinger's epiphany to have been the enabling
moment of a new specialty of medicine—interventional radiology. The basics of
Seldinger's method remain fundamental to performing most modern catheter-based
diagnostic and therapeutic procedures.

---

[3] The traditional method of puncturing the artery is to feel for the vessel's pulsation and
angle the needle so as to pass through its wall.
[4] The artery that leads from the arm into the chest.
[5] The artery along the inner side of the elbow.
[6] A noncancerous tumor of the parathyroid gland, which resides within the thyroid gland in
the neck and which can alter bone metabolism.
[7] Available at http://www.ajnr.org/cgi/content/full/20/6/1180.

The leap from Seldinger's new method for the diagnosis of abnormalities of the arteries to therapeutic procedures involved an extraordinary series of discoveries that freed a specialty previously bound to diagnosis and enabled its expansion. Today, interventional radiology extends well beyond the angiographic roots of the specialty. Percutaneous catheter-based therapies are directed at virtually every organ system and a large catalog of diseases. These procedures are guided by nearly every imaging modality. X-ray fluoroscopy, ultrasonography, and CT are the most frequently employed treatment-guidance methods. Increasingly, MRI is being use to guide the biopsy of breast masses and other hard-to-visualize tumors, as well as to guide novel, completely noninvasive treatment methods like the ultrasonic destruction of tumor masses.

## The Rise of Interventional Radiology[8]

The transition of radiology from diagnosis to treatment owes much to one man. Radiologist Charles Dotter first spoke of his vision of a new medical specialty in 1963 at a meeting of the Czechoslovak Radiological Congress:

> The angiographic catheter can be more than a tool for passive means of diagnostic observation. Used with imagination, it can become an important surgical instrument. (Roesch et al. 2003, p. 841)

Dotter made good on his statement the following year. On January 16, 1964, working at the University of Oregon, he used a catheter-based method to open an atherosclerotic[9] narrowing in the artery to the leg of an 82-year-old woman suffering from lack of blood flow. She had early life-threatening gangrene but had refused amputation. The procedure was a success, and she walked out of the hospital. The artery was still open at the time of her death at age 85.

Dotter's earliest method consisted of forcefully pushing through the obstructed artery a sequence of progressively larger catheters until the lumen (the space through which the blood flows) was reasonably restored. Dotter and others refined this technique over time as his new procedure gained currency. The physically demanding nature of the procedure caused Dotter to self-deprecatingly refer to himself and his acolytes as "body plumbers."

In fact, there was much more to early interventional procedures than simply forcing a "snake" through a clogged pipe. Emergencies occurred and required innovation—even on-the-fly experimentation. Much of what was done in the name of the patient was truly experimental and would not be acceptable practice today with modern regulations governing informed patient consent and the use of technologies not yet approved by the Food and Drug Administration (FDA). Such procedures are now referred to as *off-label* uses.

---

[8] Unless otherwise noted, the following historical commentary was derived from two sources: Ferris and Baker (1996) and Roesch et al. (2003).

[9] Atherosclerosis is by far the most common degenerative disease of blood vessels. Plaques consisting of fat, calcium, and inflammatory elements form within the blood vessel wall, narrowing or occluding the arterial lumen.

The next great advance in image-guided treatment was the invention of a catheter that had an expandable balloon on its tip. The balloon obviated the strenuous *reaming out* (a term in common usage but that Dotter abhorred) of a stretch of vessel by allowing the treatment to focus solely on the offending lesion. Expanding a balloon beyond the normal vessel lumen causes the rupture of the atherosclerotic plaque within the vessel wall and tears internal layers of the wall itself. The vessel wall maintains the newly expanded lumen as it heals.

Investigators tested a number of materials and catheter architectures to perform balloon arterial dilatations, what Dotter dubbed *percutaneous transluminal angioplasty* (PTA). The design that became the foundation for modern angioplasty was the brainchild of Andreas Gruntzig, a cardiology fellow at the University of Nuremberg. Working in his kitchen with his assistant and her chemist husband, Gruntzig molded polyvinyl chloride tubing into a usable expandable balloon catheter. The critical quality of the catheter was the ability to expand the balloon in a predictable way, with sufficient tensile strength to rupture the key elements of the arterial wall but not cause a disastrous hemorrhage outside of the vessel (Fig. 3-1).

The dissemination of balloon catheters greatly increased interest in image-guided vascular therapy, spurring the development of a host of catheter-based techniques. Radiologists Herbert Abrams and Melvin Judkins, along with cardiologist, Mason Sones, were among those who developed Seldinger-based methods for addressing coronary artery disease. Radiologists devised percutaneous methods to stop hemorrhaging by selectively delivering drugs (pharmacoangiography) to constrict bleeding blood vessels or block them off with blood clots or other substances (embolotherapy) (Fig. 3-2). Radiologists developed procedures to form shunts between the portal veins (which drain the gastrointestinal organs) and the systemic venous circulation to decompress high pressures causing bleeding from varices (dilated veins) in

FIGURE 3-1

*Series of digital angiogram images showing stent placement for superficial femoral (leg) artery (SFA) stenosis (narrowing) in a patient with leg pain while walking (claudication). (a) Selective injection of the SFA demonstrates moderate narrowing (arrow); there are some irregularities along the vessel wall farther down the leg (distally) that are too minor to be clinically important. (b) The balloon portion of the catheter (arrow) is blown up to dilate the narrowed portion of the artery. (c) A stent (concealed by contrast material) has been placed to hold open the expanded artery, restoring better blood flow to the lower leg. (Courtesy of Patrick Norton, MD, the University of Virginia.)*

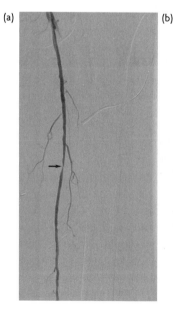
(a)

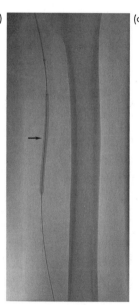
(b)

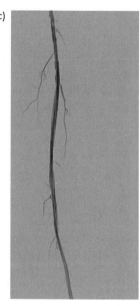
(c)

cirrhotic patients. They extended the Seldinger-based methods they had invented for the blood vessels to the treatment of biliary, urinary, and gastrointestinal tract complaints.

Today, dilatation is used mainly to prepare the artery for the insertion of a stent. *Stents* are tubular prostheses that remain in the vessel after the procedure to keep the lumen expanded. Dotter placed the first transluminal arterial stent in a patient in 1969. However, early stents too frequently occluded. Ten years passed before an inventive group of interventionalists—Swiss surgeon Dierk Maass, radiologists Julio Palmez and Cesare Gianturco, and engineer Hans Wallsten among them—designed successful expandable stents, first for the arteries and later for holding open other lumens like those of the biliary tree and esophagus. Subsequent stent designs incorporated chemical agents (drug-eluting stents) that helped to inhibit occlusions (keeping the artery from closing up again). The placement of stents has become the primary treatment for many applications requiring dilatation because of its long treatment effect.

## Modern Applications of Interventional Radiology

Numerous image-guided interventional procedures have become part of routine clinical practice. Variants of existing devices and procedures, as well as totally new ones, are being tested and doubtless will diffuse into practice over the next several years. All image-guided interventional procedures have several common elements that explain their growing popularity. The skin surface need not be opened more than about 1 centimeter (many require only a needle puncture). As a result, they can be performed as outpatient procedures or require only a short inpatient stay, typically overnight. Patients experience less pain, suffer fewer complications, and have a markedly lower risk of infection than with open surgical procedures. "It is literally surgery without a scalpel" (Rosch et al. 2003). As a result of these qualities, image-guided interventions reduce the use of expensive hospital resources and return

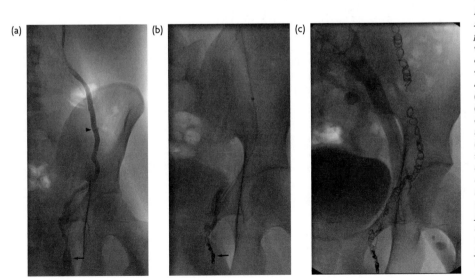

(a)  (b)  (c)

FIGURE 3-2

*Digital angiograms of a 26-year-old man with pain in the left scrotum who underwent embolotherapy for a varicocele (a benign abnormality of veins). (a) The varicocele (arrow) arises from the enlarged vein to the left testicle (arrowhead). (b) The interventional radiologist uses a catheter to place metal coils in the vein to induce clotting (arrow). (c) Radiograph of the finished procedure showing the position of the coils. (Courtesy of John Angle, MD, the University of Virginia.)*

patients sooner to productive lives, potentially saving significant overall health care and societal costs.

Like other therapies, image-guided treatments fall into two broad classes—curative and palliative (improving how the patient feels or functions when no cure is possible). To illustrate the benefits of interventional radiology procedures, here are three examples of the application of curative procedures.

- A 47-year-old woman has increasingly frequent pounding headaches. Her physician measures her blood pressure, which is found to be 195/143.[10] Subsequent blood pressure readings are all elevated but vary dramatically. Suspecting renovascular hypertension,[11] the doctor refers the woman for a CT angiogram (CTA) of the abdomen. The CTA reveals narrowing of the right main renal artery (the artery to the right kidney). In his conclusions, the interpreting radiologist recommends that the patient's doctor refer the woman to an interventional radiologist for further characterization of the lesion and, if indicated, repair.[12] The patient's doctor heeds the advice and makes the referral. The interventional radiologist inserts a catheter into the femoral artery in the woman's right groin. Under the fluoroscope, he watches the catheter as it moves upward into the midaorta. He twists the L-shaped tip of the catheter until it lodges in the orifice (opening off of the aorta) of the right renal artery. A small injection of contrast material through the catheter reveals a narrowing of the main arteries to both kidneys (Fig. 3-3). The findings are characteristic of atherosclerosis. The radiologist dilates each artery using a catheter with an inflatable balloon at its tip.[13] Finally, he fits a stent—an expandable cylinder that fits snugly against the dilated vessel wall—inside the renal artery in an effort to maintain the now-broader diameter of the vessel over a prolonged period. The patient spends 8 hours being observed in an outpatient day unit to be sure that there is no bleeding from the procedure and then goes home with instructions to take it easy for the next 24 hours. The patient's blood pressure returns to normal over several days following the procedure, both verifying the diagnosis of renovascular hypertension[14] and signaling an effective treatment.

- A 46-year-old woman sees her gynecologist for severe lower abdominal pain and irregular, heavy menstrual periods. An ultrasound scan reveals a 4-centimeter dense, mass-like focus within the wall and protruding into the cavity of the uterus (i.e., the endometrial canal), characteristic of a fibroid. Fibroids are common benign tumors of the uterus. Many fibroids are asymptomatic. However,

---

[10] The first number is systolic blood pressure (when the heart muscle is contracted); the second is diastolic (when the heart muscle is relaxed). Normal blood pressure is around 120/80, so the patient's blood pressure is quite high.

[11] The kidney is the seat of a major hormonal pathway that helps regulate blood pressure. Decreased blood flow caused by narrowing of an artery to the kidney is an unusual cause of high blood pressure known as *renovascular hypertension*.

[12] As noted in Chapter 1, radiologists require the referral of a case from a physician primarily caring for the patient, so they cannot simply make the referral to a colleague or to themselves.

[13] This is the PTA procedure.

[14] Not all renal artery narrowings cause hypertension. Most hypertension is *primary* or *essential*, meaning without an identifiable cause.

(a)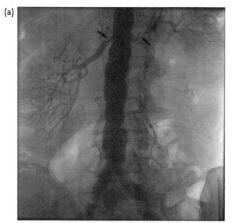

(b)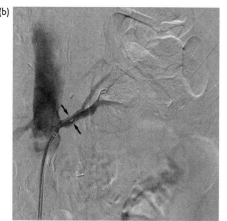

(c)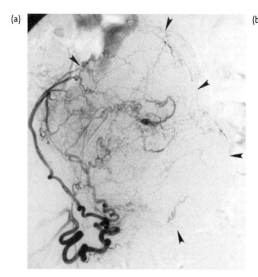

FIGURE 3-3

*Digital angiograms of a patient with diminished kidney function. (a) The aortagram shows moderate irregularity (arrows) throughout the aorta, representing diffuse atherosclerosis. Both renal arteries have significant atherosclerotic narrowings at their origins (arrowheads). (b) Left and (c) right renal arteries have been dilated and stents (faintly seen lattices with arrows) placed to hold open the expanded lumena. (Courtesy of Patrick Norton, MD, the University of Virginia.)*

(a)

(b)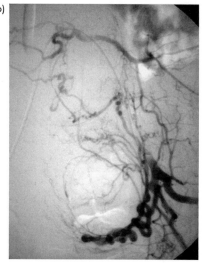

FIGURE 3-4

*Digital subtraction angiogram of the left uterine artery of a 45-year-old woman with heavy vaginal bleeding. (a) There is a large uterine mass representing a fibroid (arrowheads). (b) Selective embolization of the abnormal vessels via a catheter has blocked off the blood flow to the masses to halt further bleeding. (Courtesy of Alan Matsumoto, MD, the University of Virginia.)*

RIGHT
POST STENT

for symptomatic patients, who have pain or abnormal bleeding, the conventional treatment has been surgical fibroid removal (myomectomy) or hysterectomy. These are both open procedures that can cause a painful and lengthy convalescence. Considering all of this, the gynecologist refers the woman to an interventional radiologist for a uterine artery embolization (UAE). In this procedure, the interventional radiologist places a catheter in the uterine artery and injects a material that lodges in and blocks the small vessels in the fibroid (Fig. 3-4). Without its blood supply, the fibroid's tissues die. Its components eventually are removed by inflammatory cells and normal resorption, and the mass shrinks in size. The patient's symptoms are alleviated. Patients undergoing UAE usually spend a single night in the hospital for observation and then resume their normal activities.

- A long-time heavy drinker with a diagnosis of cirrhosis (in which fibrous scarring replaces the normal liver tissue) was found on a surveillance CT scan to have a 5-centimeter liver mass. There were no other important abnormalities identified. An ultrasound-guided biopsy confirms that the mass represents hepatocellular carcinoma (liver cancer). Because of the patient's general condition, she is considered a poor surgical risk and is referred to an interventional radiologist for an ablative (destructive) procedure. An ablative treatment for liver cancer that has shown promise involves an interventional radiologist placing an arterial catheter (as in the previous examples) into the hepatic artery, then injecting radioactive microparticles directly into the tumor circulation (Fig. 3-5).[15] The particles are larger than the diameter of the smallest tumor blood vessels, so they lodge in these vessels and emit their radioactive substance. Over a brief period the radioactivity is discharged, killing the adjacent tumor tissue but mostly leaving the healthy tissue untouched. Following the procedure, the patient undergoes periodic surveillance

FIGURE 3-5

*Angiogram of the liver in a patient with multiple metastases from an islet cell tumor (a type of cell found in the pancreas that may secrete hormones like insulin) (a) before and (b) following 90-yttrium Therasphere embolization. Theraspheres are radiation-emitting microbubbles intended to lodge in small vessels, block blood flow, and emit short-range radiation to kill nearby tumor. The angiogram is color coded to blood flow; red/yellow tones represent regions with more rapid flow than those colored in blue/green. (a) The hepatic artery (arrow) is either red or yellow in various locations, indicating high flow. The very vascular metastases (arrowheads) stand out as lighter yellow/green (faster flow) against the darker green flow through normal liver. In the postembolization image (b), the metastases are not as clearly seen because flow through the tumors is reduced and similar to flow through normal liver. (Courtesy of John Angle, MD, the University of Virginia) (See Color Figure 3-5 in the insert.)*

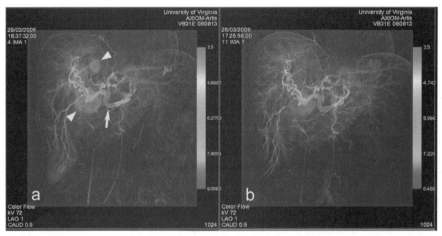

---

15 Unlike normal liver, which receives two-thirds of its blood flow from the portal vein and one-third from the hepatic artery, liver cancers receive nearly all of their blood flow from the hepatic artery.

by CT or MRI scanning with intravenous contrast material to see if the tumor has recurred (another example of imaging to monitor the effects of treatment), as signaled by the return of blood vessels to the region.

In the palliative realm, ablative treatments—which destroy abnormal tissues—are increasingly gaining currency for the local control of disease, to ameliorate symptoms, and, hopefully, to extend useful life. These less invasive treatments possess the critical advantage of minimizing the disruption of lives already shortened by terminal disease so that what remains can be lived as well as possible. There are a number of ablative therapies that are well established or currently being evaluated for the local control of cancer, exemplified by the following case study:

- A 50-year-old man with aggressive metastatic prostate cancer began to have new pain in his left lower leg. A CT scan revealed the characteristic blastic (dense) appearance of a metastasis in his left femur. The patient's oncologist refers him to the interventional radiologist for radiofrequency ablation (RFA) of the metastasis to relieve the pain. Under local anesthesia and with CT guidance, the interventional radiologist inserts into the tumor a long probe attached by wires to an external device (Fig. 3-6). When the device is activated, the probe heats up to a level that kills the tumor tissue. The patient leaves the radiology department after a short observation period. His pain decreases dramatically over the next several days.

Like any therapy, image-guided intervention has a failure rate (the percentage of time that the procedure does not produce the desired health outcome). This may be caused by an inability to achieve the therapeutic goal of the procedure (technical failure) or by the failure of the patient to respond positively. An example of the latter situation would be the patient described above whose renal artery was successfully stented had she not achieved a reduction in her high blood pressure. The failure rate varies enormously with the type of procedure being performed, the disease process to which the procedure is applied, and characteristics of individual patients

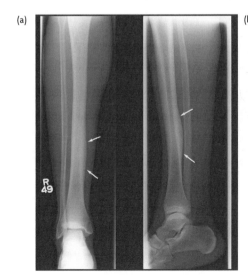

(a)

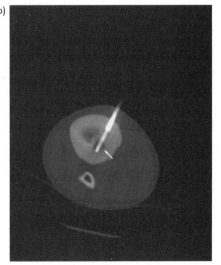

(b)

FIGURE 3-6

A 26-year-old man with pain in his right lower leg. (a) X-ray projections of the lower leg reveal a smooth, benign-appearing reaction of the tibial periosteum (the membrane surrounding the bone) indicated by arrows. (b) A probe used for radiofrequency ablation has been placed into an osteoid osteoma (arrow)—a benign tumor—to destroy the tumor and cure the patient's symptoms. (Courtesy of Michelle Barr, MD, the University of Virginia.)

(anatomy, age, the presence of diseases other than the one targeted by the procedure, and patient cooperation both with preparation and with follow-up). Complications occur, the frequency of which is specific to the procedure and the individual patient. Complications common to most image-guided interventional procedures include bleeding from an arterial needle puncture site and infection induced by a catheter.

## Progress Means Change, and Change Has Its Enemies[16]

Dotter and other early practitioners of interventional radiology met antagonism from expected quarters. Image-guided interventional procedures were most strongly resisted by the surgeons whose training and livelihood were based on open surgical procedures. In many cases, radiologists were blocked from getting hospital privileges to perform their procedures, were refused patient referrals, and were intensely scrutinized for even mild complications.

In the face of this resistance, Dotter got a lucky break. *Life* magazine came to Oregon for a story about the new Starr-Edwards heart valve[17] and heard about Dotter's innovative percutaneous procedures. The resultant article captured the drama of early interventional procedures while making Dotter a national figure in the lay press. Never shy of publicity, the flamboyant Dotter's excitement in performing an angioplasty came through brilliantly in the *Life* photographs. For the rest of his life, he came to be known by colleagues as "Crazy Charlie." More importantly, the notoriety brought an explosion of patient referrals to Dotter and other early interventional radiologists.

In the end, many of the surgeons who most resisted interventional radiology ended up incorporating the procedures into their own practices. It was not so much a matter of intellectual acquiescence as one of survival. In fact, it became clear early in the development of interventional radiology that conflict between the radiologists, who had mostly invented the techniques, and the physicians who controlled patients' management and whose practices were most threatened was inevitable.

Cardiologists believed that the new catheter-based methods represented an extension of their therapies for coronary artery atherosclerosis. Based on their control of patient referrals, cardiologists soon claimed coronary angiography and PTA for themselves. Vascular surgeons, urologists, gastroenterologists, and other specialists acquired fluoroscopic units (and, more recently, ultrasound and CT scanners) and adopted Seldinger-based methods to counter the economic threat posed by interventional radiology.

More recently, a new challenge to radiologists has emerged from an unexpected source—radiation oncologists. Until well into the 1970s, diagnostic radiology and radiation oncology were two arms of a single specialty. The commonality, of course, is that both practices are based on delivering radiant energy. Increasingly, radiation oncologists depend on advanced imaging to better direct their therapies at the abnormal cancer tissue and spare the surrounding normal organs. The improved resolution of modern CT, MRI, and PET imaging allows for much greater precision

---

[16] A statement attributed to Robert Kennedy.

[17] A prosthetic heart valve used to treat the effects of rheumatic heart disease, which frequently caused incapacitation and ultimately death.

in these tasks than previously and has facilitated the application of more precise and effective radiation treatment modalities like intensity-modulated radiation therapy (IMRT). This therapy allows for the delivery of greater or lesser amounts of radiation to different parts of tumors as needed. Radiation oncology practices are incorporating advanced imaging treatment guidance into the services they provide.

During the mid-1960s, Alexander Margulis, a gastrointestinal radiologist who was then the chair of the Department of Radiology at the University of California at San Francisco, foresaw the competition to provide image-guided treatment that has since transpired. Margulis sought to advantage his specialty at the outset by giving the new procedures the name *interventional diagnostic radiology* (later shortened to *interventional radiology*), implying its identification with radiologists (personal communication, Alexander Margulis, August 2009). In his 1965 presidential address to the Association of University Radiologists (Margulis 1967), Margulis also laid out the dictums for the new radiological subspecialty that still hold true today. Interventional radiology, he wrote, comprises:

- Manipulative diagnostic and/or therapeutic procedures controlled by imaging guidance;
- The need for specialized training, equipment, and technical skills;
- Taking responsibility for patients before, during, and after the procedure;
- Close cooperation with surgeons and others caring for the patient.

The term *interventional radiology* stuck but has never resonated with many interventional radiologists. Dotter felt that it understated the scope of the specialty. Moreover, the name ultimately did not, as Margulis had hoped, prevent nonradiologists from adopting procedures developed by radiologists and renaming the specialty to assert their ownership (e.g., *endourology* or *interventional cardiology*). Some radiologists have called for a new name that better reflects what interventional radiologists actually do (Roesch et al. 2003).

The ongoing and very active progress in interventional radiology continues to influence the organization of how and by whom image-guided treatment services are delivered. Nonradiologists' adoption of image-guided interventional procedures has forced an adaptation much like that required of the physicians originally disenfranchised by newly developed interventional radiological techniques. Interventional radiologists have recognized that they must change the way they practice to compete successfully with the *arrivistes* for patients.

As with so many important things in this field, Dotter saw the day coming and in 1968 laid out the changes that would be necessary for the long-term viability of interventional radiology. Dotter asserted that being excellent body plumbers would not be enough; interventional radiologists would have to become excellent caregivers as well. "If we don't assume clinical responsibility for our patients," he said, "we will face forfeiture of our territorial rights based solely on imaging equipment others can obtain and skills others can learn."

Interventional radiologists are, indeed, seeing fewer referrals from vascular surgeons and cardiologists. In a 2007 survey performed by the Society of Interventional Radiology (SIR), 42% of respondents indicated that they had seen deep declines from previous years in referrals from cardiologists, and 45% said the same for vascular surgeons. Most other specialty referrals were unchanged (2006–2007 SIR Socio-Economic Survey).

As a result, interventional radiologists have begun to market their services to general internists and family practitioners (the main referral sources to cardiologists and vascular surgeons), as well as directly to patients. The SIR survey showed that this new effort was paying off. Fifty-six percent of interventional radiologists reported a noticeable increase in referrals from primary care physicians; 62% indicated a considerable rise in patients directly seeking care from interventional radiologists.

But the shift required for the long-term survival of interventional radiology is both broader and deeper than simply redirecting who represents the client base. In a 2003 discourse, the authors called for interventional radiologists to pursue the following actions in defense of the long-term survival of their specialty:

- Assume responsibility for the comprehensive care of patients, including preprocedural evaluation, admissions for any procedure-related hospitalization, and postprocedural care;
- Revise the training of new interventionalists to become more focused on the unique role of therapeutic radiology, rather than considering it an add-on to diagnostic radiology training;
- Promote the recognition of interventional radiology as a distinct specialty, separate from diagnostic radiology;
- Partner with nonradiologists so that each specialist can make the best use of his or her skills to provide excellent patient care;
- Work to improve physician and lay public recognition of the existence of the specialty and its contributions to patient care;
- Continue to be innovative to keep ahead of the curve and provide new services that benefit patients;
- Perform basic and clinical research as the foundation for future practice. (Roesch et al. 2003)

These activities are underway, as reflected in the results of the 2007 SIR survey. Between 2001 and 2007, interventionalists reported an 18% increase in the fraction of the time they spent performing image-guided treatment procedures versus other practice activities (from 50% to 59% of their time). The fraction of interventional radiologists reporting that they have space allotted in their practice settings to see patients nearly doubled during the same period, from 43% to 83%. Doubtless this finding was at least partially driven by the trend of many interventional services—including PTA—to move to outpatient venues; 22% of interventional radiologists work at least some of the time in freestanding offices (versus 8% in 2001).

Many interventional radiologists now offer comprehensive services—evaluating patients for the most appropriate treatment, admitting patients to the hospital when needed, performing the procedures, and managing postprocedural care. The 2007 SIR survey found interventional radiologists spending 11% more time in evaluation and management activities than they did six years earlier (though it was still less than 10%).

Table 3-1 shows various metrics indicating that progress has been made in the transition of interventional radiology to a more hands-on patient care specialty. In sum, the data support the conclusion that competition from encroaching specialists

TABLE 3-1 *Changes in Interventional Radiologists' Activities and Resources in Becoming a Direct Patient Care Specialty: 2001–2002 versus 2006–2007*

|  | 2001–2002 | 2006–2007 |
|---|---|---|
| Percent work time spent in interventional radiology | 47% | 53% |
| Dedicated time is allotted to evaluate/manage patients | 65% | 75% |
| There is dedicated office space to see patients | 43% | 83% |
| The interventional radiologist does preprocedural office visits | 65% | 85% |
| The interventional radiologist does postprocedural office visits | 52% | 75% |

*Source*: 2006–2007 SIR Socio-Economic Survey.

has forced interventional radiologists to act less like diagnostic radiologists and more like clinicians directly involved in patient care than in the past.

For many, the transition to becoming clinicians has proven difficult. Interventional radiologists traditionally have been members of radiology groups. Many still are. However, the new demands of interventional radiology are not easily accommodated by the traditional radiology practice model. Interventional radiologists' involvement in direct patient care places more demands on their time than in the past. As a result, they are less available to "help out" by interpreting diagnostic cases when they have a free moment between interventional procedures. They now must spend that time doing intake of new patients, making rounds on hospitalized patients, and monitoring postprocedural outpatients. These evaluation and management activities pay less well than either performing interventional procedures or interpreting diagnostic imaging examinations, sometimes making interventional radiology less profitable for the group than it was in the past. Compounding the problem, as noted above, interventional radiologists require office space in which to see their patients, adding a cost that did not previously exist.

The need for new resources aside, interventional radiology is still quite profitable. Sixty-three percent of interventional radiologists report an increase in their workload over the past several years, and only 15% cite a decline.[18] As a result, interventional radiologists are in short supply (55% of all U.S. groups recruited interventional radiologists in 2006–2007[19]) and can demand from their groups very healthy salaries. Interventional radiologists had the third highest incomes among all medical specialists in the 2009 AMGA Medical Group Compensation and Financial Survey.[20] Their median income of $478,000 was roughly 10% higher than diagnostic radiologists' incomes ($438,115) and trailed only spinal orthopedic surgeons ($641,728) and cardiothoracic surgeons ($507,143) among 69 listed physician specialties. Overall, interventional radiologists' incomes increased by 9% during the period 2005–2009, consistent with general inflation.

[18] 2006–2007 SIR Socio-Economic Survey.
[19] 2006–2007 SIR Socio-Economic Survey.
[20] http://www.cejkasearch.com/compensation/amga_physician_compensation_survey.htm.

The organizational needs, money, and politics of interventional radiology have led to conflict within some traditional radiology groups. As a result, interventional radiology is a specialty in transition—one looking for a training and certification model that is conducive to attracting more individuals into the field in the future. In this regard, SIR has been militating for a new pathway (*primary certificate*) to ABR certification of interventional radiologists. The goal is to define how interested individuals can move directly into a program that is richer in therapeutic content rather than first having to become diagnostic radiologists, as things stand today.

Clinical practice models also are in transition to address how interventional radiologists must practice to be successful in a competitive environment. Most interventional radiologists still practice in single-specialty radiology groups.[21] However, various new approaches have emerged. Eighteen percent of interventional radiologists have separated from their diagnostic practices to form single-specialty interventional angiography groups. Very small fractions (1% each) have joined with vascular surgeons and cardiologists in so-called vascular centers seeking to provide more comprehensive services and access more secure lines of patient referrals.

Further disaggregation into a variety of different models is likely. Subspecialization into vascular and nonvascular interventional radiologist functions is well underway. Some interventional radiologists have joined oncology practices and cancer centers to focus their efforts exclusively on image-guided cancer treatment, which subsumes both vascular (e.g., selective arterial chemo- and embolotherapy administration directly to tumors) and nonvascular (e.g., radiofrequency tumor ablation[22]) techniques.

## Summary

Interventional radiology is now recognized by the ACR as one of the principal branches of radiology, along with diagnostic radiology, nuclear medicine, and radiation oncology. Interventional radiology employs image-guided percutaneous methods to treat patients effectively but less invasively than was previously required by open surgical techniques. As a result, patients undergoing interventional radiological procedures tend to experience less discomfort, have less severe complications, and return to full function more rapidly.

Interventional radiology began with the invention of techniques for diagnosing and treating arterial abnormalities. Today there are interventional radiological treatments applicable to nearly all organ systems and many diseases. The evolution of interventional radiology continues with regard to both treatment methods and the training and organization of the field. As discussed in Chapter 9, new methods under development use penetrating radiant energies to treat patients without breaking the skin surface. Future training pathways will focus less on a foundation of diagnostic radiology, as they do currently, and more on needed clinical expertise and greater experience in performing procedures. Interventional radiologists are adopting new

---

[21] 2006–2007 SIR Socio-Economic Survey.
[22] A technology that applies heat directly to a tumor by percutaneously placing a probe within the tumor mass under imaging guidance.

practice models designed to ensure reliable pathways for referrals and the ability to maintain their historical incomes.

The invention of imaging-guided, catheter-based therapeutic methods extended the reach of radiologists from diagnosis to treatment and infringed on the procedures offered by other medical specialists. As such, interventional radiology has been perhaps the most disruptive component of a highly disruptive specialty. The struggle among various specialists to perform interventional procedures is reforming the organization of medicine. The conflicts over imaging "turf" will be discussed in much greater detail in Chapter 7.

## References

2006–2007 SIR Socio-Economic Survey. Fairfax, VA: Society of Interventional Radiology, 2008.

Ferris EJ, Baker ML. Vascular and interventional radiology. In: McClennan BL, ed. *A History of the Radiological Science: Diagnosis*. Reston, VA: Radiology Centennial 1996:271–288.

Margulis AR. Interventional diagnostic radiology — a new subspecialty. *AJR Am J Roentgenol.* 1967;99:761–762.

Roesch J, Keller FS, Kaufman JA. The birth, early years, and future of interventional radiology. *J Vasc Intervent Radiol.* 2003;14:841–853.

# 4

# The Risks of Medical Imaging Examinations

*Marion Willow had been having morning bouts of abdominal pain. The pains had recurred for nearly a week, with no relief in sight. Sometimes a bowel movement helped, but not always. It was not the first time this had happened, but this episode was a little different. Previously, the symptoms had always disappeared after only a few days.*

*Marion's symptoms slowly subsided. However, even though she was feeling better, she began to think about what the problem could be. The more she thought about it, the more concerned she became that the pain might return—or worse, that it might be a sign of something more serious. She made an appointment to visit her family physician.*

*Dr. Janelle Halpern sized up Marion as she listened to her story. She felt pressured by the fact that she had so little time for each patient—a "performance metric" monitored by the hospital that had bought her practice a couple years before. So, as politely as possible, she tried to urge Marion to get to the point. What Dr. Halpern saw was an obese woman in her mid-30s who had too much time on her hands. Brief questioning confirmed her conclusion that Marion's sedentary lifestyle and a fondness for lunchtime cheeseburgers and evening martinis might encourage bouts of constipation, which she felt were almost certainly responsible for her symptoms.*

*Dr. Halpern had just begun to lay out a regimen of lifestyle changes and laxatives, as needed, that she felt would be effective when Marion interrupted her.*

*"Doctor," Marion said. "I'm sure you're right, but isn't it possible that I have something more dangerous? I didn't tell you this, but my mother had a cousin who died of colon cancer. Couldn't this be colon cancer?"*

*Dr. Halpern paused a moment to consider what Marion was saying. "No, I really don't think so. Your symptoms are classic for intermittent constipation. You're very young to have colon cancer, and you had no blood on the stool guaiac test the nurse took. As for your mother's cousin, he wouldn't really count as a close relative."*

*"Still, Doctor, I'm worried. Isn't there something we can do to be sure? I read on the Internet about this new test that uses a CT scanner to take pictures of the inside of the colon. Couldn't I have one of those?"*

*Dr. Halpern looked at her watch. She picked up the intercom telephone and dictated the information required to request a CT colonography from the local hospital's radiology department.*

*The insurance company will never approve this for signs of constipation, she thought. She would have to punch it up a bit. Dr. Halpern directed the office administrator to write in the space on the requisition for the indication for the exam "Change in bowel habits." She hoped that she was doing the right thing. She had already tried to be honest with the patient. What other choice did she have?*

As illustrated by this brief fictional (but all too common in real-life) tale, patients have a great deal to say about the medical testing they receive (Pham et al. 2009; Wilson et al. 2001). Most patients' and physicians' desire to eliminate even minimal levels of diagnostic uncertainty, in concert with today's greater availability of information via the Internet, has led to more imaging evaluations than ever before. Any medical testing involves both potential benefits to the patient and risks of harm. Medical tests should only be performed when the potential to improve the patient's health outweighs the risk of an adverse outcome.

Specific diagnostic and interventional imaging studies pose different types and levels of risk of harm. The referring physician can minimize the risks of imaging by requesting imaging only when it is truly indicated and, in consultation with a radiologist, selecting the most appropriate examination for the patient. This professional interaction is the best assurance patients have that the imaging exams they receive are both necessary and represent the best choice for their situation.

It is not possible for us to describe all the possible harms of individual studies. This chapter deals with several common classes of risk associated with medical imaging tests—the potential for misinterpretation, the risks associated with diagnostic levels of radiation, the administration of contrast agents, and risks unique to MRI.

## The Risks of Misinterpretation

As you have already seen, the images produced by modern imaging technologies are quite extraordinary. The anatomical detail displayed is exquisite, sometimes allowing the depiction of abnormalities as small as 1 millimeter. Looking at these images may lead you to believe that the results of imaging are inevitably accurate. Unfortunately, this is not the case. The process of imaging diagnosis requires the interaction of fallible machines and fallible humans with complex, difficult-to-interpret clinical evidence. Even under the best circumstances, there is the potential for error in diagnosis. Thus, diagnostic error is the most common risk to patients undergoing diagnostic imaging. In fact, a popular expression among radiologists is "The only radiologists who are never wrong are the ones who no longer interpret exams."

Errors in interpretation are more likely to occur when the quality of the images is poor. Most patients take it for granted that those who operate imaging devices maintain state-of-the-art equipment and that the technologists who obtain the images are well trained and properly supervised. Unfortunately, this is not always the case. Indeed, providers' financial incentives work in exactly the opposite direction. With few exceptions,[1] insurers, including the Medicare program, have historically made no distinctions concerning the age or technical capacity of imaging equipment in their payments. Providers are paid exactly the same fee for exams generated on old, outmoded, or poorly maintained equipment[2] by a multipurpose office assistant as for an exam performed on a state-of-the-art device by a licensed imaging technologist.[3]

As a result, the quality of images can vary dramatically, and poor–quality imaging can lead to errors (Kolata 2008). Certification of a facility by a nationally recognized accrediting body, like the ACR or the Intersocietal Accreditation Commission is the best indicator that the images produced by the facility will be of sufficiently high quality to allow an accurate professional interpretation. Some private insurers and, beginning in 2012, the Medicare program will require accreditation of facilities (doctors' offices, freestanding imaging facilities, and hospital outpatient imaging departments) that apply for payment for imaging services. This is a sensible policy change that should dramatically reduce or eliminate shoddy and ineffective imaging.

Even with high quality imaging, however, honest errors in interpretation can occur. To diminish the likelihood of misinterpretation, radiologists simultaneously try not to overlook an abnormality (an error of omission, known in the trade as a *miss*) and to avoid incorrectly declaring the presence of a lesion that does not exist (an error of commission, sometimes referred to as an *overcall*). An abnormality can be missed either when the radiologist does not see the lesion (a detection error) or sees it but decides that it will not affect the patient's well-being (an error of characterization). A miss might mean losing a chance to treat a condition earlier in its course when there is a better chance for cure. Overcalling a lesion that is not actually present usually involves more testing and the risk of either unnecessary invasive procedures like biopsies or incorrect treatment.

Any effort to increase the detection of true abnormalities may result in overcalling abnormalities that do not, in fact, exist. The converse also is true. Internally resetting one's interpretative judgment to a lower level of sensitivity to avoid overcalling may result in a greater number of misses. Because there is a trade-off, radiologists must develop a reading style that they believe achieves a beneficial balance for their patients. The trade-off is different for each radiologist and, depending on the radiologist, may even vary among different imaging interpretation tasks.

Partly consciously, partly without thinking about it, radiologists develop an interpretation style that internalizes the trade-off between errors of omission and errors of commission as they proceed through their radiology training. Their style may continue to evolve as they practice throughout their careers. Some radiologists are consistent in their approach, while others consciously vary their interpretive style

---

[1]  A rare example is a requirement that the imaging receptor for PET scanners meet specific qualifications.

[2]  In fact, there are powerful economic incentives for imaging operators to run their equipment into the ground, past the point where the equipment is paid for and/or fully depreciated, because scanning is more profitable at that point.

[3]  Imaging technologists train for at least two years; they train at least a year more to become qualified in an advanced technology like CT or MRI.

according to the type of examination and the clinical indication. For instance, when the clinical suspicion of an abnormality is higher or when missing an abnormality might have graver consequences (e.g., for a CT exam of a patient suspected of having lung cancer), the radiologist may purposely shift the way he or she reads the images to avoid missing any possible lesions, even at the expense of incorrectly identifying some abnormalities. In the opposite situation, when the preexamination probability of serious disease is lower or when missing an abnormality will have less impact on the patient's health, the radiologist may wish to purposely avoid overcalling abnormalities and setting off a cascade of unnecessary additional imaging (Blackmore and Terasawa 2006).

A number of factors influence the choice of trade-offs that radiologists make between not missing and overcalling abnormalities. In our experience, a dominant consideration for many radiologists is the fear of legal liability. Like most people, many radiologists tend to overestimate the risk of rare events that have very serious negative outcomes. The risk of being sued for any individual case is actually very small. Nonetheless, radiologists will read tens of thousands of exams over a lifetime, so the fear of being sued at some point in their career is not irrational. Radiologists know that they are much more likely to be sued for a missed abnormality that results in perceived patient harm (e.g., a missed breast cancer, resulting in delayed diagnosis and treatment) than for reporting a lesion that does not exist and having it subsequently disproven by further testing or a negative biopsy. Many radiologists also fear the embarrassment of a radiologist colleague or a referring clinician pointing out a missed abnormality, the nightmare scenario that every radiologist has experienced during his or her training.

Finally, there are important individual differences in training and experience that affect how accurately physicians interpret imaging exams. Research on the differences in interpretive accuracy between nonradiologists—who may receive little formal imaging training—and radiologists will be discussed further in Chapter 7. However, there is even variability among radiologists.

The training period required for radiologists to qualify for ABR certification examinations is one year of internship and four years of residency. The great majority of radiologists add one to three additional years of subspecialized fellowship training in a specific modality or in the diseases of a particular organ system. However, only a fraction of those who undergo fellowship training spend the majority of their time in practice in their subspecialization; the majority enter general practice. While research is scant, the expectation is that radiologists who obtain additional training in a modality or organ system and focus their practice on their area of subspecialization will have better diagnostic performance on the specific set of exams and clinical indications comprising their area of concentration.

All of these influences potentially affect performance according to the type of exam and the organ system imaged. The accuracy of all diagnostic imaging depends on the interaction of a device that produces images and a physician who interprets them. All medical imaging requires skill in both generating the images and interpreting them to optimize accuracy. However, some imaging methods are more dependent on the skill of the interpreter than others.

The prime example of an operator-dependent imaging technology is ultrasonography. Compared to the other major technologies we have described, where a machine automatically produces images, ultrasound imaging is directed by a physician or technologist aiming an ultrasound-emitting and receiving transducer. It takes both skill and training to image the entire area of interest reliably without skipping across important territory. A minute flick of the wrist dramatically alters what the operator sees. The images also tend to be "noisier" (i.e., the structures are less clearly seen) compared with those of CT and MRI and, hence, more difficult to interpret. Ultrasonography images the patient from any angle, which can be disorienting. Unlike MR and CT images, ultrasound images are isolated segments of anatomy, so the lack of context can be confusing. As a result of all of these factors, the quality of ultrasound imaging and interpretation varies more than that of other modalities. It takes considerable training and experience to use the technology accurately, especially for the detection and diagnosis of smaller and more occult abnormalities.

Interestingly, because ultrasonography units have become less expensive and more portable, an increasing number of primary care and emergency physicians are incorporating ultrasonography into their office practices. However, inexperienced operators may be more susceptible to both overcalls and misses, which put their patients at risk. Furthermore, downstream referrals to investigate inconsequential or spurious findings have the potential to increase imaging costs unnecessarily. Eventually, training programs in primary care will evolve to help fill this competency gap, but until they do, the subtlety and complexity of this modality will challenge the unskilled physician employing office-based ultrasonography.

Regardless of the technology, the difficulty of identifying and recognizing the significance of subtle abnormalities and generating diagnoses on the toughest diagnostic dilemmas generates uncertainty even among the most skilled radiologists. This uncertainty is reflected in radiologists' reports to the referring physicians in their use of terms like *possibly* or *probably* to describe the likelihood of the presence and characterization of an important lesion. The less confident a radiologist is about either the findings or the diagnosis, the more concerned he or she may be about legal action. The lower the radiologist's tolerance for uncertainty, the more likely he or she is to recommend follow-on imaging studies to reduce that uncertainty. For some cases, suggesting to the referring physician that he or she order additional imaging studies is good patient care. For others, it leads to the performance of unnecessary examinations. The difficulty in differentiating between the two circumstances is responsible for some of the overuse that policymakers and payers attribute to medical imaging.

## The Hazards of Ionizing Radiation

All medical imaging examinations employ some form of radiant energy. For example, MRI uses radiofrequency waves to interrogate the anatomy of a patient contained within an intense magnetic field. Ultrasonography detects the reflections of very-high-frequency sound waves from the interfaces of normal and diseased tissues. Within the range of doses recommended for diagnostic studies, no harms to patients have been identified from either of these types of radiation so long as the patient does not have a specific contraindication.

The same cannot be said for the ionizing radiation of X-rays and the emissions of radionuclides injected into the body. Ionizing radiation is the basis for plain radiography, fluoroscopy, CT scanning, and nuclear medicine imaging, including PET. Ionizing radiation induces physical changes in tissues as the energy passes through them. The increased use of medical imaging—particularly CT scanning and nuclear cardiology—has been the major contributor to a sevenfold increase in the exposure of Americans to ionizing radiation since 1980. Indeed, with its massive installed base of all imaging equipment, the United States is responsible for 12% of the radiological examinations and 50% of the nuclear medicine examinations performed annually worldwide (Mettler et al. 2009).

Prolonged interventional procedures like the treatment of complicated vascular abnormalities under either fluoroscopic or CT guidance can produce, in rare instances, enough tissue injury to result in skin burns. The risk of such complications depends on the amount of time during the procedure when the X-ray tube is actually generating radiation and the intensity of the radiation (larger patients may require more intense radiation to achieve diagnostic quality and are at greater risk for acute radiation injury).

The risk also may be greater for patients being treated by physicians who are less well trained in the risks of radiation. Radiologists are the only specialists who receive comprehensive training about the risks of ionizing radiation, and on their certifying ABR examinations, they are tested on the biological effects of radiation and radiation-induced injury. Nonetheless, specialists like cardiologists, vascular surgeons, and gastroenterologists increasingly are performing X-ray–guided interventional procedures.

Beyond acute radiation injury, during the past few years there has been an intense media focus on the long-term effects of cumulative radiation exposure from diagnostic imaging exams (especially CT) causing the excessive development of cancers. As a result, the general public has become more concerned about the perceived increasing risk of the eventual development of cancer associated with the growing use of diagnostic imaging using ionizing radiation. In a recent study of nearly 1 million individuals in five major U.S. cities, 69% had at least one study involving ionizing radiation during 2005. Nineteen percent received what the authors termed "moderate" cumulative radiation doses from multiple exams, while 1.9% received high and 0.2% very high cumulative doses, respectively. Nuclear medicine and CT exams accounted for over 75% of all radiation received by the study population (Fazel et al. 2009).

The subject has gained considerable attention in both the professional literature and the lay press, with one publication suggesting that 1%–2% of all future cancers in the United States will be caused by diagnostic radiation (Brenner and Hall 2007). Another study, evaluating the roughly 70 million CT scans performed in 2007, projected about 29,000 new cancers developing in relation to those scans over the individuals' lifetimes, with nearly half (14,000) associated with scans of the abdomen and pelvis (Berrington de Gonzalez et al. 2009). The growing use of CT for pediatric patients has received particular attention, both because the more rapidly dividing cells of children are more susceptible to mutations caused by radiation and because cancers have more time to develop over their longer expected lifetimes.

That diagnostic levels of ionizing radiation raise the risk of carcinogenesis (i.e., the development of cancer) is broadly accepted, but it is not without controversy (Mezrich 2008). The main counterargument is that the toxic effect of occasional low-dose radiation is cleaned up by scavenger cells and internal genetic repair mechanisms to ensure proper function. Those who believe that diagnostic levels of radiation are not harmful point to the fact that people living in locales with higher naturally occurring background radiation show no increase in their cancer incidence or mortality rates compared with those living in areas with normal levels of background radiation (Nair et al. 2009; Tao et al. 2000).

The carcinogenic effect of diagnostic radiation has not been measured directly. Instead, its scientific foundations lie in laboratory observations and in the aftereffects of the Hiroshima atomic bomb blast of World War II. Survivors exposed to a single massive dose of radiation showed a much greater frequency of blood-related cancers like leukemia and solid tumors. Clearly, this is a very different circumstance than repetitive low-dose exposure over a long period of time, as occurs with CT scanning.

Nonetheless, the majority of radiation scientists and radiologists subscribe to what is known as the *linear-no threshold model*, first introduced in 1972 and since then repeatedly reviewed and reaffirmed by the Advisory Committee on the Biological Effects of Ionizing Radiation (Advisory Committee on the Biological Effects of Radiation 1972). According to the committee, the biological effect of radiation in any amount is cumulative, and the effect builds with each new dose of radiation. The clinical upshot of this construct is that:

- Even low doses of ionizing radiation add some small risk of carcinogenesis over time;
- The risk of carcinogenesis increases linearly with the amount of ionizing radiation received (i.e., the higher the dose per exam and/or the greater the number of exams, the greater the incremental risk).

The parts of the body exposed to radiation and the age of the patient are also believed to affect the risk of developing a cancer. Tissues in which cells normally divide actively (i.e., reproduce at a higher rate), like ovaries and testes, are more susceptible to radiation-induced genetic errors that eventually lead to cancer. Similarly, children, adolescents, and young adults have both more actively dividing cells in more tissues and more years ahead of them during which radiation-damaged tissues might develop malignancies (Brenner et al. 2001). Finally, ionizing radiation may act synergistically with other risk factors—like smoking cigarettes or possessing certain cancer-promoting genes (like BRCA)—to increase significantly the risk of developing a cancer.

This does not mean that rapidly regenerating tissues and young people should not receive ionizing radiation–based imaging exams. Rather, there should be special consideration of whether the immediate benefit outweighs the long-term risk and whether there is an alternative, equally effective diagnostic modality in which the radiation dose could be lowered (or, ideally, eliminated entirely) and produce the same benefits.

Because radiation-induced mutations leading to the development of cancer are rare and because cancers may take decades to develop, it would take an enormous population, many years, and a great deal of money to confirm or disconfirm the effects of diagnostic levels of ionizing radiation on cancer rates in the U.S. population. For the present, prudence suggests that the use of exams employing ionizing radiation be limited to situations where the benefit to the patient exceeds the potential for harm. This means that plain X-ray examinations, fluoroscopy, CT scanning, and nuclear medicine studies should be performed only when there is a good reason. The chosen exam should be the one most likely to clarify the patient's problem and result in appropriate therapeutic decisions. Finally, the exam should use the lowest possible dose of radiation that will provide sufficient diagnostic content to benefit the patient. This is particularly critical. As an extreme example, a patient with symptoms of pneumonia having a CT scan of the chest would receive an effective radiation dose of 7 mSv (the equivalent of two years of a normal background dose of radiation in our environment); in most cases, a chest X-ray (0.1 mSV) providing one-seventieth of the dose would produce the necessary diagnostic information (http://radiologyinfo.org).

The need to act sensibly in employing ionizing radiation means that it is critically important both to measure the dose of radiation being administered and to understand the implications of the exam. A recent study makes it clear that radiologists have a long way to go in this regard (Smith-Bindman et al. 2009). The authors found an enormous range in the administered radiation dose based on the part of the body being scanned, the specific imaging protocol, and the institution where the scan was performed. In what seems an almost ironic understatement, the authors conclude that radiation doses vary greatly and that there is a need for better standardization across imaging facilities according to the clinical indication.

Concerns over the possible cumulative effects of diagnostic ionizing radiation have helped shape imaging guidelines in Western Europe since the 1990s. However, in the United States, the risks of radiation have received little attention until the past few years. A collaboration of medical societies has responded with the "Image Gently" program aimed at reducing ionizing radiation exposure in children (Goske et al. 2008). Promotion of this program has had the additional benefit of increasing the profile of the potential risk of ionizing radiation more generally. The American College of Radiology (ACR) and the Radiological Society of North America (RSNA), the two largest and most powerful U.S.-based radiology organizations, recently charged a joint task force with increasing public awareness of and suggesting control mechanisms for the problem of excess diagnostic radiation in adults. The upshot has been the initiation of a program analogous to the pediatric Image Gently program, called "Image Wisely." The ACR also has initiated a national registry [the Dose Index Registry (DIR)] to track radiation exposure as part of its National Radiology Data Registry (NRDR).[4]

A 2007 ACR panel listed 37 strategies to control levels of imaging-related radiation (Amis 2007). As of 2010, 30 of the 37 recommended initiatives have been completed or are in progress.[5] One response to these initiatives is that device manufacturers have begun to develop operating modes for CT scanners that can produce diagnostic-quality studies with less radiation than previously (Mahesh and Hevezi

---

[4]  http://nrdr.acr.org.
[5]  Personal communication, Penny Butler, American College of Radiology, March 2010.

2009). New federal regulations require manufacturers to include on their scanners the capacity to measure the radiation dose to patients for reporting in their medical record (Neumann and Bluemke 2010). Newer CT scanners may offer the option of intermittent radiation transmission during scanning.

Operators of CT scanners also play an important role. The most direct approach to radiation reduction is to lower the amount and/or power of the radiation (known in the trade as the mAs and kVp). It is also important to image only the areas of interest, without overlap into adjacent body parts or organs. Imaging protocols for specific clinical applications help to limit radiation exposure by avoiding unnecessary exposures.

To be effective in reducing the radiation dose, imaging services providers must decide for which patients to operate their scanners in dose-reduction modes. Employing any of these approaches usually means a trade-off in reduced image quality. Obese patients present a particular problem in this regard and may actually need increased radiation dose levels to achieve diagnostic images. The issue, however, is not the "prettiness" of the images but whether the quality of the resultant images remains sufficient to enable the highest diagnostic accuracy.

## Adverse Events Related to Iodinated Contrast Agents for CT and Radiography

For many examinations using X-rays, the diagnostic information is increased by using a contrast agent containing iodine. Common applications employing iodinated contrast material include catheter arteriography, injections through catheters to demonstrate abnormal passages (called *sinuses* or *fistulas*), and CT scanning of almost any part of the body. Indeed, by far the most common use of iodinated contrast material is for CT scans. Most contemporary CT scans employ contrast material to increase the differences in shades of gray between tissues and thereby improve the detection and characterization of abnormalities (Fig. 4-1).

For CT, the contrast material is injected intravenously, usually into a vein in the patient's arm. The venous circulation takes the contrast agent to the right side of the patient's heart, through the lungs, and back to the left side of the heart, where it is propelled throughout the body via the arterial circulation. The contrast agent

FIGURE 4-1

*A CT scan performed (a) without and (b) with contrast material. In the noncontrast scan, the organs look generally the same and few internal features are seen. In the contrast-enhanced scan, there is better differentiation of structures. The liver (L), spleen (S), aorta (A), and pancreas (P) are much better evaluated, as are numerous arteries and veins. A small, inconsequential hemangioma (benign growth—arrow) is well seen in the right lobe of the liver on the contrast-enhanced scan but is invisible on the noncontrast scan. (Courtesy of Mathew Bassignani, MD, the University of Virginia.)*

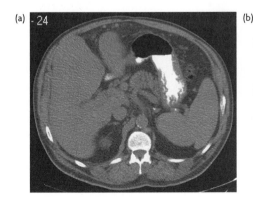

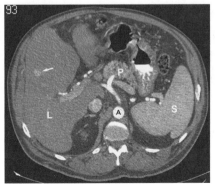

traverses first the large arteries—the aorta and aortic branch vessels to the major organs—then smaller and smaller vessels until it reaches the capillary beds of various tissues like the kidneys, liver, intestines, and muscle, providing a distinction between more and less vascular tissues. Many tumors and inflammatory abnormalities like abscesses have highly vascular components, which, when filled with the contrast material, look whiter, or more dense, than normal tissue; other abnormalities are less vascular than normal tissue and appear darker, or less dense. Either way, the abnormal feature stands out against the background of normal tissue. In persons with normal kidney function, the contrast material is excreted from the body almost entirely by the kidneys.[6]

Two main risks are associated with iodinated contrast material—allergic reactions and, for patients with poor kidney function, acute renal failure. Since the introduction of a new generation of contrast agents in the early 1990s, serious allergic-type reactions to contrast material have become very rare (one in hundreds of thousands of doses). Even such minor reactions as hives and shortness of breath are relatively uncommon.[7] The chance of a reaction is increased for patients who have other allergies and, most significantly, for patients who have reacted to a previous injection of contrast material. Such patients may be pretreated with a regimen of steroids and antihistamines and can safely undergo closely monitored CT exams. In cases warranting particular caution, patients may be encouraged to have a different imaging procedure not requiring iodinated contrast material, like ultrasonography or MRI.

The other major complication of iodinated contrast administration is acute renal failure. Acute renal failure is a sudden, often at least partly reversible worsening of kidney function (Fig. 4-2). Clinically significant acute renal failure due to iodinated

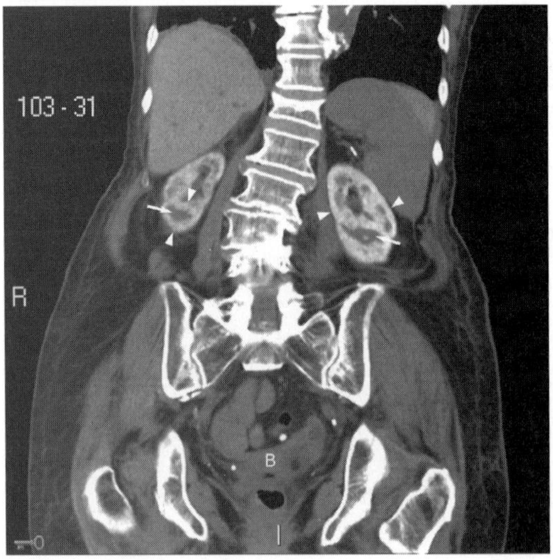

FIGURE 4-2

*Contrast-enhanced CT scan reconstructed in the coronal projection (as though you were facing the patient). The kidneys are small. The contrast, injected two hours previously, is held up in the cortex along the rim of the kidneys (arrowheads). Excretion into the medulla (arrows point to examples), the kidney collecting system, and the bladder (B) is delayed, indicating decreased renal function. The constellation of findings is characteristic of acute renal failure. (Courtesy of Mathew Bassignani, MD, the University of Virginia.)*

[6]  In patients with kidney failure, the liver excretes much of the contrast material, but this takes much longer.
[7]  Patients may feel nauseated or vomit, but this is not considered an allergic reaction.

contrast agents is almost always limited to patients who already have poor kidney function.[8] For this reason, most radiology departments require performance of a simple blood test, from which renal function can be estimated, prior to the patient's exam. Patients below a certain level of renal function can either be hydrated as a precaution (if their renal function is only slightly abnormal), have their CT study without contrast material (valid for certain clinical indications), or be referred for other imaging studies that do not require iodinated contrast material.

## Adverse Events Related to Gadolinium-Based Contrast Agents for MRI Exams

Initially, when MRI was introduced in the 1980s, a major advantage of the new technology relative to CT was that it did not require contrast agents to show important distinctions between normal and abnormal tissues.[9] In fact, the majority of MRI exams are still performed without contrast material. However, for a large number of clinical applications, contrast enhancement using gadolinium-based contrast agents[10] offers the same diagnostic advantages for MRI as iodinated agents do for CT—that is, they improve the distinction between normal and abnormal tissues (Fig. 4-3). The biological distribution and excretion of gadolinium agents are virtually identical to those described for iodinated agents. In normal individuals, the agents are almost entirely excreted by the kidneys. Contrast reactions occur, but serious reactions are even rarer for gadolinium contrast material than for iodinated agents. What's more, gadolinium contrast agents do not produce acute renal failure in patients with compromised renal function at recommended dosages.[11] As a result, until recently, it was common practice to refer patients with poor kidney function for MRI, rather than contrast-enhanced CT, to avoid this complication.

FIGURE 4-3

(a) *Noncontrast MRI scan of the upper abdomen and lower thorax showing the liver (L), heart (H), and spleen (S). (b) Following contrast administration, the organs are better defined and a multifocal liver mass can be seen (arrows). (Courtesy of Mathew Bassignani, MD, the University of Virginia.)*

(a)

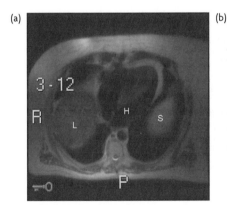

(b)

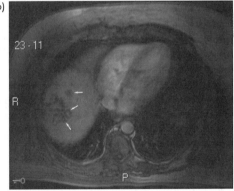

---

[8] Since many of these patients have numerous medical problems, some authorities question whether it is really the contrast agent causing the problem or the other comorbidities.

[9] Magnetic resonance imaging produces intrinsically higher contrast resolution.

[10] Gadolinium is a paramagnetic element. Gadolinium agents are small molecules binding gadolinium to an organic matrix.

[11] Higher than recommended doses do create a risk of inducing acute renal failure.

What changed this practice was the description of a serious new condition—nephrogenic systemic fibrosis (NSF). It was first reported after the turn of the twenty-first century (Cowper 2008). Once recognized, cases of NSF were reported with increasing frequency, consonant with both greater recognition of the syndrome and greater use of gadolinium-enhanced MRI (Kuo and Abu-Alfa 2008). As can best be determined, given the little time clinicians have been aware of NSF, the condition affects only those with severely diminished renal function. Nephrogenic systemic fibrosis manifests as diffuse fibrotic changes in both superficial soft tissues like skin and critical internal organs. Patients present with skin changes, muscle contractures, or multiple failing organs resulting in severe disability or death. Changes may occur weeks or months after gadolinium contrast material administration. No treatment has been proven effective for the condition.

In recognition of the risk to patients with poor renal function, the FDA has required manufacturers to give a *black box* warning to providers administering gadolinium contrast agents. The high recognition of the risk associated with gadolinium-based contrast agents has led to a dramatic fall in the number of new cases, so the incidence of NSF is now almost nil.[12]

## Risks Associated with the Performance of MRI

Magnetic resonance imaging devices generate high magnetic fields. For many years, the predominant field strength has been 1.5 Tesla. Imaging facilities are now moving to more powerful magnets—predominantly 3 Tesla—to improve the quality of images and to image smaller and more subtle abnormalities.

As mentioned earlier, for the great majority of patients, no dangerous biological effects have been ascribed to MRI scans performed using recommended techniques at current clinical magnetic field strengths. Although there has never been any proof that having one's molecules temporarily jumbled by a high-strength magnetic field has lasting adverse effects, the myth continues to exist. However, there can be adverse effects for the unwitting. For example, it is unwise to ignore the posted warnings in the area around MRI scanners delimiting the magnetic field. To do so risks the possibility of erasing the magnetic strips on one's credit cards or freezing the delicate movement of a Piaget watch.

More seriously, reports describing the potential hazards of and precautions for the use of MRI scanners are extensive.[13] There have been reports of injury and even death from flying ferrous (iron- and steel-containing) objects inadvertently carried into the scanning room by patients or providers.[14] A vast array of objects have found their way into the bore of MRI scanners—from medical instruments and oxygen tanks to janitorial mop buckets and mail carts. Better-enforced quality assurance measures in hospitals and imaging centers have greatly reduced the frequency of such accidents.

Providers of MRI scans also must concern themselves with ferrous objects inside patients' bodies. Metalworkers whose eyes may have been penetrated by iron

---

[12] Personal communication, Jeffrey Weinreb, MD, June 17, 2009.
[13] For example, http://www.mrisafety.com/list.asp.
[14] http://www.simplyphysics.com/flying_objects.html.

particles can suffer serious eye damage if they undergo MRI. Ferrous surgical clips can move under the influence of the strong magnetic fields. In some cases, they may even slip off vessels and put the patient at risk of organ damage or hemorrhage. Increasingly, companies are developing and producing MRI-compatible surgical instruments and clips, and surgeons prefer to use them.

Exposure of electromagnetically controlled devices to the radiofrequency waves of MRI can reduce the reliability of the devices' operation. Initially, having a pacemaker (Fig. 4-4) was considered an absolute contraindication to an MRI exam. It is clear from simulated testing that high magnetic fields do lead to erratic and unintended electrical stimulation, which might be potentially hazardous to patients with pacemakers (Bassen and Mendoza 2009). Surprisingly, however, clinical experience has shown that there is rarely a problem with scanning these individuals. Nonetheless, more conservative practitioners advocate that a cardiologist and a "crash cart"[15] be nearby while the exam is taking place.

Well-run hospitals and imaging facilities address these risks by obtaining thorough medical, surgical, and occupational histories. If there is anything to suggest that the patient is at increased risk, the patient may undergo an X-ray examination to confirm the presence of metallic objects. Concern over the detection of a potentially harmful implant is cause for reconsideration, either delaying or canceling the MRI exam and initiating alternative imaging considerations.

A final risk of performing MRI relates to the heating that occurs with radiofrequency energy deposition in the body. The MRI devices depend on radiofrequency energy emitted through a coil placed on the skin surface to generate images. Higher-field systems, like modern 3 Tesla scanners, deposit more energy than lower-field systems. The FDA sets standards for allowable radiofrequency deposition,[16] which must be followed by manufacturers. Nonetheless, accidental excessive

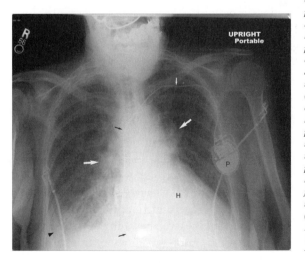

FIGURE 4-4

*Chest radiograph of an 82-year-old patient in congestive heart failure. The heart (H) is large. The pulmonary vessels are engorged (large white arrows). There is fluid in the pleural space (arrowhead), which commonly accompanies heart failure. The pacemaker (P) is buried in the soft tissues of the left chest, and the pacing wire (small black arrows) leads from the pacemaker into the right ventricle. (Courtesy of Mathew Bassignani, MD, the University of Virginia.)*

[15] A crash cart stores supplies and medications needed to support a patient who "crashes," that is, suffers respiratory and/or cardiovascular compromise.

[16] http://www.fda.gov/cdrh/ode/guidance/793.pdf.

radiofrequency deposition rarely has caused burns to the skin surface and internally. The risk of overheating is enhanced when the patient has a ferrous-containing implant. There is a growing trend to develop and use implants that are less susceptible to radiofrequency heating (Bottomly 2008).

## Summary

What was said at the beginning of this chapter is so important that it bears repeating. Any medical testing—including diagnostic imaging examinations—has both potential risks and benefits. Individuals should undergo imaging only in situations where the benefits outweigh the risks. Therefore, appropriate imaging is performed in consideration of the patient's signs and symptoms, physical condition, special susceptibilities to harm, and the potential impact that imaging might have in reducing diagnostic uncertainty, detailing the extent or recurrence of disease, and revealing important complications of treatment.

The role of imaging in reducing uncertainty is a particular point of contention. Imaging is most valuable when uncertainty about the cause of illness is in the middle ground. To amplify, exposing a patient to the risks of imaging makes little sense when the cause of the patient's suffering is clear. Similarly, the benefit-to-risk ratio is low when imaging is used to test for a rare and unlikely diagnosis. Yet, imaging is commonly used in both circumstances for a number of reasons:

- Many patients have come to expect medical imaging and demand it of their physicians;
- Physicians are trained to provide more rather than less care even if less care is more appropriate;
- Much of the evidence basis for the most effective use of imaging is ambiguous;
- Physicians wish to reduce their uncertainty as much as possible because:
  - Aspects of their training encourage them to "be sure";
  - They may be concerned about embarrassment by colleagues;
  - They fear litigation that focuses more aggressively on missing something important rather than causing harm by being too careful.
- Physicians may own imaging equipment, like CT and MRI scanners, and have a financial incentive to perform marginally necessary examinations.

The risks of medical imaging relate to both the performance of the examination and its interpretation. The quality of imaging varies greatly among providers. Poor-quality imaging or interpretation by physicians who are not trained and credentialed in image generation, management, interpretation, and reporting increases the risk of adverse outcomes for patients. The risks of harm associated with missing significant lesions and incorrectly calling normal structures abnormal are especially great for the most operator-dependent exams such as ultrasound. As much as possible, patients should recognize the balance of risks and benefits associated with the imaging exams their physicians recommend. They should ask their physicians appropriate questions to assure themselves that any imaging exam they undergo is warranted, properly performed, and interpreted by physicians who are well trained and qualified to perform their examination.

# References

Advisory Committee on the Biological Effects of Ionizing Radiations. *The Effects on Populations of Exposure to Low Levels of Ionizing Radiation*. Washington, DC: National Academy Press, 1972.

Amis ES, Butler PF, Applegate KE, et al. American College of Radiology white paper on radiation dose in medicine. *J Am Coll Radiol*. 2007; 4:272–284.

Bassen HI, Mendoza GG. In-vitro mapping of E fields induced near pacemaker leads by simulated MR gradient field. *Biomed Engineer Online* 2009,8:39. Available at http://www.biomedical-engineering-online.com/content/8/1/39/abstract.

Berrington de Gonzalez, Mahesh M, Kim K-P, et al. Projected cancer risks from computed tomography scans performed in the United States in 2007. *Arch Intern Med.* 2009;169:2071–2077.

Blackmore CC, Terasawa T. Optimizing the interpretation of CT for appendicitis: modeling health utilities for clinical practice. *J Am Coll Radiol*. 2006;3:108–114.

Bottomly PA. Turning up the heat on MRI. *J Am Coll Radiol*. 2008;5:283–285.

Brenner DJ, Elliston CD, Hall EJ, et al. Estimated risks of radiation-induced fatal cancers from pediatric CT. *Am J Roentgenol*. 2001;176:289–296.

Brenner DJ, Hall EJ. Computed tomography—an increasing source of radiation exposure. *N Engl J Med*. 2007;357:2277–2284.

Cowper SE. Nephrogenic systemic fibrosis: an overview. *J Am Coll Radiol*. 2008;5:23–28.

Fazel R, Krumholz HM, Wang Y. Exposure to low-dose ionizing radiation from medical imaging procedures. *N Engl J Med*. 2009;361:849–857.

Goske MJ, Applegate KE, Boylan J, et al. The Image Gently Campaign: working together to change practice. *AJR Am J Roentgenol*. 2008;190:273–274.

Kolata G. The pain may be real, but the scan is deceiving. *New York Times*, December 8, 2008; available at http://www.nytimes.com/2008/12/09/health/09scan.html?emc=etal.

Kuo P, Abu-Alfa A, eds. Special issue: nephrogenic systemic fibrosis. *J Am Coll Radiol*. 2008;5:21–57.

Mahesh M, Hevezi JH. Slice wars versus dose wars in multi-row detector CT. *J Am Coll Radiol*. 2009;6:201–202

Mettler FA Jr, Bhargavan M, Faulkner K, et al. Radiological and nuclear medicine studies in the United States and worldwide: frequency, radiation dose, and comparison with other radiation sources—1950–2007. *Radiology*. 2009;253:520–531.

Mezrich R. Are CT scans carcinogenic? *J Am Coll Radiol*. 2008;5:691–693.

Nair RR, Rajan B, Akiba S, et al. Background radiation and cancer incidence in Kerala, India—Karanagappaly cohort study. *Health Phys*. 2009;96:55–66.

Neumann RD, Bluemke D. Tracking radiation exposure from diagnostic imaging devices at the NIH. *J Am Coll Radiol*. 2010;7:87–89.

Pham HH, Landon BE, Reschovsky DE, et al. Rapidity and modality of imaging for acute low back pain in elderly patients. *Arch Intern Med*. 2009;169:972–981.

Smith-Bindman R, Lipson J, Marcus, R, et al. Radiation dose associated with common computed tomography examinations and the associated lifetime attributable risk of cancer. *Arch Intern Med*. 2009;169:2078–2086.

Tao Z, Zha Y, Akiba S, et al. Cancer mortality in the high background radiation areas of Yangjiang, China, during the period between 1979 and 1995. *J Radiat Res (Tokyo)*. 2000;41 (suppl):31–41.

Wilson IB, Dukes K, Greenfield S, et al. The patients' role in the use of radiological testing for common office practice complaints. *Arch Intern Med*. 2001:161:256–263.

# 5

# Economic Consequences of Successful Innovation: The Imaging Boom

*By the time Robert arrived in the hospital's emergency room parking lot, he was barely able to walk, let alone drive. Robert was a 38-year-old stockbroker, in excellent physical condition, who led a very active life. The pains had begun about three hours earlier while he was out running. He dismissed them as a "stitch" in his side, but they recurred and grew worse after his run had finished. Each time the pain returned, it was more intense. Finally, it became unendurable, and he drove with great difficulty to his community hospital's emergency room. Doubled over in pain and sweating, Robert wobbled to the emergency room entrance. He explained to the triage person that he was experiencing stabbing pain in his abdomen and was on the point of passing out. He was taken to a cubicle, where the doctor who examined him immediately had blood drawn to look for possible infection and started intravenous (IV) fluid administration. She further directed that Robert be prepped for an abdominal CT scan.*

*Ninety minutes later, the CT scan was underway. The radiologist who interpreted it found an inflamed appendix. Robert was informed of the reason for his pain and was relieved that it could be dealt with expeditiously. Two hours later he underwent emergency surgery, having the appendix removed by laparoscopy.*

*A process that two decades ago would have taken most of a day and exposed Robert to the risk of a ruptured appendix and a possible agonizing death from a rampant abdominal infection took place in less than four hours. Robert was back home in 36 hours, weakened by the experience but raring to be back out on his favorite running trail. He gratefully paid the $1000 patient portion of the cost of the nearly $15,000 episode when the hospital bill arrived.*

When someone appears in the emergency room with stabbing abdominal pain, the possibilities are numerous and frightening. Robert could have been suffering from a leaking abdominal aortic aneurysm, a bowel obstruction, acute ulcerative colitis, severe gas, or various other conditions. Today, the diagnostic path for this problem is clear and direct: obtain as soon as practical an abdominal CT scan (Fig. 5-1).

Thirty years ago, the diagnostic course of a patient like Robert would have been both riskier and more costly—a physical examination, perhaps followed by exploratory surgery if the physical findings were ambiguous. Exploratory surgery would have revealed Robert's inflamed appendix, but in many patients with similar symptoms nothing was found. In fact, in a high percentage of cases, the exploration did not provide a definitive answer. The patient was exposed to the possible complications of anesthesia, the risk of a postsurgical infection, an extended hospital stay, and a painful convalescence with no therapeutic benefit.

Abdominal CT for unexplained abdominal pain in the emergency room has replaced a much more invasive and costly diagnostic routine. How many of us would return to that 1970s world voluntarily? Figure 5-2 shows that exploratory

FIGURE 5-1

*Contrast-enhanced CT scan through the pelvis of a 22-year-old man. (a) Axial scan showing the enhancing, thickened wall of the appendix (arrows) and the air and fluid contained within it, which are indicative of appendicitis, and (b) sagital scan (arrows). (Courtesy of Mathew Bassignani, MD, the University of Virginia.)*

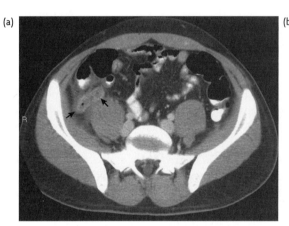
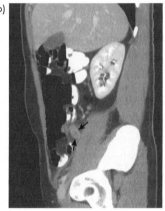

FIGURE 5-2

*Exploratory surgery volume trends. Laparotomy and thoracotomy rates declined continuously during 1993–2006. Source: Lee D. GE Healthcare (2009). Reprinted with permission.*

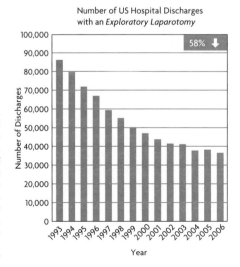
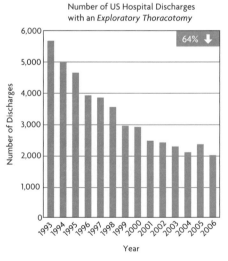

abdominal surgery (laparotomy) declined from 85,000 cases in 1993 to about 35,000 in 2006, and exploratory lung surgery (thoracotomy) declined from 5500 cases in 1993 to 2000 in 2006, about a 60% reduction in both cases.[1] How much of this decline was the direct result of the substitution of diagnostic imaging is unknowable, but it certainly is a sizable fraction.

There are other invasive diagnostic procedures that have virtually disappeared thanks to advanced medical imaging. One that has been replaced by CT of the brain and that will not be missed by anyone is pneumoencephalography. Pneumoenecephalography was an excruciatingly painful procedure that involved pumping air into the narrow subarachnoid space between the skull and the brain and then spinning the patient in a rotating chair to see if the air outlined a tumor on the surface of the brain. New procedures like CT colonography, CT angiography, and MR pancreatography[2] similarly may eventually replace more invasive procedures like colonoscopy, catheter-based angiography, and endoscopic pancreatography,[3] respectively.

At one level, this is good both for patients and for society. No one would question these benefits were it not for the rapid increases in imaging spending over the past 15 years. The controversy stems from the widespread belief that imaging technology is being used in many situations that provide little benefit for patients. Economists and health policy specialists cite multiple reasons: a thin evidentiary basis for ordering many imaging exams; great variability in practice patterns; the fear of malpractice suits; and inappropriate economic incentives for physicians to self-refer for imaging examinations. These and other economic issues will be explored in this chapter.

## A Problematic Success Story

Imaging has become a more than $170 billion business in the United States alone (Jonathan Sunshine, personal communication, December 2009).[4] Over 687 million imaging procedures were performed in the United States in 2008 (see Table 5-1)—more than two for every man, woman, and child in the country. In any other sector of the U.S. economy, the growth of imaging as an industry would be viewed as a smashing success.

[1]  Personal communication , David Lee, General Electric Healthcare, January 12, 2009.
[2]  Magnetic resonance pancreatography is a noninvasive test using MRI to display the pancreatic ducts in order to diagnose pancreatic cancer, pancreatitis, and other conditions of the pancreas.
[3]  Endoscopic pancreatography requires that a scope be placed through the nose or mouth, down the esophagus and past the stomach, into the first portion of the small bowel, called the *duodenum.* The main duct that carries secretions from the pancreas spills into the middle of the second portion of the duodenum. The endoscopist injects contrast material into the duct to display the main duct and its branches as a means of diagnosing abnormalities. Complications include rupturing the structures traversed by the scope and inducing pancreatitis with the contrast injection.
[4]  This is an intermediate estimate of the cost of radiology services billed to public and private insurers only for the year 2007. It does not include capital expenditures for imaging equipment or supporting information technology infrastructure, nor does it include public or private research and development in imaging and related information technology.

TABLE 5-1 *U.S. Imaging Utilization by Modality (Based on Procedure Counts for Part B, Non-Managed Care Medicare Enrollees)—2008*

| Modality | Part B Non-HMO | All Medicare | All Population | Per 1000 Persons |
|---|---|---|---|---|
| CT | 22 million | 29 million | 87 million | 287 |
| MR | 7 million | 9 million | 26 million | 86 |
| Ultrasound | 40 million | 53 million | 159 million | 522 |
| Interventional | 10 million | 13 million | 40 million | 131 |
| Nuclear medicine | 10 million | 14 million | 41 million | 135 |
| PET | 1 million | 1 million | 2 million | 8 |
| X-ray, total including mammography | 84 million | 111 million | 332 million | 1091 |
| All diagnostic radiology | 174 million | 229 million | 687 million | 2259 |

*Source*: Analysis of Medicare's Physician Supplier Procedure Summary Master file, 2008 and extrapolations, by Rebecca Lewis, American College of Radiology Research Department.

In health care, however, imaging is viewed both by the policy community and by those who pay for care as a problem—a clinical franchise growing out of control. After pharmaceutical spending (presently in a decade-long deceleration), spending on medical imaging is perhaps the most visible cost reduction target for government and the businesses that ultimately pay for health care.

High-technology imaging involving CT, MR, and PET has become a frequently blamed culprit for the nation's ongoing health cost problem. Computed tomography and MR scanning represent about 15% of the total volume of all medical imaging but more than half of the cost (GAO 2008b). Use of these two modalities, the high-technology workhorses of imaging, grew for the better part of a decade at the rate of 15% to 17% a year until 2007 and has been for 20 years the leading edge of industry growth. Although this growth rate appears to have slowed since 2007 (Moran 2009), coincident with the economic downturn and increasing insurer scrutiny, imaging remains a highly visible target for cost reduction.

Given the many examples of how medical imaging has made health care safer and more effective, what is the problem with using more imaging? The questions begged by imaging's controversial growth are complex:

• How much of the use of imaging is clinically appropriate and necessary?
• What fraction of patients receiving imaging are being examined for reasons other than good clinical care—like fear of a lawsuit or the desire for financial gain?
• Why has dramatic technological progress not reduced the cost of imaging, as it has for other technologies like personal computers and electronics?
• Why do we continue using seemingly duplicative older imaging modalities when newer, faster, and more accurate modalities are available?
• Is society getting good value from its substantial investment in imaging technology?

The controversy over the cost of imaging has its roots in our convoluted and dysfunctional health care payment system. Health care is not, in the main, a consumer-driven activity, where knowledgeable customers pay the bill directly. According to McKinsey, consumers pay only about 15% of the nation's outpatient bill (Farrell et al. 2008). Consumers pay only about 3% of the nation's hospital bills (Hartman et al. 2009), where one-quarter of outpatient imaging takes place (GAO 2008a).

Like nearly all of medicine, imaging is paid for largely with "other people's money" (OPM)—by employers through private health plans and by taxpayers through Medicare and Medicaid. Of course, every penny of that money is actually *our* money, processed through a gigantic money-laundering mechanism. When we pay our taxes or, in fact, pay for almost anything, a sizable fraction of that amount represents the cost of health care. The use of OPM leads directly to a moral hazard problem (discussed extensively in Chapter 7) by creating an other-worldly suspension of normal economic forces. Specifically, the moral hazard is that patients can seek care without bearing most of the cost. This increases the likelihood that patients will seek more care, even when it may not be beneficial.

A succession of policy analyses from such diverse sources as the congressionally appointed Medicare Payment Advisory Commission (2005) and the Government Accountability Office (GAO) (2008a) have identified imaging as a problem technology for the nation's Medicare program. The question of how to control the growth in imaging costs will take on new urgency as government considers how to change our health care payment system following the enactment of the 2010 health care reform legislation. So, how did things get to where they are today?

## How Is Imaging Paid For?

A powerful driver of growth in the imaging industry (and of medical costs in general) has been the piecework system of fee-for-service payment for physician services, by far the dominant payment mechanism in the United States. This system contains powerful incentives for providers to do more imaging work, since the more units of service they produce, the more they earn. The vast majority of imaging payments, whether from private insurance or public programs like Medicare, comes to providers—hospitals, physicians, and imaging centers—via fee-for-service.

The largest payer for health care in the United States is the federal Medicare program, which covers roughly 43 million people, 35 million of whom are over 65 years of age.[5] Medicare payment is critical to the hospitals and practitioners who perform imaging services because Medicare beneficiaries are their largest pool of customers. Hospitals rely on Medicare for more than 28% of their revenues (Hartman et al. 2009). Specialists who are the most dependent on imaging for their diagnostic work—cardiologists, oncologists, orthopedic surgeons, and vascular surgeons, for example—have a disproportionate number of older patients in their waiting rooms. As Table 5-1 shows, though Medicare beneficiaries represent less than 15% of the U.S. population, they account for one-third of imaging procedures.

[5] Though the press and sometimes politicians confuse Medicare with the entire U.S. health financing system, Medicare represents only a little over 20% of total health spending (about $425 billion in FY2009) (U.S. Office of Management and Budget 2009).

Medicare is influential for several other reasons. Though private health plans cover about 160 million Americans (almost four times as many as Medicare), they tend to follow Medicare's lead in covering or not covering a particular clinical service. In addition, many private health plans use Medicare's payment rates as a benchmark for how much they pay for the same service. Private insurance payments almost always exceed those of Medicare, but the amount varies considerably by payer and region of the country.[6] Medicare's processes for determining coverage and payment are public and researchable (although some Medicare policymaking relies upon recommendations from private advisory bodies chartered by medical professional groups). Medicare denial of coverage for a technology provides cover for individual private health insurers to resist similar pressure from providers and manufacturers. On the other hand, Medicare approval for coverage is often the gateway to broader acceptance by private insurers. Private health plan executives are politically sensitive, as well as sensitive to criticism by their large corporate customers and subscribers. Most do not wish to damage their firms' already controversial public images or alienate customers by being more restrictive in coverage and payment than the public standard set by Medicare.

## Medicare's Arcane Program Structure

Unlike ancient Gaul, which was divided into merely three parts,[7] Medicare is divided into four. Two of those parts are ancient and venerable, dating from the 1965 inception of the program. Part A, modeled on the original Blue Cross plans of the 1930s, pays for inpatient hospital care and is funded in part by the payroll tax deducted from our paychecks every month, supplemented by general federal tax revenues. Since 1983, Medicare has paid for inpatient hospital imaging technical costs (e.g., the actual imaging process; see below) as part of a fixed payment for all the services in a hospitalization, though each physician who sees the patient (as well as the patient's radiologist) still bills Medicare separately for services he or she provides and receives a separate fee. Medicare's control over inpatient imaging payment helped propel a lot of imaging into the hospital's outpatient department, where the costs were less subject to control, or out of the hospital altogether into imaging centers or physicians' offices.

Part C of Medicare, which was added in 1982, provides beneficiaries the option of being covered by their private health plans, which contract with the Medicare program through a highly controversial framework of public subsidy. Part D of Medicare is the new prescription benefit plan passed in 2003 during the Bush administration.

Part B of Medicare, in which enrollment is voluntary, is most germane to the subject at hand. Part B originally paid principally physicians' fees, like the private Blue Shield plans on which it was modeled. But as outpatient care has diversified and grown more important, Part B has expanded to include not only physician care but

---

[6]  Since private payers individually negotiate the rates they pay providers, large hospital systems and physician groups with significant bargaining power can demand and be paid more (often a lot more) for imaging (Allen and Bombieri 2008) than smaller hospitals or independent freestanding imaging centers.

[7]  As described by Caesar in his *Gallic Wars*.

also hospital outpatient care, services provided in freestanding imaging and surgical facilities, outpatient cancer treatment, durable medical equipment, and home health care. As a result, Part B cuts a wide swath across a powerful group of constituents, including hospitals, surgeons, subspecialty and general practice physicians, medical device and product manufacturers, home care and rehabilitation providers, and the imaging industry. The politics of managing Part B are chaotic and multifaceted, and the cast of characters seems to grow daily.

Part B pays for individual units of care (e.g., doctors' visits, outpatient surgeries, laboratory tests, imaging studies) after the care has been provided. Until the early 1990s, Part B paid physicians' fees for imaging studies based on their "customary, prevailing and reasonable" (CPR) charges. Physicians not only controlled the volume of services they provided but, in many cases, could set their charges for each service. Providers and manufacturers still talk wistfully but inaccurately about Medicare "reimbursement" (like a teenager who filled up Dad's car and expects to be made whole), a linguistic holdover from the days of the so-called charge-based CPR payment.

In fact, Medicare does not reimburse anyone; it pays fixed prices through an almost incomprehensibly complex fee schedule. As CPR payment became unaffordable in the late 1980s due to rampant cost increases, the federal government developed a Part B fee schedule based upon an arcane and highly complex formula. The fee schedule is based on something called the Resource Based Relative Value System (RBRVS), which assigns to each of the thousands of procedures paid for by Medicare a value based on its complexity and input costs relative to other services.[8] Each relative value unit (RVU) is multiplied by a dollar amount (the conversion factor) to determine how much Medicare pays for that procedure. The total amount is then adjusted for geographical differences in the expense of providing the service. Almost all private payers have adopted the RBRVS schedule but apply different conversion factors and modifiers.

For outpatient imaging services billed under the Medicare physician fee schedule (rather than billed through the hospital), Medicare payment has two components: a much larger *technical component* intended to compensate providers for the cost of acquiring and maintaining imaging equipment, as well as the service costs for actual acquisition of the images, and a smaller *professional component* for the physician's oversight, consultation, and interpretation of the images. Both components are based upon the RBRVS methodology discussed above. However, the technical component is where the money is (as it is for any medical service with a high equipment cost). For an MR scan, the technical component of payment may be five or more times the professional component. Physicians who own their imaging equipment may bill separately for each component or bill a combined *global fee.*

The technical component is larger because it covers the high cost of acquiring the equipment (historically a $1 to $3 million capital investment for advanced

[8]  For those who wish to learn more than they ever wanted to know about this methodology, the American Medical Association maintains a Web site for physicians and their office staffs about RBRVS. See http://www.ama-assn.org/ama/pub/physician-resources/solutions-managing-your-practice/coding-billing-insurance/medicare/the-resource-based-relative-value-scale.shtml.

technologies like CT, MR, or PET) plus the costs of performing an imaging procedure (technicians, facilities, scheduling, and reporting). Medicare technical payments for imaging have tended to remain at the relative value levels originally set in the early 1990s. This is despite marked advances in imaging technology that have lowered imaging session times and enabled dramatic improvements in throughput. Financial innovation has also lowered the barriers to purchasing the equipment and spread the cost over longer time periods. Because equipment costs are fixed, once an operator has covered both fixed costs and variable costs like staffing, any increase in volume leads to greater profitability. The resultant escalating profit per scan is a major incentive to acquire scanners for hospitals, physicians, and other business entities.

The Centers for Medicare and Medicaid Services (CMS), the agency that administers Medicare, reviews survey data on provider practice costs gathered by the American Medical Association and other professional societies on a regular basis. All technical and professional values for billing codes undergo review no less than every five years. However, there is considerable gaming of the review system, which has had the effect of maintaining payments at a high level or increasing them, even as productivity increased.

## Putting Part B on a Diet

Part B is financed in part (specifically 25%) by Medicare beneficiaries themselves, but the majority of funding is from general federal revenues—the source of intense congressional concern. Thus, Part B is heavily subsidized by (mostly younger) taxpayers. People who voluntarily enroll in Medicare Part B after age 65 (or when they become disabled) pay a *premium,* in effect a user fee, every month.[9] In addition, beneficiaries pay a nominal deductible but a 20% copayment for any services they use (which can be a great deal for serious illnesses because the amount is not capped). This would pose a very significant risk for Medicare beneficiaries, except that 85% of them have nearly first-dollar supplemental insurance (privately purchased, employer based, or Medicaid), shifting most of the economic risk of seeking care to a broad insurance pool and also the federal taxpayers who fund current Medicare outlays (Moon 2006).

The transition to RBRVS in the early 1990s failed to contain the growth in Part B spending, largely because it failed to control, or might even have helped contribute to, the increasing volume and complexity of outpatient physician services. So Congress, in the Balanced Budget Act (BBA) of 1997, imposed a cap on the rate of growth of Part B physician spending, tying allowable growth in physicians' fees to the per capita gross domestic product (GDP), a crude measure of the economy's output. This methodology is termed the *sustainable growth rate* (SGR).

However, the growth in overall U.S. health care spending has historically outstripped GDP growth by about 2.5% per year and, not surprisingly, continued to do so after a brief pause under BBA. The SGR cap on the Medicare Part B physician fee schedule was akin to putting an iron dog collar on a rapidly growing puppy. Instead of catalyzing a reorganization of medical practice or a constructive dialog about how

---

9  The premiums are set by statute to equal 25% of the total cost of the program and rise as the program's cost rises, basically every year.

to contain Part B costs, SGR mandated that Congress make politically inflammatory across-the-board Medicare Part B physician fee cuts almost every year for the past decade to fit spending within the cap.

Because of intense lobbying by physicians and patient advocacy organizations, and because of the threat that fee cuts would lead to providers refusing to treat Medicare beneficiaries, Congress has faced a "Perils of Pauline"—style political crisis every year in this decade. Congress let the mandated fee reductions stand only once, in 2002. Every time Congress rides to the rescue without changing the formula, it simply pushes the need to cut Part B fee schedule spending into later years and deepens the hole in the program's finances. The pothole is now over $300 billion deep[10] (Congressional Budget Office 2008), requiring future savings/payment reductions that will never be realized, in effect a large "bad mortgage" on the federal balance sheet.

Imaging has played a special and unwelcome role in these crises. Although imaging remains a relatively small fraction of total health care expenditures, its rate of growth has alarmed federal budget-makers. Imaging spending per beneficiary rose twice as fast as overall physician services expenses in Part B from 2000 to 2005 Figure 5-3.

High-technology imaging services such as CT and MR rose at a rate 4 to 5 times general medical inflation during the same period (GAO 2008a). Under SGR's cap, the effect was to increase pressure on overall physician spending by consuming a greater than expected share of the limited resources within the cap.

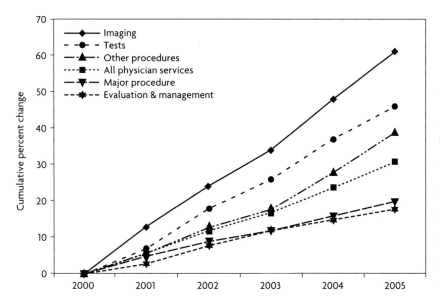

FIGURE 5-3

*Medicare physician services per beneficiary, 2000–2005. The rate of growth in imaging utilization has outpaced that of all other physician-directed services during the period. Source: MedPAC (2006). Note: Includes only services paid under the physician fee schedule.*

---

[10] The Congressional Budget Office in 2008 estimated the 10-year cost of abolishing the SGR caps and "simply" freezing physician fees for a decade (not a real-world assumption) at $308 billion. To abolish the caps and update physicians' fees to medical inflation for a decade would cost $439 billion. To do this *and* hold beneficiaries harmless from any increases in their Part B premiums for a decade would cost a staggering $556 billion. This latter amount is more than half of the expected 10-year cost of the health care reforms enacted by Congress in March, 2010.

The excessive growth in imaging spending has caused agitation in the physician community. Under the SGR methodology, payment for any new technology reduces the resources available to fund payments for other physician services. This is true regardless of the benefits it creates for patients. The introduction of an expensive surgical procedure that cured Alzheimer's disease would have an effect similar to that of medical imaging. People would clamor for access to it. Costs to the program would escalate. Medicare would pay for the greater costs, while most of the benefits realized in reduced anguish to patients and their families would occur off the Medicare balance sheet. Since the funding available for Medicare Part B physicians' fees has been artificially capped, the additional surgical fees for the newly popular Alzheimer's disease procedure would, in effect, come out of the pool of fees paid to the rest of the physician community.

## Swimming Upstream to Get Paid: The Path to Riches for New Medical Technology

To reach the promised land of payment by the Medicare program—and hence private insurance payment—a new technology must surmount a series of regulatory hurdles that can be likened to a system of dams and fish ladders. While one would like to say that only the hardiest salmon make it upstream to breed and only the fittest technologies achieve health insurance coverage, the reality is that there is a great variety of pathways through the ladders. There is no "correct" route through this system. The main "fish ladders" for a new technology are:

1. Meeting FDA premarket review requirements;
2. Obtaining a Medicare billing code;
3. Securing a Medicare Coverage Determination (e.g., the service is "reasonable and necessary," according to Medicare);
4. Securing a Medicare payment rate.

*FDA Regulation*    The FDA is charged with assuring that new devices, radiotracers, and drugs (including contrast agents) entering the medical marketplace are safe and effective.

The FDA approval process for devices is *risk-based*—the higher the perceived risk of a device, the more rigorous the review. The requirements for FDA clearance of devices differ, depending on whether a similar device is already being marketed (i.e., there is a *predicate* device). In cases where there is a predicate device, the manufacturer may be assigned an expedited route to approval via what is known as the *510K notification pathway*. The FDA has the prerogative of requiring the company to submit clinical research data as part of their 510K notification, depending on the risk posed by the innovation. If there is no predicate technology or if there is potentially high risk to the public the company (i.e., the *sponsor*) may be required to undergo a more stringent (and expensive) review process involving a premarket approval (PMA) application.

Higher-risk devices are labeled Class III technologies and must undergo the PMA process. About 10% of all medical devices are subjected to this type of review. In some cases, the FDA may decide that the technology has evolved to the point where even though one or more predicate devices are already on the market, the risks associated with the technology, or with novel applications of the technology, require this higher level of scrutiny.

With both 510K notifications and PMA applications, there is considerable interaction between the companies and FDA staff on the design of the research necessary to achieve approval. In fact, the process is more collaborative than is generally realized. However, the FDA only provides guidance. The companies make their own decisions on the type of research they conduct to file either a 510K or PMA application. Once the application is filed, however, the FDA has the final say on whether the application is approved, enabling the product to be marketed.

Drugs and biological agents, including imaging contrast agents and radiotherapeutic compounds, follow a developmental path qualitatively similar to that of devices (Hoffman et al. 2007), though with different regulatory schemes and evidentiary requirements. The demands of testing and regulatory approval tend to be more exhaustive for drugs than devices, requiring a longer and more expensive course to approval. The time and cost of bringing a new imaging contrast agent to market depend greatly on whether it is a *tracer* (effective in nano- or picomolar amounts), like 18-FDG (used for PET scanning) and most other radioactive agents, or a contrast agent (for MRI or CT), which requires larger dosages and has the potential for a greater biological effect on the patient.

Despite the close collaboration between the FDA and drug and device manufacturers, there are considerable tensions. With the stakes as high as they are, there will inevitably be dissatisfactions. Trade groups representing the companies and the companies themselves commonly charge the FDA with being capricious in developing its review policies, as well as in delaying the consideration and approval of new therapies. Consumer advocates often argue the opposite—that the process is too lenient and insufficiently sensitive to potential patient risks. The political currents that wash across this process tend to come in cycles of loosening or tightening of FDA scrutiny.

A prominent example of how this has played out with one class of medical devices is digital mammography. Digital mammography is a relatively new technique that uses X-rays to generate an electronic image displayed on a television monitor rather than on film. The advantages are that the image can be manipulated in an infinite number of ways to better show certain anatomical structures and that it can be viewed simultaneously by many providers, even in different parts of the world.

Early trials demonstrated value to this modality in comparison with conventional film mammography, but the data were not sufficiently generalizable to assure its safety and effectiveness. In particular, some of the published research led the FDA to be concerned that the technology produced higher false-positive rates (calling abnormalities when they did not exist) that would lead to a precipitous rise in the number of unnecessary breast biopsies. The American College of Radiology Imaging Network (ACRIN)[11] convened researchers and representatives of the National Cancer Institute (NCI), FDA, and CMS to design a convincing multicenter trial.

[11] ACRIN is a clinical trials cooperative group funded by the NCI and charged with conducting clinical trials of diagnostic imaging and image-guided treatment. One of the authors (BJH) was the founding principal investigator and chair.

The result was the 50,000-woman Digital Mammographic Imaging Screening Trial (DMIST). The NCI funded this large trial, which showed the equivalence of digital mammography and film mammography for most women and the superiority of digital mammography for women who were young, perimenopausal, or had dense breasts.

Despite the positive result, it took significant patient advocacy effort, a push on the part of the interested device manufacturers, and a lengthy period of time before the FDA proposed guidelines to down-classify (i.e., impose less stringent regulatory barriers on) future digital mammography devices for approval. Years after the publication of the DMIST results, the new guidelines still have not been implemented. Despite the approval of a number of digital mammography systems (i.e., there are now predicate devices), a new digital mammography device remains Class III, requiring the applicant to undergo the arduous and expensive PMA process. In November 2009, the FDA's external advisory panel on digital mammography again advised the agency to down-classify digital mammography to Class II.

*Medicare Coverage and Payment*     Once a medical innovation successfully negotiates the FDA review process and a procedure code has been established for it, the next step is to secure coverage by the Medicare program, as well as a payment rate.

For many new products, this is a relatively straightforward and rapid process that may not even require a formal coverage decision. For others, it may be a multi-million-dollar, multiyear process involving attorneys, regulatory filings, administrative and peer review processes, committee meetings, and, not infrequently, congressional lobbyists and patient advocates. For a new technology, the process can be accomplished in as little as nine months or as long as several years. The arcane details of this process are beyond the scope of this book, but few fully understand it and almost no one—Congress, the industry, the profession, or patients—is happy with it (Lewin Group 2000).

Medicare coverage determinations are not as centralized as many laypersons believe. Medicare has, since its inception, outsourced its claims management and payment to local contractors. These contractors are now called *Medicare administrative contractors* (MACs)—mainly regional health plans, which, in most cases, decide independently whether to pay for a new service through what is known as a *local coverage decision* (LCD). Alternatively, MACs can simply begin paying the claims for use of the new technology using an existing procedural billing code. Though the MACs have some limited discretion, payment levels tend to be set by the federal agency, CMS, that manages Medicare payment policy. There are presently 15 local contractors for basic Medicare services and 4 more for durable medical equipment (DME). Each is a potential fish ladder for the technology manufacturer and its advocates to surmount.

Due to limited federal staff and out of respect for local differences in medical practice, relying on local coverage decisions of Medicare contractors has been the historical norm for technology payment. CMS [and its predecessor agency, the Health Care Financing Administration (HCFA)] had limited involvement. This situation is changing, however, as the stakes become higher, and CMS has added dozens of staff to review coverage policy. Increasingly, technologies that pose a significant cost risk to the agency are reviewed centrally. These reviews may cause CMS to issue a *national coverage determination* (NCD), particularly if LCDs differ in outcome. Usually, NCDs are far-reaching in their implications for a technology and are, in principle, subject to both political and administrative constraints. For the agency to impose empirical cost/benefit tests to justify a Medicare coverage decision exposes it to politically inflammatory charges of *rationing*. Nonetheless, the concern about cost clearly lurks in the shadows as federal agencies consider whether to cover a service (Raab and Parr 2006).

The process is also vulnerable to political influence, as with a 2008 decision by Medicare to withdraw a controversial NCD that would have limited payment for CT angiography under pressure from a consortium of industry, professional, and patient advocacy groups (Appleby 2008) or a 2009 decision to deny payment for CT colonography for colon cancer screening ("Radiology Benefits Managers" 2009).[12]

## Increasing the Rigor of Imaging Coverage and Payment Determinations

There is a strong belief in the Washington health policy community that the Medicare coverage and payment determination process ought to be more rigorously evidence-based. In other words, many believe that the fish ladder system ought to be redesigned and consolidated. Complaints by congressional and policy community critics include the following: the present Medicare process is too decentralized; there is too much variation among the MAC contractors; evidentiary hurdles are too low; payment and coverage decisions are not effectively coordinated; evidence of cost effectiveness is not formally considered in either coverage or payment levels; and all providers are paid the same amount, regardless of quality or outcomes. Neither the FDA nor CMS consistently require evidence of the impact of diagnostic technology on patient outcomes and manufacturers do not provide that evidence, leaving the burden to fall on practitioners.

It seems logical and straightforward to study the effect of using medical technologies both on the health of patients and on the overall cost of caring for them before deciding whether and how much Medicare should pay for them. This would provide the necessary information to make Medicare coverage and payment decisions on a more scientific basis. During the first few weeks of the Obama administration, Congress passed the American Relief and Recovery Act of 2009 (ARRA), which allocated $1.1 billion to support "comparative effectiveness research" (CER) with precisely this objective in mind.

CER seeks to determine which among a choice of medical actions provides the greatest benefit to patient care and health outcomes. For therapeutic interventions, such comparisons are often straightforward. But CER is complicated for imaging by the special circumstance that imaging is just one link in a chain of diagnostic and therapeutic actions that determine patient outcomes (Fig. 5-4). There is variability in the treatment pathways patients follow after a diagnosis is made. This complicates

---

[12] For an excellent review of how complex this process is, it is worthwhile to read Steven Pearson's superb case study on evaluating a promising emerging imaging modality, CT colonography, a noninvasive imaging alternative to the cringe-inducing invasiveness of colonoscopy (Pearson et al. 2008).

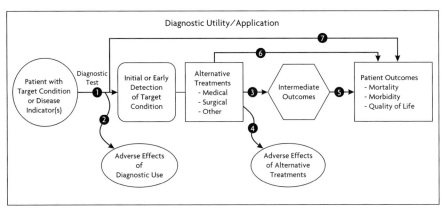

FIGURE 5-4

*Causal chain: the
role of diagnosis in
patient outcomes.
Numerous diagnostic
and treatment decision
points determine the
value of imaging
to patient health
outcomes. Source:
Adapted from Harris
RP, Helfand M, Woolf
SH, et al. Current
methods of the U.S.
Preventive Services
Task Force: A review
of the process. Am J
Prev Med. 2001;20
(3, Suppl 1):21–35.
Reprinted with
permission.*

1. Is a particular diagnostic test accurate for the target condition?
2. Does diagnostic use result in adverse effects or harms?
3. Do treatments change intermediate health outcomes (e.g., cholesterol levels, tumor size)?
4. Do treatments/health interventions result in adverse effects?
5. Are changes in intermediate outcomes associated with changes in health outcomes?
6. Does treatment improve health outcomes?
7. Is there direct evidence that diagnostic use improves health outcomes?

the work of health services researchers in evaluating the impact of imaging on patient care and makes it expensive to do so.

Crucial complexity is also introduced into this process by the fact that imaging technology is being continually improved, with a view toward greater precision and accuracy. Imaging technology is continually changing, largely through many small, often unpublished research studies and the proprietary research activities of the imaging industry. All of this variability and change challenges conventional methods for evaluating health outcomes and societal impact and increases the costs of performing clinical trials of effectiveness.

Granted then, medical imaging poses unique methodological and cost issues for traditional comparative effectiveness trials. On the other hand, the old ways of relying on small, nongeneralizable studies promoting diffusion and eventual coverage without rigorous evidence of societal value are unsustainable.

## The Remarkably Dense Installed Base of Imaging Technology

Except for Japan, the United States has the densest and most complex imaging infrastructure of any major country in the world. There were over 10,300 fixed CT scanners of varying vintage and over 7800 fixed MRI scanners in 2007 serving a country of 300 million people (Gail Prochaska, IMV Medical Information, personal communication, February 4, 2010). According to a McKinsey analysis (Farrell et al. 2008), the United States has approximately a 50% higher density of CT scanners per million people and triple the MRI density of the average of the 24 advanced countries that belong to the Organization of Economic Co-operation and Development (OECD). Most OECD countries control both the diffusion of imaging technology and payment for that technology through the political and/or budgetary process.

The United States also has higher utilization rates per million people than most other countries (Fig. 5-5), and payment rates are far higher in the United States than in comparably developed nations. As discussed above, these payment rates create powerful incentives for both the purchase and use of the technologies.

As Figure 5-6 shows, the U.S. high-technology scanning infrastructure has grown in spurts. The cycles you see in these exhibits were produced by two interacting factors: the evolving state of the technology and the federal government's policy and payment environment. Impending political or regulatory changes, particularly the threat of price controls or of systemic health reform, have historically had a chilling effect on high-technology imaging equipment sales.

Computed tomography scanners were introduced in the early 1970s. After initial explosive dissemination, overwhelmingly inside hospitals, the federal government instituted a process to review hospital capital spending called *Certificate of Need* (CoN). Initially, CoN fell under Section 1122 of the Social Security Act, but was subsequently strengthened in the Health Planning and Resources Development Act

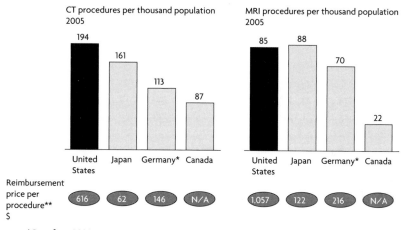

FIGURE 5-5

*Per capita high-technology scanning and utilization costs. U.S. patients receive more imaging and physicians are paid more for imaging than those in other developed countries. Source: McKinsey Global Institute (2008). Reprinted with permission.*

\* Data from 2004.

\*\* Reimbursement prices are for 2008 for all countries. All prices are for public reimbursement for an abdominal CT or MRI.

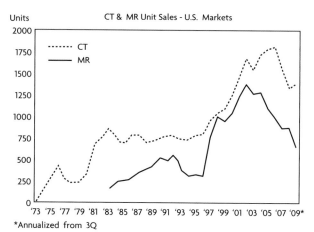

\*Annualized from 3Q

FIGURE 5-6

*U.S. high-technology scanning growth. The sales of advanced imaging equipment are associated with policies that either encourage or discourage investment in scanning capacity. Source: National Electrical Manufacturers Association (2010).*

of 1974. The purpose of CoN was to slow the advance of high-capital-cost technologies and hospital capital spending.

Computed tomography acquisition as well as hospital bed expansions were the main regulatory targets of the federal law. However, since a national review program was too complex to administer, CoN implementation was left to the individual states under the 1974 statute.

Some states with active CoN programs conducted elaborate reviews based on community need to attempt to contain the technology's growth. Massachusetts, for example, initially limited CT acquisition to five hospital providers in the Commonwealth. To some extent, this strategy succeeded in temporarily cooling technology acquisition in stringently regulated locales, with the effect of channeling the scanners approved to politically powerful hospitals. Other states chose to minimize regulation. In California, for example, there was almost a frontier attitude toward entrepreneurism. The number of CT installations accelerated as new imaging applications were introduced. Finally, politically powerful providers captured the process in a number of states and used it to keep new entrants out of their markets. As federal health planning was defunded by the Reagan administration, CoN continued in some states while sunsetting in others.

As CoN complicated hospital capital expansion, including imaging equipment acquisition, manufacturers of imaging equipment turned to potential nonhospital purchasers of their products. In part to take advantage of growth opportunities in the less regulated physician office and ambulatory setting, as well as in overseas markets with very low payment rates for imaging, imaging technology firms reengineered their products to make them more affordable and easier to operate. The key advances that led to rapid diffusion were miniaturization; simplification of operations, which reduced the skill levels of staff required to operate the equipment; and improved speed and resolution, enabling the expansion of imaging applications.

In combination with the lucrative technical payments for advanced imaging, these innovations made it practical for physicians and entrepreneurs to place advanced imaging modalities in outpatient settings. As MRI became commercially available in the early 1980s, it followed a pattern of diffusion similar to that of CT (Hillman et al. 1987). However, magnetic resonance imaging moved more rapidly into less regulated freestanding imaging centers.

In the mid-1990s, the combination of the prospect of health care reform under the Clintons and the impact of Stark legislation restricting referrals to facilities owned by physicians temporarily cooled the industry's growth. Figure 5-6 shows that both equipment sales and growth in scanning volumes subsided for several years during this period. When this threat faded, CT and MR resumed their former rapid pace of dissemination.

By the late 1990s and into the early twenty-first century, CT had entered a new era of speed and resolution with the introduction of spiral and then multidetector CT. Higher power 3T MRI scanners became commercially available, enhancing the ability of the technology to detect small and subtle abnormalities. Software innovations also improved the reconfiguration and display of images.

Despite the physician payment reforms of the early 1990s and the institution of prospective payment for hospital outpatient imaging in the late 1990s, the use of both CT and MR grew dramatically until the federal government cut technical payments to offices and freestanding imaging centers as part of the Deficit Reduction Act (DRA) of 2005. This crackdown produced an unprecedented 11% reduction in federal spending for high-technology imaging in the first year the reductions were implemented (even though scanning volume continued to grow, though at a much slower rate than before the cuts) (GAO 2008b). The DRA reductions had a chilling effect on opening new imaging centers, but they did not immediately reduce overall imaging capacity (SDI Health 2008).

As freestanding and physician-owned imaging facilities adjusted to the realities of lower payment rates, hospitals felt less competitive pressures to match nonhospital technology and imaging equipment sales collapsed (see Fig. 5-6).

*Does Supply Create Demand for Imaging Services?* There are numerous hypotheses that attempt to explain why imaging has grown so rapidly in the United States and elsewhere in the modern world. The most obvious factor has been the benefit these technologies provide to patient care. However, economic influences have also played an important role. The marketing of advanced imaging equipment has been highly organized and effective. In some policy analysts' view, increased clinical capacity of any sort—whether hospital beds, operating suites, clinicians, drugs, or CT and MR scanners—has the almost magical "if you build it, they will come" effect of generating increased utilization (Fisher 2007). As shown by Wennberg's Dartmouth health policy group, regions of the country, states, and even cities with large amounts of clinical capacity, on average, generate higher utilization and health care costs than areas with lower capacity (Dartmouth Institute 2008).

Recent analyses by McKinsey of the 23 OECD countries confirm the association between scanner supply and utilization at the country level. In the United States, the correlation between growth in scanner density and scanning use is almost perfect (with a correlation coefficient approaching 1.0) at a high confidence interval for both CT and MR (Fig. 5-7). But correlation does not mean causation. The machinery does not, by itself, have some supernatural power to attract patients and money. Rather, as explained in the following section and elsewhere in this book, a complex mix of economic and cultural factors are working in concert to increase the use and cost of imaging examinations.

*Imaging's Contribution to Profit: The Allure of Technical Payments* Certainly the companies that create these remarkable technologies expect to generate an economic return for developing and manufacturing them. Those who purchase the devices and provide services need to generate a return on their investment as well. Advanced medical imaging has been reliably and highly profitable in both inpatient and outpatient settings.

Indeed, the most profitable hospital services are not the hotel and nursing services most people think about when they think about a hospitalization. Rather, they are the ironically named *ancillary services*, such as imaging and laboratory studies. Imaging is not ancillary to hospital operating profits. Rather, imaging has become the core of the hospital franchise. Hospitals generate a remarkable three-quarters of their operating profits from elective outpatient services—imaging, surgery, rehabilitation, laboratory analyses, and so on (Farrell et al. 2008). A very large fraction of

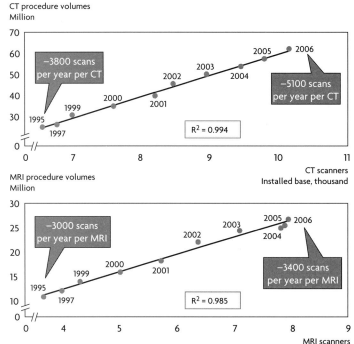

FIGURE 5-7

*U.S. high-technology
scanning capacity
versus volume. The use
of advanced imaging is
almost perfectly corre-
lated with the capacity
to generate scans.
Source: McKinsey
Global Institute
(2008). Reprinted with
permission.*

those profits are derived from imaging studies. The Advisory Board estimated that outpatient imaging contributed over $24 billion in hospital profits in 2007, almost triple the contribution of cardiology, the next most profitable hospital service (Radiology Business Journal, 2010).

For outpatient services, the current payment rates for advanced imaging originated in the transition to the RBRVS payment system. Radiology was only one of two disciplines to develop their own RVU methodologies and a relative value scale for professional services for all imaging procedures (anesthesia was the other) prior to the development of the federal RBRVS. This prescient exercise, led by the ACR, rigorously analyzed the clinical effort and practice expense devoted to the almost 800 imaging procedure codes covered by Medicare to support the development of a fee schedule for the specialty (Moorefield et al. 1993). These ACR-developed radiology RVU values were later integrated into the new Medicare RBRVS fee schedule.

As imaging payment transitioned to RVU-based fees for professional payment, imaging professional fees were reduced modestly.[13] Imaging technical fees, on the other hand, remained very attractive—on average, between three and five times the professional payments, depending on the modality—and grew more so as advances in technology increased imaging's capabilities. Higher scanner throughput and providers' focus on improving operational efficiency allowed more scans to be completed per day. Since the RBRVS cost input for buying and maintaining the scanners was set at an assumed 50% utilization of capacity, greater throughput meant lower cost

---

[13] Personal communication, Sunshine, January 2009.

and greater profit per scan. As discussed in Chapter 7, 2010 health care reform legislation effectively reduced technical payments for advanced imaging by increasing what was perceived to be a too low assumption of scanner utilization.

The high technical fees proved very attractive to physician specialists who rely upon imaging extensively, like cardiologists, urologists, vascular surgeons, and orthopedists. These and other clinical specialists increasingly acquired advanced imaging devices for their offices (Levin et al. 2004), taking advantage of a loophole in the Stark Medicare anti-fraud legislation which generally prohibits physicians from referring their patients to facilities in which they have a financial interest (discussed further in Chapter 7). By purchasing advanced imaging equipment, these physicians were able to charge technical fees for services that were formerly performed in hospitals. Imaging became an increasingly important contributor to their practice income. As an example, according to the GAO, American cardiologists derived 36% of their income from imaging studies in 2006, a 50% increase from the year 2000 (GAO 2008a).

The incorporation of imaging equipment into physicians' practices allows physicians to charge for the technical component alone or a global fee that includes both the technical component and the professional fee for interpretation of the exam. Owning imaging equipment enables physicians to compete directly with hospitals for this lucrative business. The incentive for physicians to acquire imaging for their office practices was enhanced by the fact that, until DRA payment reductions went into effect in 2007, nonhospital outpatient imaging providers were actually paid higher technical fees than hospitals for some imaging studies, despite having a lower overhead, more limited hours of operation, and fewer charity patients. According to the GAO, imaging volume grew twice as fast in the physician office setting as it did in hospital outpatient departments from 2000 to 2005 (GAO 2008a).

*Economic Incentives Play a Major Role*　There is compelling, if circumstantial, evidence that a lot of imaging use is financially motivated. Nonradiologist physicians have a powerful economic incentive to refer their patients for imaging to their own office-based facilities (i.e., self-referral). A cottage industry of legal advisers has emerged to help physicians and other entities profit either directly or indirectly from imaging examinations, circumventing the spirit, if not the letter, of antifraud regulations. The profusion of clever legal strategies for sharing profits from the technical fees of medical imaging with referring physicians—as detailed in Chapter 7—will impress, then anger, the lay reader.

These income-sharing arrangements have the effect of paying referring physicians for their imaging referrals, contravening the intent of Medicare fraud and abuse laws that forbid paying kickbacks to physicians in exchange for referring Medicare patients. Many hospitals have been forced by financial necessity to share their imaging profits through joint ventures with physicians who would otherwise move their patients to freestanding facilities in which they have ownership interests. These joint ventures have had the effect of giving physicians an incentive to increase patient imaging studies in hospital-controlled facilities.

Inappropriate financial incentives doubtless motivate many unnecessary imaging services. The costs of all these complex ownership arrangements are embedded in Medicare and private payer spending. McKinsey estimated that physician dividends from ambulatory facility investments—in surgical and rehabilitation facilities, as well as imaging facilities—amounted to approximately $8 billion in 2003 (Angrisano 2007).

These and other findings prompted a further tightening of Medicare's restrictions on imaging economic arrangements in 2008, some of which will be implemented during 2009–2012.

*The Contribution of Malpractice Risk*   A physician's decision to order imaging studies may be powerfully influenced by concerns over medical-legal liability. Indeed, a 2008 Massachusetts Medical Society survey of its members found that 28% of imaging studies may be ordered solely because of malpractice concerns.[14] There is an extensive literature on the economic consequences of tort liability in medicine. A searching review of the impact of malpractice concerns on imaging utilization is beyond the scope of this book. Suffice it to say that the present tort liability system punishes "missing" a health- or life-threatening abnormality far more than uncovering and pursuing a meaningless finding. The pressure to avoid being sued creates a powerful incentive for clinicians to conduct overly thorough workups as a means of reducing even minimal diagnostic uncertainty.

When accused in a court of law for failing to diagnose an important condition that has led to patient harm, clinicians are measured against a *community standard* of overlapping and repetitive testing. Part of the problem is that juries seeking a measuring rod for appropriate thoroughness find limited empirical evidence to justify a particular diagnostic pathway. In the absence of good research data on what is an appropriate patient evaluation in a given clinical circumstance, courts rely on lay judgments (powerfully influenced by emotional appeals to juries) of what constitutes allowable uncertainty in diagnosis and the perceived alleged harm done to individual patients.

The numerous estimates of the cost of defensive medicine vary greatly. One widely cited study suggested that the cost of defensive medicine in the United States, based on data from 1984 to 1990, was about $50 billion a year (Kessler and McClellan 1996). By updating these costs to current dollars, adding estimated direct costs of malpractice insurance premiums and damage awards of $30.3 billion in 2006, McKinsey estimated that the United States could be spending as much as $150 to $190 billion more than needed due to defensive medicine. This is not a small sum in a more than $2 trillion health system (Angrisano 2007). On the other end of the spectrum, a recent CBO analysis suggesting that the costs of defensive medicine are more limited. The CBO review concluded that capping jury awards and other changes in the present system would save, at most, one-half of 1% of current medical costs—only about $12.5 billion in 2009 expenditures (CBO 2008). Somewhere between the Kessler–McClellan study and the CBO review estimate most likely lies the truth. The costs are non-trivial and avoidable.

Because physicians' behavior is so difficult to study, these estimates should be taken with a grain of salt or as a stimulus for more careful analysis. Physicians' claims that tort liability forces them to practice defensive medicine are undercut when these same physicians own imaging equipment and profit from referring their patients for

---

[14] http://www.massmed.org/AM/Template.cfm?Section=Professional_Liability&CONTE NTID=23557&TEMPLATE=/CM/ContentDisplay.cfm.

testing. While malpractice reform would alleviate some of the pressure for order-ing medically unnecessary tests, tort reform alone would not banish inappropriate imaging. Like self-referral, malpractice exposure may be an important enabling fac-tor in imaging's rapid growth, but it is not the primary driver.

*Is There a Substitution Effect in Imaging?*   In most other sectors of the economy, when a new technology appears, legacy technologies that do the same thing less well usually disappear. There are some notable exceptions, such as the remarkable persistence of the fax machine in the Internet age, but for the most part, we do not even notice the disappearance of things like electric typewriters, Sony Walkmen, or personal digital assistants (PDAs) without cell phone access that no longer generate social value.

That is frequently not the case with medicine. When a new diagnostic technol-ogy appears, it takes at least a few years, and often longer, for the outmoded method to vanish from practice. The new approach augments the diagnostic toolbox rather than pushing legacy technologies out. Some have argued that this is a function of marketing. Manufacturers continue to profit from selling legacy technology and, to an extent, old and new products compete with one another even within the same company's product offerings. It may take some time before formal guidelines appear detailing the appropriate use of the innovation, leading to changes in professional practice. As a result, in the health care system, there are many electric typewriter technologies sitting on physicians' desks alongside their computers, and they fre-quently end up using both.

A recent study of CT angiography (CTA) provided an example of how the advent of a new imaging technology may be more additive than substitutive of existing technologies. One use of CTA is as a less invasive substitute for the traditional inva-sive test, catheter-based angiography, for dissecting aortic aneurysms.[15]

Catheter-based angiography involves threading a catheter from an artery in the leg to the site of a potential rupture and injecting contrast material into the aorta to be examined by conventional X-ray. The invasive procedure carries patient safety risks, including the risks of infection, bleeding, and allergic reaction to the contrast medium (the last risk is shared by CTA). It is also more time-consuming, more uncomfortable for patients, and more costly to perform.

When Baker et al. (2008) examined Medicare records, they estimated that for every 100 abdominal CTA patients, there were about 68 who ordinarily might not have received either a CTA or a catheter angiography, 15 are people who would have received a catheter angiography but now receive a CTA instead, and 16 others who receive *both* CTA and catheter angiography (italics added). Computed tomography angiography did not generate significant new follow-on costs related to repairing the dissecting aneurysms (only about 1.1 cases per 100 scans), suggesting that while CTA significantly increased the number of procedures, it added little to uncovering more disease. Because CTA is noninvasive and readily available, however, patient and clinician resistance to its use is minimal, and the population of individuals receiving

---

[15] An aneurysm is a potentially fatal rupture between layers of the wall of the aorta that descends from the heart through the abdomen.

the test (many with only minimal indications) has widened, while the value of the test remains uncertain.

Too much should not be inferred from a single study. However, absent a robust and compelling evidence-based justification for using a new test, both research and historical experience suggests that new technologies that can shed additional light on a complex medical problem will simply be added to an already crowded toolbox and be demanded by patients and referring physicians who are aware of it. The evidence that could lead to exclusion of older and less capable technologies needs to be developed, taught in medical school and residency training, and incorporated more rapidly into the medical culture. The propensity of new imaging technologies to add to, rather than substitute for, existing technologies assuredly plays a key supporting role in the growth of imaging spending.

*The Real Culprit: The Impossible Quest for Medical Certainty*   The primary driver of the overly aggressive use of diagnostic testing is the typical physician's discomfort with clinical uncertainty. This approach is a core element of the culture of medical practice instilled in young people during their medical training. It will continue to be the principal driver of the marginally necessary and unnecessary use of imaging regardless of the level of imaging payments, the permissible ownership arrangements for imaging equipment, the advent of tort liability reform, and other policy issues.

Clinicians in the United States have been taught in their training to find the cause of a patient's complaint, resources be damned. Interns and residents who are learning to manage the care of their patients do not want to be exposed to the withering glare of their chief resident or faculty physician and asked why they did not perform a particular test. Young physicians are too often taught to test regardless of how small the chances are that the test will reveal the cause of the patient's complaint. The negative findings, their superiors often argue, still contribute to the learning experience. There is also more than a little "up the organization" attitude in the clinical faculty's guidance of trainees. Because teaching hospitals are so vast and decentralized, the trainee or faculty adviser has no economic incentive to make responsible use of the institution's (and ultimately the public's) resources. Only in rare instances are trainees acculturated in a system of diagnostic minimalism. In most medical training settings, the message from one's elders is unambiguous. Figure out what's wrong with the patient right now, and let the hospital administration sort out the costs later.

This aspect of medical culture has been caricatured in the popular television drama *House*, which features a brilliant and implacable medical diagnostician who tests his patients to the *n*th degree. Though rarely so extremely, most physicians bring some element of this attitude to medical practice. We believe that the culture of contemporary medical practice—incubated in medical school and residency training and flowering afterward—may be the most powerful driver of aggressive imaging use, even more powerful than the compelling economic incentives.

In support of this opinion, a recent research study cast some doubt on the saliency of several of the "usual suspect" drivers of imaging volume growth and added to the suspicion that broader cultural factors in the medical practice world are at work. The study analyzed the use of CT and MR imaging studies in a large staff model health maintenance organization (HMO) (Group Health of Puget Sound) over a 10-year period (1997–2006). The setting for this study was very important because Group Health's physicians are salaried, and their compensation does not increase by ordering additional tests. Indeed, because Group Health is an *integrated* health system—that is, an insurer as well as a direct provider of care—unnecessary testing actually damages the organization's profitability. In other words, the incentives of HMO payment are precisely the reverse of the prevalent fee-for-service system described in this chapter, punishing rather than rewarding marginal and unnecessary medical spending.

The Group Health imaging study found "rising use of imaging services among health maintenance organization (HMO) members, closely paralleling the trends found in the traditional fee-for-service Medicare or privately insured populations" during the study period. Per capita use of CT increased 14% per year during the study period, use of MR by 26% a year, and ultrasound studies by 40% a year (Smith-Bindman et al. 2008).[16] Imaging studies examined in this research were confined to those ordered by Group Health's salaried physicians and excluded studies ordered in geographic regions covered by fee-for-service contractors.[17]

The authors speculated that increased availability of CT and MRI capacity inside Group Health and pent-up demand for studies may have contributed somewhat to the growth. They also theorized that fee-for-service utilization patterns that Group Health clinicians learned in medical school "could affect clinical practice standards that extend into the managed care setting." Because Group Health has historically offered a rich benefit design with limited patient cost sharing., patient demand for high-technology imaging (for whom the use is largely free) and a physician concern about malpractice liability might have contributed to the growth. The authors also suggested that improvements in imaging technology, such as the advent of the multidetector CT discussed earlier, as well as imaging's increasing usefulness in monitoring the effectiveness of cancer therapy, might have encouraged volume growth in the absence of economic incentives.

This single research study does not absolve the above-listed usual suspects—supply-generated demand, the attractiveness of imaging technical payments, self-referral incentives, the institutional and practitioner profit motive, and fear of malpractice—from blame for imaging's singular growth. What the Group Health study suggests is that "single-bullet" theories are insufficient to explain the extraordinary rise in the use of medical imaging. A multiplicity of factors is at work. Perhaps most importantly, clinicians are trained to use all the tools available to them to help their patients eliminate the threatening uncertainty of disease. New imaging developments have put increasingly powerful tools at the clinician's disposal to do exactly that in more clinical situations than ever before.

---

[16] It is worth pointing out that while the rate of rise Smith-Bindman and her colleagues found in high-technology imaging use at Group health might compare to that of the fee-for-service world for the time period they studied, it was from a far lower historical base of utilization. Health maintenance organizations like Group Health are, in general, much more conservative in their use of clinical resources, including imaging, than the traditional fee-for-service community.

[17] Personal communication, R. Smith-Bindman, University of California, San Francisco, June 1, 2009.

## How Have Health Insurers Responded?

As discussed above, the DRA slowed (at least temporarily) the growth in Medicare imaging expenditures by slashing nonhospital outpatient imaging technical payments. Private health insurers have followed suit by implementing similar technical fee reductions. Private payers also have repurposed an old stand-by managed care technique to control imaging expenses — requiring prior authorization for advanced imaging studies or hiring radiology benefits management (RBM) firms to control imaging volumes.

Prior authorization requires that physicians ordering a test provide clinical justification that matches the insurer's or RBM's standards for acceptable use. In the absence of clinical justification, the health insurer will not approve payment for the study. This approval loop has the effect of introducing a costly bureaucratic hurdle into the ordering process, and sometimes delays. Preauthorization may even deny appropriate care.

Prior authorization by RBMs now covers an estimated one-half of all privately insured patients ("Radiology Benefits" 2007) whether patients are aware of it or not. Some of the RBMs claim that they have produced an impressive flattening of the upward trend of imaging use, denying as many as 15% of requests for imaging studies. A recent study by Mitchell and LaGalia found that RBMs succeeded in reducing CT use by 9%–14% in the first year and MR use by 8%–15%. However, two of the three plans studied saw rebounds in use in the second year, presumably as clinicians adapted by changing either their ordering patterns or their clinical justifications to anticipate RBM review questions (Mitchell and LaGalia 2009). In one of the large RBMs, surgical specialties tended to have low single-digit denial rates, while some primary care physicians, like family practitioners, had 20% or higher denial rates (Allen 2008). How many of the initial denials are later overturned by clinicians providing additional justification for their orders is unknown.

Even given the significant initial denial rates, most observers believe that prior authorization might have more pervasive effects indirectly, through the *sentinel effect* (the concern that Big Brother is watching) and the *hurdle effect* (busy physicians dread the drain on their and their staff's time imposed by prior authorization). The sentinel and hurdle effects serve to discourage marginal as well as some appropriate requests for examinations. But these effects are virtually impossible to measure, perhaps somewhat akin to measuring the effect of those famous garlic amulets that purport to protect persons from vampires.

Having dealt with the volume side of the expense equation, the private insurers and RBMs have begun to work at reducing the cost per unit of service by assembling panels of *preferred imaging providers* who accept substantial discounts from their customary charges in exchange for additional referrals from the health plans that RBMs represent. There are some communities (Phoenix, Arizona, for example) where RBMs have been able to achieve discounts in technical and/or professional payments as great as 50% by limiting their imaging panels to only those facilities accepting the lower payments.[18] Markets with high densities of scanning capacity might be fertile territory for significant reductions in unit payment through RBM

---

[18] Personal communication, Keith Pitts, January 2009.

market pressure, compounding the effects of the Medicare payment reductions discussed earlier.

For many medical specialties, patients would complain about being steered away from their previous doctor by a health plan or review organization. However, the invisibility of the radiologist, discussed in Chapter 1, makes this more feasible for imaging. Patients usually do not have a personal relationship with the imaging centers or radiologists who perform high-technology scans. In most urban and suburban communities, there are many convenient locations that provide imaging services. Some health plans may eventually further reduce patient resistance to using the services of the lowest-cost imaging provider by lowering the patients' copayment if they visit the centers that agree to accept the discounted rates.

In some sense, prior authorization represents a step back into the past for the private insurance system. The criteria by which imaging referrals are denied are not always transparent. Moreover, the process tars every orderer of imaging services for the abuses of a few, even though some RBMs claim to have narrowed their review focus to habitual overutilizers, sparing those with more modest ordering patterns (i.e., they are given what is sometimes known as a *gold card*). However, RBMs create an inescapable set of problems: their criteria for approving exams are proprietary and may be capricious; delays for patients and time lost from patient care are inevitable; and there are increased administrative costs for both insurers and medical practices.

The administrative burden of responding to health insurers' requests for documentation and microscopic oversight of clinical practice has already imposed huge costs on the nation's practitioners. According to a study published in 2009, the typical American physician spends 43 minutes per workday fulfilling data requests, haggling over claims, credentialing, and requesting authorizations and approvals of various kinds, at a cost to society of $21 to $31 billion a year (Casolino et al. 2009). RBMs add to this cost burden and are a 1970s solution to a twenty-first-century problem. Despite this, perhaps out of frustration with the ineffectiveness of other approaches, the GAO has recommended extending RBM surveillance to all Medicare patients referred for imaging studies. To date, no such action has been taken.

## Information Technology Provides an Alternative

There are alternative and less costly approaches to solving this problem, incorporating modern clinical information technology with embedded appropriateness criteria based on the best available scientific evidence. The radiology departments of the main Partners Hospitals in Boston—the Massachusetts General and Brigham and Women's hospitals—have built sophisticated radiology order entry and decision support systems that require physicians referring their patients for imaging studies to supply the clinical justification for their orders in order for them to be processed. The order for an imaging study may not actually be scheduled by the radiology department unless the supporting clinical information for the requested exam is determined to be adequate. This clinical justification is essential to ensure that an imaging study is warranted, that the correct studies are done, and that the studies are billed to insurers properly. The information provided also ensures that the referring physician has pursued alternative, less costly diagnostic approaches, if appropriate, before ordering an expensive scan.

The major differences from the RBM approach are several: The information rationalizing the exam must be provided to the people who would be performing the examination inside the normal (but now automated) consultative loop rather to a financially interested third party. The criteria used to determine appropriateness are transparent in the way they are developed and applied. Consultative advice from radiologists is available both online and in person for referring physicians if they have questions about the most appropriate diagnostic course. All of these exchanges are documented and retained in the radiology department's information system to justify the ultimate diagnostic course chosen and to track the effects on reducing unnecessary imaging. Since the request for imaging services is handled at the point of service by colleagues, there is less opportunity for patients to encounter delays or cancellations.

Both Partners' "intelligent" radiology order entry systems were judged sufficiently rigorous by Massachusetts' major health plans—Blue Cross and Blue Shield, Tufts Health Plan, and Harvard Pilgrim Health Care—that they exempted both hospitals from external RBM reviews. In other words, the plans considered this home grown but rigorous self-policing of clinical appropriateness to be more efficient and effective than third-party review. Evaluations of the performance of the systems have documented improved efficiency of the imaging process, as well as provision of the most appropriate care supportable by scientific evidence. Referring physicians' questions were answered the first time, requests for duplicate examinations decreased, and there were substantial savings in reduced imaging expenses.[19]

The Partners' systems took years to develop and provide a glimpse of a future with more appropriate imaging care. However, there are a number of barriers to adoption. Relatively few radiology departments or imaging centers have this level of technical sophistication in their information technology (IT) infrastructure. Commercial systems exist, but only a minority of physicians practice in a setting where there is a completely electronic system for ordering and scheduling imaging studies.

This electronic decision-support approach also requires an essential, but potentially jarring, cultural shift in the relationship between radiologists and their referring physicians. At Brigham and Women's Hospital and Massachusetts General Hospital, implementation required extensive dialog between the radiology staffs and their referring physicians to develop the system's specifications and consensus that radiologists should provide counsel and even deny inappropriate radiological examinations. As with most IT systems, successful implementation requires a cultural shift as well as a technological one.

Nonetheless, it is likely that sophisticated imaging ordering systems of this type will proliferate, and it will become progressively less necessary to impose external entities like the RBMs on the referral process for radiological studies. Patients will benefit from fewer delays in receiving appropriate care. There will be fewer impositions on the time and energy of physicians and less administrative overhead. Departments and imaging centers that make these IT investments might well be able to stake a claim to higher payment levels from health insurers, since they will reduce

---

[19] Personal communications, James Thrall and Ramin Khorasani, November 2008.

administrative expense by making it unnecessary to hire RBMs to vet imaging referrals. In 2008, CMS commissioned a demonstration project to attempt to measure the effects of these IT-based solutions on ordering patterns under Section 135b of the Medicare Improvements for Patients and Providers Act (MIPPA).[20]

## Summary: Society's Larger Question

The forgoing discussion begs one overriding question: Is American society receiving value for money for the use of these remarkable but costly diagnostic tools? There is no simple "yes" or "no" answer to this question. The past 40 years have provided a remarkably fertile climate for experimentation and refinement of the imaging tool set. These technologies have alleviated suffering and saved lives. In the course of doing so, imaging technology has developed to the point where it has altered the ecology of medical practice.

If one examines the history of medicine, as Sir William Osler first observed a century ago, medicine's diagnostic power has consistently preceded its ability to cure disease. That has certainly been the case with diagnostic imaging. Imaging's accuracy and ability to resolve clinical uncertainty will continue to improve. The question society must ask is, how much does lowering uncertainty by a small fraction change the care patients receive or improve the quality of their health? Given the urgent emphasis on reducing health care costs, the answer may depend more on economic than clinical priorities.

Given that this is likely the case, how can society encourage the more thoughtful use of imaging technology while continuing to improve it? This almost certainly will require a greater degree of scientific rigor in evaluating the usefulness of imaging procedures. But it will also require a better balancing of economic risk and responsibility among patients, referring physicians, radiologists, and those who create, maintain, and operate imaging's infrastructure.

How better to integrate scientific information on clinical effectiveness into the payment process, end financially motivated imaging, and correct the balance of economic risk to payment so as to eliminate waste and abuse will be addressed in the final chapter of this book. Our recommendations will not please everyone. But a more thoughtful approach to developing and fostering the growth in imaging could lead to both better societal value and improved patient welfare.

## References

Allen GA. MedSolutions, Inc. Presentation to the GE Healthcare Market Drivers Summit, January 29, 2008.

Allen R, Bombieri M. A healthcare system badly out of balance. *Boston Globe*. November 16, 2008. Accessed on May 13, 2010.

http://www.boston.com/news/local/articles/2008/11/16/a_healthcare_system_badly_out_of_balance/.

[20] See the CMS Web site for details on this project at http://www.cms.hhs.gov/ DemoProjectsEvalRpts/MD/itemdetail.asp?filterType=none&filterByDID=-99&sort ByDID=3&sortOrder=descending&itemID=CMS1222075&intNumPerPage=10.

American Medical Association. Physician resources, solutions for managing your practice. http://www.ama-assn.org/ama/pub/physician-resources/solutions-managing-your-practice/coding-billing-insurance/the-resource-based-relative-value-scale.shtml. Accessed on May 13, 2010.

Angrisano C, Farrell D, Kocher B, et al. *Accounting for the Cost of Health Care in the United States*. McKinsey Global Institute, January 2007.

Appleby J. The case for CT angiography: how Americans view and embrace new technology. *Health Aff*. 2008;27:1515–1521.

Baker LC, Atlas SW, Afendulis CC. Expanded use of imaging and the challenge of measuring value. *Health Aff*. 2008;27:1467–1478.

Casolino LP, Nicholson S, Gans DN, et al. What does it cost physician practices to interact with health insurance plans? *Health Aff*. 2009;28:533–543.

Congressional Budget Office (CBO). *Budget Options, Vol. 1, Health Care*. December 2008, 112–113.

Dartmouth Institute for Health Policy and Clinical Practice. Tracking the care of patients with severe chronic illness. *The Dartmouth Atlas of Healthcare*, 2008. http://www.dartmouthatlas.org/atlases/2008_Chronic_Care_Atlas.pdf. Accessed on May 13, 2010.

Farrell D, Jensen E, Kocher B. Accounting for the Cost of U.S. health care: a new look at why Americans spend more. McKinsey Global Institute, December 2008.

Fisher E. Pay for performance: more than rearranging the deck chairs. *J Am Coll Radiol*. 2007;4:879–885.

Hartman M, Martin A, McDonnell P, et al. National health spending in 2007: slower drug spending contributes to lowest rate of overall growth since 1998. *Health Aff*. 2009;28:246–261.

Hillman BJ, Neu CR, Winkler JD, et al. The diffusion of magnetic resonance imaging scanners in a changing health care environment. II How experiences with X-ray computed tomography influenced providers' plans for magnetic resonance imaging scanners. *J. Technol Assess Health Care*. 1987;3:554–559.

Hoffman JM, Gambhir SS, Kelloff GJ. Regulatory and reimbursement challenges for molecular imaging. *Radiology*. 2007;245:645–660.

Kessler DP, McClellan MB. Do doctors practice defensive medicine? *Quart Rev Econ Finance*. 1996;111:353–390.

Khorasani R. Role of information technology in improving the quality of care in radiology: an overview. *J Am Coll Radiol*. 2005;2:1035–1036.

Levin DC, Rao VM, Parker L, et al. Who gets paid for diagnostic imaging, and how much? *J Am Coll Radiol*. 2004;1:931–935.

Lewin Group. Outlook for Medical Technology Innovation, Report #2: *The Medicare Payment Process and Patient Access to Technology*. Washington, DC: Advanced Medical Technology Association, 2000.

Massachusetts Medical Society. Investigation of defensive medicine in Massachusetts. Informational Report I-08, November, 2008. http://www.ncrponline.org/PDFs/Mass_Med_Soc.pdf. Accessed February 12, 2010.

Medicare Payment Advisory Commission. Report to the Congress: Medicare payment policy. March, 2005. http://www.medpac.gov/documents/Mar05_EntireReport.pdf. Accessed November 24, 2009.

Mitchell JM, LaGalia RR. Controlling the use of advanced imaging. *Med Care Res Rev*. 2009;20:1–13.

Moon M. *Medicare: A Policy Primer*. Washington, DC: Urban Institute Press, 2006.

Moorefield JM, MacEwan DW, Sunshine JH. The radiology relative value scale: its development and implementation. *Radiology*. 1993;187:317–326.

Moran Company. Trends in imaging services billed to part B Medicare carriers and paid under the Medicare physician fee schedule 1998–2008. Report prepared for the Access to Medical Imaging Coalition, October, 2009.

Pearson SD, Knudsen AB, Scherer RW, et al. Assessing the comparative effectiveness of a diagnostic technology: CT colonography. *Health Aff.* 2008;27:1503–1521.

Raab G, Parr D. From medical invention to clinical practice: the reimbursement challenge facing new device procedures and technology—Part 2: coverage. *J Am Coll Radiol.* 2006;3:772–777.

Radiology benefits managers offer Medicare cost-saving option for imaging. Gray Sheet, July 2, 2007. www.thegraysheet.elsevierbi.com. Accessed February 16, 2010.

Radiology Business Journal. Implications of reform for hospitals: subtle or seismic? February/March 2010, pp. 12–14.

SDI. *Diagnostic Imaging Center Market Report.* Yardley, PA: SDI Health, 2008.

Smith-Bindman R, Miglioretti DL, Larson EB. Rising use of diagnostic medical imaging in a large integrated health system. *Health Aff.* 2008;27:1491–1514.

U.S. Government Accountability Office (GAO). *Medicare Part B Imaging Services. Rapid Spending Growth and Shift to Physicians Offices Indicate Need for CMS to Consider Additional Mangement Practices. Report to Congressional Requesters* (GAO 08–452). Washington, DC: GAO, 2008a.

U.S. Government Accountability Office (GAO). *Medicare Imaging Payments. Medicare: Trends in Fees, Utilization and Expenditures Before and After Implementation of the Deficit Reduction Act of 2005. Letter to Congressional Requesters* (GAO 08–1102R). Washington, DC: GAO, 2008b.

U.S. Office of Management and Budget, Executive Office of the President. *Budget of the United States FY2010.* Updated Summary Tables. Washington, DC: U.S. Office of Management and Budget, May 2009, p. 6.

# 6

# Digital Pioneers: Globalization and Corporatization

*The year 1972 was an auspicious one.*

*In 1972, Richard Nixon was running his doomed, Watergate-tainted campaign for reelection. The nation remained mired in Vietnam. Elton John's "Rocket Man" and Curtis Mayfield's "Superfly" were playing on the radio. IBM 360 mainframes stalked the earth, feeding on vast decks of IBM punch cards. Bill Gates was a junior at Lakeside School in Seattle, sleeping in the school's computer center.*

*In 1972, the authors of this book were preparing to embark on their careers. One (JG) was living in an apartment with bars on the windows on Chicago's South Side, using a manual Olivetti Lettera 32 to type his doctoral dissertation on erasable bond paper. The underlying data were stored in a 2-foot-high deck of 5-by-7-inch file cards on which he'd taken down and organized his research. The other (BH) was playing out the string of his medical student education. By day, he was seeing patients on elective clinical rotations at Strong Memorial Hospital in Rochester, New York. By night, he was earning a little money interpreting blood smears, catching the odd hour of sleep on a stretcher in the emergency room.*

With the introduction of CT scanning in 1972, diagnostic radiology arrived at the digital revolution before anyone else in medicine, or for that matter, before most of society. However, CT as a digital technology stood in virtual isolation. The information CT captured far outstripped the electronic means of storing, transmitting, or making use of it.

To interpret the scans and share them with colleagues, radiologists printed out the images on film, slice by adjacent slice, 8–24 slices to a sheet. They read them the same way they read conventional X-rays, squinting sequentially at tiny images displayed on a light box until every one of them had been viewed. The films were stored with the rest of the patient's films in manila file folders. These files frequently were lost by the film file room staff, or hoarded by referring physicians or house staff, and were thus often unavailable when needed for patient care. Hospitals stored the CT scanner's digital output on hard-to-access magnetic tape reels and typically purged the tapes after a few months.

Radiology has come a long way since those early days. Advanced radiology departments are operated wholly by digital technology. Many other medical disciplines are actively working toward this goal. This chapter describes how radiology became, through digitization and the electronic transmission of images over the Internet, a global medical specialty. Digital networking using the broadband Internet has yielded enormous efficiencies in the practice of radiology. It transformed radiology into a 24/7 activity unbounded by physical location. It also benefited the health system by extending access to imaging expertise to previously underserved locales. However, the "digitization" of imaging also has been highly disruptive of traditional radiology practice. This chapter describes how the digital era is changing the economic and organizational structure of the discipline.

## Rules for Radiology

In *The World Is Flat* (Friedman 2005), Thomas Friedman talked about the explosive moment when an array of complex technological enablers converged to flatten the world's economy. These enablers include ubiquitous high-performance personal computers, affordable bandwidth and data storage, database management tools, new workflow tools, and the global Internet backbone. These technologies, in turn, have catalyzed new digital business models that help organize and distribute information to reach billions of potential new customers.

In medicine, this digital convergence happened first in imaging. Radiology, at its core, is a discipline of frustrated engineers and tinkerers. Radiologists realized that the full potential of digital imaging could not be realized unless they could create the means to store and share digital images. Their journey toward harnessing the potential of digital imaging began in the early 1980s, long before the Internet, high-capacity data storage, and digital communication networks. Radiology's development of and adaptation to digital technology laid the groundwork for its emergence as the first global medical discipline and for the explosive growth in imaging that has followed. Moreover, developments in digital image capture, transmission, and interpretation have promoted profound organizational changes in how radiology is practiced.

To fully realize the potential of digital imaging, it was essential to create data standards that could be applied uniformly across different types of digital devices and that were independent of the manufacturer. Data standards are the rules that enable digital information to pass through networks from devices to users in comprehensible and usable fashion and to be retained and managed in large-capacity databases. The developers of these standards foresaw that images would be transmitted through high-speed institutional networks (intranets) and be communicated among facilities on the Internet.

Some people think of the Internet as a physical infrastructure, which it is—vast server farms of Internet service providers such as Google and Amazon. However, what has enabled the Internet to function and grow exponentially is a simple and powerful hierarchy of rules, specifically TCP/IP (Transmission Control

Protocol/Internet Protocol) that define how Internet messages are managed and transmitted across the network (Cerf and Kahn 1974).[1] These rules define the logic of cutting messages into packets to be disassembled and reassembled across the Internet. The rules were designed to be flexible and have shown a robust ability to scale up as Internet traffic has burgeoned.

To create the analogous digital standards in imaging required collaboration among the physicians, physicists, and engineers who would further develop CT and a fractious collection of competing CT vendors. In 1983, the ACR launched a collaborative effort with the National Electrical Manufacturers Association (NEMA) to create technical standards that would permit better management of CT images (Hammond and Cimino 2006). Without these standards, it would have been impossible for radiologists to do research, extend and improve the technology, or establish technologies that could improve CT interpretation.

Manufacturers of CT technology were not anxious to come to the party. Most of them entertained visions of dominating a lucrative new market and had little incentive to collaborate. Most manufacturers entertained the vision of a "walled garden" of imaging devices, storage mechanisms, peripherals such as displays, and software that supported and communicated with that vendor's products. However, prompted by the professional radiology community, the FDA, which regulates medical devices, applied gentle leverage by suggesting that the alternative to voluntary collaboration might be regulatory action (personal communication, Steven Horii, April 2009).

The initial goals of the first ACR/NEMA working groups were modest: to create standards that enabled different manufacturers' equipment to connect physically to storage devices (in this era, nine-track magnetic tape recorders) and communicate standard digital messages to the storage medium (point-to-point). The result was a crucial beginning: a consensus on the common physical connection (e.g., cable) between machines and storage devices (through a 50-pin connector) and an agreed-upon structure for tagging and organizing strings of imaging data that could be communicated through cable connections and stored on tape.

This first standard, called ACR/NEMA v.1.0, was made public in 1985. A second version was released in 1988, which enabled better communication with display devices and more detail about the output (the digital representation of the images) from the imaging devices themselves. The first two ACR/NEMA standards did not anticipate data networks or database management; the physical infrastructure to enable this did not exist in the mid-1980s.

The first ACR/NEMA standards represented the beginning of a complex and highly productive collaboration between the profession of radiology and industry that produced one of medicine's most important and highly developed data

---

[1] These rules were created by software engineers and architects originally charged by the Defense Advanced Research and Projects Agency (DARPA) to build a secure and survivable information architecture for nuclear weapons command. After a decade's refinement, TCP/IP was adopted as the data standard for all computer communications inside the U.S. Department of Defense in 1982. Today, TCP/IP is the core rule set for a flexible and indispensible worldwide communications network. See Clark (1988) for a history of the development of these standards.

standards: DICOM (Digital Information and Communication in Medicine).[2] High-capacity local communications networks such as Xerox's Ethernet emerged in the early 1990s, and data storage advanced to the point where a more refined and complex standard was required (Kahn et al. 2007).

## Anywhere, Anytime Images

The existence of DICOM and the emergence of enhanced digital and communications technologies paved the way for the development of complex data systems to manage, store, and communicate digital images. These data systems are called PACS (Picture Archiving, Communication, and Storage) systems. The PACS systems made it possible to dispense with printing CT and MR images to film. Rather, images could remain in digital form throughout the entire use cycle, be transmitted from the device to any location on the network to be interpreted on high-resolution workstations, and then stored in an easy-to-retrieve form in digital data archives (Greenes and Brinkley 2006).

The goal of PACS was not only to eliminate the physical storage of images in manila files—which required a great deal of supporting manpower and was, at best, unreliable—but also to make medical images and their interpretations more accessible to radiologists and referring physicians. With PACS, images could be made available anywhere the data system could be connected. Radiologists could work from remote offices, or from home, or from hotel rooms overseas, for that matter, rather than in hospital reading rooms. Referring physicians did not have to go down to a dank hospital basement to retrieve films or consult with the radiologist. By replacing everything done by film except the actual image acquisition (which must be digitized for everything else to work), PACS revolutionized the role of imaging in medical practice.

The PACS systems became the first high-capacity data systems in most hospitals. Under pressure from their radiologists, many hospitals purchased PACS systems long before they had digitized internal communications, such as e-mail, or installed an electronic health record (EHR). Initially, PACS systems were bounded by the hospital or by the locations of the radiology group that served the hospital. In other words, they were local area networks (LANs). The third version of DICOM addressed this shortcoming. Released in 1992, this version was explicitly intended to facilitate imaging management across data networks. This third version, crucially, recognized TCP/IP—the Internet messaging protocol—as the organizing principle for communicating digital images across networks, and was released more than three years before Netscape broke open the Internet to broad popular use.

Thus, imaging professionals adopted the same digital standard that facilitated the explosive growth of the Internet years before the Internet's dramatic expansion. This crucial decision positioned radiology to become the first of medicine's disciplines to "go global." Thanks to DICOM and to TCP/IP, images could be transmitted to colleagues anywhere around the globe so long as there was broadband Internet access, high-resolution workstations to display the images, and competent radiologists to

[2] Those interested in learning more about DICOM should read Oleg Pianykh's (2008) excellent technical guide for users.

read them. DICOM turned imaging studies from something physically solid, residing on film, into something much more liquid and movable.

Ironically, the same development of standards and technology that has been so beneficial to radiologists has catalyzed what may become an irreversible economic process of converting diagnostic radiological interpretation into a commodity. The convergence of all these technology enablers—digital standards, networks, imaging equipment, storage and retrieval software—has made possible a distributed business model of imaging interpretation called *teleradiology*.

Tom Friedman's *The World Is Flat* envisioned vast rooms full of radiologists in India reading scans ported to them from America. Called by some "sweatshop radiology," the phenomenon was one of Friedman's most compelling examples of the globalization of complex knowledge work. "Thank God I'm not a radiologist," he wrote (given the evolving state of the newspaper business, he concluded entirely too optimistically, "There will be no outsourcing for me"). Friedman's implication was that if you could replace your local American radiologist with someone earning $25 an hour halfway around the world, nobody's job was truly safe.

## The Dawn of Telemedicine

Remote interpretation of radiological images was not the first application in the broader field of telemedicine (Brennan and Starren 2006). Beginning in the late 1970s, cardiologists began monitoring electrocardiographic (ECG) telemetry of heart electrical activity remotely through dedicated telephone lines and advising local physicians on the management of critically ill heart patients. However, the bandwidth and interpretative skill required to evaluate ECG tracings pale by comparison to those required to transmit and interpret a radiological image.

Teleradiology was effectively impossible before the development of worldwide access to the broadband Internet. Digital imaging files are large and bulky. A typical MR scan file is about 150–500 megabytes. So, the fiberoptic boom of the 1990s, which ringed the world with fiberoptic data conduits, created the essential enabling infrastructure for the emergence of teleradiology. Another critical precondition was the ability to extract and transmit images from the hospital or radiology group and stream them to a remote location over broadband networks, a comparatively mundane technical challenge. Finally and most critically, to practice teleradiology, one needed trained radiologists who were interested in a new kind of radiological practice wherein image interpretation could be performed in their homes or in vast imaging "bunkers" or "warehouses" around the world.

Globalized teleradiology had particular appeal to increasingly stressed U.S. radiologists for night and weekend interpretation. By outsourcing "off-hours" work to teleradiologists in other countries, U.S. radiologists could sleep while their colleagues in Barcelona or Sydney or another location worked during daylight hours. Outsourced teleradiology also benefited referring physicians, their patients and hospital emergency departments, since teleradiology often enabled faster off-hours responsiveness to consultative requests.

Though shortages of radiologists were common during the 1990s, increases in the size of residency programs later in the decade created a new surge of young radiologists. Some Generation X and Generation Y radiologists were receptive to this adventurous new style of practice. However, several barriers limit the "offshoring" of U.S. image interpretations.

- Most importantly, Medicare and most private insurers will not pay for interpretations that originate overseas. As a result, companies offering offshore teleradiology provide only "preliminary" interpretations to guide immediate clinical care. U.S. based radiologists must overread these night and weekend exams—usually the next day—and submit their charges.
- States' licencing laws consider the point of origin of the exam (i.e., where the patient is imaged) to reside in their jurisdiction. Thus, any teleradiologist must be licensed in the state where the imaging exam was performed. To address this requirement, teleradiology companies usually license their radiologists in every state in which they hold a contract.
- Hospitals usually require even remote physicians to be credentialed in their institution if imaging is performed in their imaging facilities. Teleradiology companies must manage the administratively burdensome credentialing process for each hospital for which their radiologists interpret images.

As a result, while offshore preliminary interpretation services still exist, the business has blossomed into myriad forms. Indeed, in just a decade, teleradiology has grown to become a $6 billion global business, according to TechNavio, an industry intelligence firm ("Teleradiology" 2009). The teleradiology world is populated by 2 large, publicly held companies and almost 30 privately held companies, as well as many private practice radiology groups and academic radiology departments in medical schools.

Teleradiology is fundamentally altering the economic landscape of radiological practice as traditional radiology groups—often supported by their hospitals—have taken advantage of ubiquitous and increasingly inexpensive "after-hours" coverage to improve their physicians' lifestyles and fill gaps in staffing. A 2007 study revealed that roughly 50% of U.S. practices were outsourcing at least some of their imaging to teleradiology companies (Kaye et al. 2008). Increasingly, teleradiologists based in the United States are assuming a larger share of the market by working nighttime hours to provide definitive interpretations that obviate the need for the morning overreads. Outsourcing of imaging interpretation on the less desirable shifts has become so pervasive in U.S. radiology practice that radiology groups not offering after-hours and weekend teleradiology coverage have difficulty filling vacant professional positions, as many younger radiologists do not wish to be burdened with after-hours or weekend call coverage responsibilities.

While extending its geographic reach, however, teleradiology has destabilized a successful profession, giving rise to concerns about the "commoditization" of radiological practice. Once one establishes the principle that some images can be interpreted offsite, it is remarkable how high the percentage of total imaging work-flow (not just on evenings and weekends) can follow directly. This essential fact about teleradiology has undermined the income stability of established radiology groups and placed at risk radiologists' long-term exclusive contracts with hospitals. As teleradiology has developed, the boundaries between teleradiology and onsite coverage have become highly fluid.

The logical endpoint of competition over imaging is glimpsed with the creation of an online auction market for teleradiology intepretation. The company which created it is called Telerays (http://www.telerays.com). Telerays announced at the beginning of 2009 an eBay-like auction site that permitted those who require radiological interpretation to bid out their work and award spot contracts to individual radiologists or radiology groups who bid the lowest for providing the services. Telerays charged the winning bidder a 15% fee for arranging interpretative services. While still in its testing phase, the Telerays online auction is a logical extension of the teleradiology concept that frees hospitals and other consumers of imaging services from exclusive contracts with radiologists. Telerays also gives the buyer the economic leverage to lower the price of consultation.

The company began full-scale operations in the first quarter of 2009. It remains to be seen how robust and deep the spot market is for interpretative services. If it prospers, it will be the first fully functioning, Internet-based auction market for professional medical services. To the chagrin of conventional radiology groups, this is another "first" for radiology. From DICOM (3.0) to Telerays was only a 16-year journey.

## The Flight of the NightHawk

Teleradiology became identified with what business analysts call the *first mover* in this space: NightHawk Radiological Services, founded by an entrepreneurial radiologist, Paul Berger, his son, and a young colleague in 2001. NightHawk's corporate headquarters were in the wilds of Coeur d'Alene, Idaho, though with recent management changes, the company has relocated to Arizona. So thoroughly did NightHawk dominate the market in off-hours teleradiology services during the early years that *nighthawk* has become the generic name for off-hours remote interpretation. In other words, NightHawk became the Xerox of the teleradiology business.

Berger began working in the 1990s to cover night and weekend readings for multiple radiological sites from a traditional service center in his Long Beach, California, practice. He quickly learned that the demand for such services required a more robust, geographically dispersed network of radiological consultants. From this original vision has emerged a $170 million business, with 128 affiliated radiologists who contract with NightHawk to practice in four service centers: Sydney, Australia; Zurich, Switzerland; Austin, Texas; and San Francisco, California. All of these radiologists were trained and are licensed in the United States, for reasons discussed above. From these sites, NightHawk serves 790 radiology groups, which, in turn, cover some 1560 hospitals in the United States. Some 78% of NightHawk's income is derived from preliminary interpretations provided during off-hours.[3] Each of NightHawk's affiliated radiologists is licensed, on average, in 36 states and has privileges in some 560 hospitals. The company went public in 2006 and is presently traded on the NASDAQ exchange. There is one publicly traded competitor,

[3] See NightHawk radiology website at http://wwwnighthawkrad.net/index.php, accessed online December 14, 2009.

Virtual Radiologic, with approximately 60% of NightHawk's revenue base (but half again the market capitalization as of this writing).[4]

When a remote radiological consultation is required, radiology technicians can request a NightHawk interpretation by telephone, fax, or e-mail. The sending hospital forwards the image file to a NightHawk server, where a technician prepares the file and forwards it to be interpreted by a NightHawk radiologist. The NightHawk interpretation is then edited, packaged, and forwarded to the requesting facility, with a follow-up call to make sure that the facility received it.

NightHawk frightened and, at the same time, galvanized the entire imaging industry. As NightHawk and its imitators rapidly discovered, the barriers for entry to this business are minimal, and competitors piled in. Radiology groups of a sufficient size began internalizing nighthawk coverage, creating their own service centers and hiring radiologists to staff them. As noted above, insuperable regulatory barriers block the entry of the most feared competition from inexpensive Indian or Chinese radiologists. However, domestic regional and national competitors added teleradiology offerings to their menu of hospital coverage. Younger radiologists, as well as older radiologists moving to partial retirement, provided a ready workforce for teleradiology companies. The work enabled radiologists to control their schedules better and to locate where they wished.

To respond to competitive pressures, NightHawk expanded its service offerings in 2006 by merging with American Teleradiology to include final interpretations, as well as business management services for radiology groups (NightHawk's main client base). After experiencing earnings difficulties at the beginning of 2008, NightHawk's stock price plummeted. In the spring of 2009, Berger resigned his chairmanship and dissolved his relationship with the company he had founded over philosophical differences with the new corporate management. His resignation letter read, in part: "...the Company has embarked on business and strategic initiatives which in good conscience I cannot support and do not wish to be part of going forward."[5]

## The Inland Empire

Some larger radiology groups have incorporated teleradiology operations into their practices in order to extend the geographic reach of the group and facilitate expansion of its volume of services. Expanding volume is important to groups, since the real dollar payment per case for imaging interpretation has not grown since the mid-1990s and electronic efficiencies have greatly improved radiologist productivity over the same period of time (Monaghan et al. 2006). One example of the involvement of traditional radiology groups in teleradiology is privately held Inland Imaging of Spokane, Washington. Rather than being its principal business, teleradiology has

---

[4]  See Virtual Radiologic Corporation (NASDAQGM: VRAD), Yahoo!Finance, accessed online December 14, 2009 at http://finance.yahoo.com/q?s=vrad

[5]  http://markets.on.nytimes.com/research/stocks/fundamentals/drawFiling. asp?docKey=137-000119312509128756-2JH3691HTJN3EEQT22VPLUP9AL&docFor mat=HTM&formType=8-K.

been an important lever for Inland in developing regional hospital relationships and supporting the practice of a large, tightly linked radiology group.

In 1998, a small entrepreneurial radiology group joined with two other groups in Spokane and the dominant local hospital system, the Sisters of Providence, to create Inland Imaging. This much larger group now had the capacity to cover multiple hospitals in Spokane and the surrounding region. Rather than fighting the merger, the Sisters of Providence regional management actively encouraged and supported it, taking an equity position in the group's network of freestanding outpatient imaging centers and its nascent software company. The radiology group operates the hospitals' outpatient imaging centers, which are organizationally indistinguishable from the hospitals' outpatient imaging operations.

Inland covers two large Sisters of Providence hospitals, the regional tertiary center Sacred Heart Hospital, and the Holy Family Hospital. Inland also developed coverage arrangements with 10 small community hospitals radiating from Spokane into Idaho, Montana, and eastern Washington. Inland entered the teleradiology business in 1993, covering a small hospital in Moses Lake, Washington. Inland then developed coverage arrangements with two large multispecialty group practices in Seattle. Inland also reached out to cover imaging services for a hospital in faraway Phoenix, Arizona, affiliated with Banner Health, employing four onsite radiologists based in Phoenix coupled with the infrastructure the group used to cover its own Spokane-based operations.

As a consequence of all these relationships, Inland has grown to $100 million in annual revenues. With its 60 radiologists and 400 employees, Inland Imaging was the fifteenth largest radiology group in the country in 2009, according to a survey by the *Radiology Business Journal* (White 2009). In contrast to NightHawk's teleradiology-based economic model, most of Inland's revenues come from 13 hospital coverage contracts and a network of Spokane imaging centers that it has joint ventured with the Sisters of Providence. Inland has developed a proprietary suite of business management and PACs software, maintained by an in-house IT staff of 40 people. This infrastructure positions Inland to expand its management and teleradiology services to other radiology groups. That Inland is privately held shields the company from the glare of investor scrutiny and the pressure of quarterly earnings expectations. Its business model relies on hospital partnerships, stable hospital-based imaging payment rates, and favorable equipment leases to supply its capital.

## To Infinity and Beyond

Academic radiology departments also have taken dominant roles in teleradiology and the emergence of geographic coverage networks. Coincident with the 1992 DICOM standards, the Department of Radiology at the Massachusetts General Hospital began developing e-consultation with health systems in the Middle East (the United Arab Emirates, Lebanon, and Saudi Arabia), enabling overseas physicians to seek second opinions on diagnoses. By 1994, this experiment led to telecommunication of radiology and pathology results and live videoconferencing between clinical teams at Mass General and colleagues 6000 miles away.

This pioneering work led to the formation in 1997 of a consortium of leading U.S. medical centers, including Duke University, Johns Hopkins Medical Center,

Wake Forest University, and the Cleveland Clinic, as well as their Harvard teaching hospital affiliate in Partners Healthcare, the Brigham and Women's Hospital in Boston, to broaden access to second opinion e-consultation for overseas physicians and patients. This consortium created an international teleconsultation company called WorldCare.[6]

The business premise of WorldCare was that the Internet would enable physicians worldwide to transmit imaging and pathology studies and electronic versions of patient records to faculty physicians practicing in the consortium hospitals. Consortium specialists would render second opinions on the clinical problems of overseas patients and recommend treatment plans based on those opinions. In addition, the hope was that the electronic relationship would eventually serve as a portal for direct patient contact. Building upon multi-continental collegial relationships between U.S.-based and overseas physicians, patients might travel to the member institutions for more comprehensive care (though no data on the extent of actual visits created by virtual consultation were available). WorldCare was thus an early entrant into the burgeoning field of medical tourism (however, one directed into, rather than out of, the United States). WorldCare has now reached physicians and patients in 30 countries and rendered over 15,000 patient consultations, generating between $6 and $7 million in annual revenues.[7]

For WorldCare, teleradiology represents an important tool for growing and shaping the critical consultative relationships that support both the expanding patient care base required for medical education and the generation of new knowledge. The development of referral and consultative relationships across a broad geographic area is strategically important to academic health centers. The teaching and research missions of these complex enterprises are not fully self-supporting, requiring that moneys be shifted from clinical service revenues to sustain them. Expanding the clinical franchise requires reaching out to community-based physicians and hospitals across populations numbering in the millions.

The Massachusetts General Hospital[8] radiology department, under the leadership of its entrepreneurial chairman, James Thrall, is in a fundamentally different and more diverse business than NightHawk or a large regional radiology practice such as Inland Imaging. The MGH is a 900-bed academic medical center, which supports the highly complex multispecialty practice of physicians who also teach Harvard medical students, train residents and fellows, and conduct basic science and applied clinical research.

The department's total revenues from all sources were approximately $249 million in 2009, of which approximately $83 million represented the department's professional fee collections. Another $65 million was provided by sponsored research

---

6  Present consortium members include the two Partners Hospitals in Boston (Mass General and the Peter Bent Brigham), Duke University, the Mayo Clinic, and UCLA, and their respective clinical faculties.  See the WorldCare Web site for more details: http://www.worldcare.com/NewFiles/company.html. Accessed on December 14, 2009.

7  Personal communication, James Thrall,  Massachusetts General Hospital, December 2009.

8  The Massachusetts General Hospital, a principal teaching affiliate of the Harvard Medical School, is often referred to as Mass General or MGH, which some ironically translate as "Man's Greatest Hospital."

projects funded by the NIH, other government agencies, and industry.[9] The department is a leading international research site for extending the major imaging modalities into more definitive diagnosis for complex diseases, especially cancer and coronary artery disease. The department combines an on-site hospital presence with teleradiology to operate a network of community-based imaging centers in metropolitan Boston, as well as maintain coverage relationships with local community hospitals.

The department's regional role has not been without controversy, however. Mass General's remote imaging practice has created conflict with local radiologists in their extended referral region. In 2007, Mass General entertained the idea of a combined teleradiology and "feet on the ground" contract to provide comprehensive radiology services for Rhode Island's 359-bed Kent Hospital. A local radiology group that would have been displaced from that role complained to the hospital's management and the local press. Mass General withdrew from the Kent affiliation. However, the conflict unlocked deep-seated fears among the nation's radiologists. If it could happen at Kent, what would keep some other giant from doing the same thing to them?

## Teleradiology Destabilizes Hospital/Radiology Group Relationships

Because night and weekend coverage represents a significant part of the service relationship between radiology groups and hospitals, radiology groups choosing to outsource their after-hours coverage assume a risk. The hospital may become happy enough with the outsourced service to consider terminating the radiologists' contract.

Recognition of this risk has chilled the enthusiasm for outsourcing imaging work to teleradiology companies during the past few years, diminishing their growth rates.[10] Nonetheless, the opportunity afforded hospitals by the easy availability of teleradiology has not gone unnoticed. Some hospitals have seen teleradiology as a means of displacing established independent radiology groups that have underperformed or caused economic or political problems for the hospital administration. Alternatively, hospitals may see replacing their group with salaried radiologists augmented by a teleradiology company as a means of gaining greater control over one of their major profit centers. Recent incidents involving hospitals and radiologists have put seemingly secure local radiology groups on notice that the contractual grounds on which they stand are shaky at best. Some radiology groups have lost long-standing contracts.

A highly publicized example is the case of Consulting Radiologists Corporation (CRC) of Toledo, Ohio. For over 60 years, CRC provided exclusive radiology services to three hospitals managed by Mercy Health Partners under what one partner termed a "gentleman's agreement." According to one of CRC's partners, with 19 days' notice, Mercy informed CRC that it was replacing the group with combined teleradiology and "feet on the ground" staffing provided by California-based Imaging Advantage. Members of the local 19 radiologist group were offered the

[9] Personal communication, James Thrall, December 2009.
[10] Personal communication, Jonathan Sunshine, ACR, November 2009.

possibility of *locums tenens* (e.g., temporary) contracts by the hospital for an indefinite period, but all declined.

CRC argued that the hospital had illegally bypassed its own medical staff and executive committee in canceling their contract, but to no avail. The hospital publicly charged the group with poor performance; the group denied that was the case and demanded evidence. In the end, Imaging Advantage had difficulty fulfilling the contract and outsourced some of the work to NightHawk Radiology.[11] Because NightHawk founder Paul Berger resigned his position on the Nighthawk board of directors within days of Imaging Advantage taking over the Mercy radiology service in June 2008, there has been speculation that the CRC affair may have been the precipitating event.

Another conflict between an established radiology group and a powerful local hospital in Orlando, Florida, attracted national attention in 2008. When negotiations deadlocked over a contract extension between the Florida Regional Medical Center and its long-standing radiology group partner, Florida Radiology Associates (Wiley 2008), FRA canceled their contract, presumably as a means of hastening the hospital's return to the bargaining table. The move prompted the hospital to begin hiring some of the group's 47 associates and supplementing service by outsourced teleradiology. Florida Radiology Associates, once one of the largest radiology groups in the state, ceased business operations in the aftermath of these events.

A final example serves as a cautionary tale showing that even radiology groups acknowledged by the hospital to be providing exemplary service are not safe. The story involving Sutter Health—by far the dominant health system in northern California—and Radiological Associates of Sacramento Medical Group Inc. (RAS)—one of the country's largest and most entrepreneurial radiology groups[12]— starts out like the Orlando tale. Difficult negotiations between the hospital and its radiology group for the past several decades broke down. However, this time, it was the hospital that announced its determination to end the contract.

According to Sutter spokeperson Dr. Cecilia Hernandez, "RAS is a fine group of physicians—and we do have respect for their clinical abilities—but their vision is very different from ours . . . . Sutter's goal is to improve quality, timeliness, and effectiveness—and over time, to make our services more affordable" (Robertson 2009). The meaning of Hernandez's statement is, no doubt, purposely ambiguous but may have had something to do with RAS's diversification into radiation oncology and other services that might be perceived to be competitive with Sutter. Sutter plans to employ its own radiology group, supplemented by teleradiology services supplied by Radisphere National Radiology Group (formerly Franklin and Seidelmann), under the aegis of its professional foundation. The hospital system has hired Mark Martin, the same consultant who advised Florida Hospital in their split with FRA, to help them be ready by April 2010 to assume the services currently provided by RAS at their five hospitals.[13]

---

[11] Personal communication, Yogesh Patel, MD, October 2009.
[12] Founded in 1917, the group has more than 900 employees, including about 90 radiologists, nuclear medicine physicians, and radiation oncologists.
[13] Personal communication, Fred Gaschen, December 2009.

As evidenced by the Toledo, Orlando and Sacramento examples, the options prof-fered by imaging companies combined with teleradiology have become a wedge in the complex and highly charged interplay between hospitals and radiology groups. Along with the reductions in non-hospital imaging technical payments previously detailed, teleradiology has helped shift the balance of power in this often tense relationship in favor of the hospitals. The case studies also show how hospitals can choose to exercise this power to their financial and organizational advantage.

By outsourcing radiology services on their own terms, hospital administrators can more directly control the radiologists who work for—rather than with—them under new agreements. Hospitals also may see abandoning their relationship with their radiology group as a financial opportunity. By billing insurers for the global fee (technical plus professional fees) and outsourcing exams to a teleradiology com-pany at a rate lower than the payment, hospitals can establish a new revenue stream. Finally—and this may be particularly relevant to the case of Sutter/RAS—hospitals may be preparing for the day when they must once again assume financial risk as part of proposed bundled, system-wide payments.

Hospitals learned during the managed care era that loose contractual relation-ships with physicians often resulted in unmanageable costs. Hospital administra-tors might prefer tighter control of physicians' activities in order to be profitable under future risk-bearing payment systems.[14] With a new round of technical com-ponent cuts for nonhospital outpatient centers and physician offices mandated for 2010–2112, the shift in power in favor of hospitals is likely to continue.

## Corporate Imaging Takes Off

Teleradiology has been one of two major forces moving radiology toward consoli-dation into larger corporate enterprises. The other has been the decentralization of imaging away from hospitals into physicians' offices and freestanding imaging cen-ters. This process began in the early 1990s, when manufacturers began selling more office-friendly high-tech imaging devices and developed more accessible sales and leasing strategies aimed at broadening their markets. A rise in mobile imaging (scan-ners placed in vans and moved from site to site to service hospitals whose patient base could support scanning only a few days per week) and the new prominence of freestanding imaging centers fundamentally changed the business of medical imaging. Indeed, the largest corporate actors in the imaging business are imaging center operators, rather than professional practices.

The outpatient imaging business has gone through several cycles of growth and contraction over the past 20 years. Expansionary federal and private insurance pay-ment policies encouraged the growth of imaging capacity in the 1980s and early 1990s, and then again in the early 2000s (see Fig. 5-5 in the previous chapter). Both private investors and the major equipment vendors provided a great deal of the capi-tal to finance the creation of new imaging outlets. After dramatic growth in the num-ber of physician-owned imaging centers in the 1980s, the sector rolled up in a series of corporate mergers in the wake of the 1992 Stark II legislation, which forbade

---

[14] Personal communication, Larry Liebscher, December 2009.

physicians from billing for services provided by freestanding imaging centers in which they or their family held an ownership interest.

As physician partnerships divested their facilities to comply with the Stark legislation, two large publicly traded firms filled the void—U.S. Diagnostics and Medical Resources, Inc., each with over 100 centers. These firms' enthusiastic purchases, at escalating prices, resulted in heavily leveraged companies that could not sustain their cost structures. Both crashed when the 2005 DRA reduced technical payments for advanced outpatient imaging (Burkland 2008).

Currently, the two largest companies in the imaging business primarily operate freestanding imaging centers. One of these, Alliance Healthcare, based in Newport Beach, California, originated in mobile CT and MR scanning. Unlike the other corporate radiology businesses discussed in this chapter, Alliance does not rely on teleradiology income. However, the company has been a beneficiary of the general trend toward consolidation fostered by the digitization of the imaging business and its relationships with hospitals, which have benefited from the cuts in technical payments to their outpatient center and office-based competitors.

In 2009, publicly traded Alliance expected combined revenues to exceed $500 million. As the center of gravity of imaging moved into the outpatient arena, rather than competing with hospitals, Alliance operated imaging centers in partnership with hospitals, offloading hospitals' responsibilities for both capital support and management of outpatient imaging (not a traditional hospital core competence). Alliance manages 469 MR, CT, and PET/CT units in 120 fixed-site imaging centers (most of which are on or adjacent to hospital campuses) across the United States. The company's most rapidly growing business is intensity-modulated and image-guided radiation therapy (IMRT/IGRT)—in 2009, a $50 million business the company expects to double in the next few years.[15]

Because Alliance's hospital partners bill Medicare the technical fees for the services in Alliance's imaging centers under hospital prospective payment rates (i.e., not the RBRVS physician fee schedule discussed in Chapter 5), the company was largely sheltered from the DRA payment cuts that sharply reduced payments to freestanding imaging centers. To the extent that health reform and the present economic downturn negatively affect hospital capital availability, companies like Alliance could play a larger role in extending and maintaining imaging infrastructure for hospitals, because hospitals might choose to focus their capital spending on other areas, such as IT and facilities development.

Alliance's principal publicly traded comparable company (with about the same revenues - over $500 million in revenues), RadNet, has concentrated its business outside of hospitals' economic "force field" in independent freestanding centers. RadNet is the largest operator of freestanding imaging centers in the United States, with 164 facilities. In 2006, RadNet acquired a major imaging center operator, Radiologix, whose facilities were based mostly on the East Coast, diversifying away from the brutally competitive and oversupplied California market. Many of RadNet's facilities are linked via teleradiology to regional reading centers staffed by radiologists in tightly linked radiology groups.[16]

---

[15] Personal communication, Paul Viviano, June 2009.
[16] see RadNet's website: RadNet, Inc, corporate at http://www.radnet.com/index.php. Accessed December 14, 2009.

## Will Corporations Dominate Imaging and Radiology Practice?

What happens to imaging payments will have a strong influence on how far and how fast imaging moves toward corporatization. The recent wave of consolidation in the outpatient imaging industry in response to the 2005 DRA is instructive in this regard. The DRA damaged the economic performance of outpatient imaging centers dependent on RBRVS fee schedule technical payments. At this writing, it is far too early to tell how much additional impact the 2010 reductions in imaging technical fees mandated in the health care reform bill will further affect the cash flow and operations of outpatient imaging facilities.

The Deficit Reduction Act had only a modest impact on most radiologists' incomes. According to a recent ACR survey, the average radiologist derives 82% of his or her income from billing the professional fee (Moser and Hastreiter 2009). Since the DRA did not reduce professional fees for interpreting the images, radiologists in academic practice, those whose practices focused mainly inside and around hospitals, and others without ownership interest in scanners saw no adverse effect on their incomes. The 53% of radiologists who own equipment in freestanding centers or office-based scanners and receive technical payments were adversely affected to varying extents based on the level of their ownership and their degree of collaboration with hospitals.

As discussed in Chapter 5, imaging remains in the crosshairs of federal policymakers seeking to contain the cost of Medicare spending. Cuts to imaging payments currently scheduled for 2010–2012 threaten to reduce the profitability of both the technical and professional components but are much more weighted to reducing technical payments. These planned reductions will place pressure on radiology groups and imaging companies alike to consolidate their operations as a means of developing economies of scale, improving their competitive advantage, and leveraging negotiations with private insurers.

The upcoming payment changes might trigger a further wave of consolidation of ownership of imaging centers and place more pressure on radiology groups who own their own equipment. They also will pressure nonradiologists, such as orthopedic surgeons and cardiologists, who derive an increasing fraction of their income from technical fees for performing imaging examinations, by reducing the attractiveness of owning their own radiological equipment. Many nonradiologists with marginal scanning volumes may find themselves unable to support expensive equipment leases and withdraw from imaging practice. Finally, the new cuts in imaging payments will likely extend the sales drought in imaging equipment that began in 2007 as the first wave of DRA cuts hit the industry.

The Australian experience in corporate consolidation of radiology practice is viewed by some in the radiologist community as a potential bellwether for the future organization of imaging in the U.S. In Australia, with a population of about 26 million, more than 70% of radiologists practice as the employees of just four companies. The country experienced a rapid corporate roll-up of radiology practices in the wake of efforts by the Australian government to contain the growth in its imaging expenditures. This consolidation took place in the late 1990s, coincident with the ultimately unsuccessful attempts in the United States by so-called physician practice management firms (PPMs) to roll up physician group practices. The U.S. PPM sector crashed in 1998, eventually liquidating some $12 billion in publicly traded market capitalization (Reinhardt 2000).

On the professional side, U.S. radiology practice remains extremely fragmented. According to the ACR, there are approximately 30,000 radiologists in practice in the United States, approximately 15%–20% of whom practice in academic medical centers. A recent survey by the *Radiology Business Journal* showed that there was exactly one community-based radiology practice employing more than 100 radiologists. The tenth largest group employed only 65 full-time equivalent radiologists (White 2009).

The extent of economies of scale or coordination in professional radiology practice is unclear. Larger groups appear to have comparative advantages over smaller groups in both business and clinical information technology, the capacity to offer subspecialty consultation both in-market and remotely, and the capacity to offer work schedule flexibility to young radiology recruits. Mastering and integrating digital information both in management and in professional practice may give larger radiological practices important practical advantages over smaller groups. However, how these advantages translate into sustaining physician compensation in the face of possible fee reductions, and in the ability to retain and leverage capital expense, remains to be established.

In this regard, it is significant that the Australian corporations are now suffering the same fate as have U.S.-based imaging facilities firms.. That is, they have over-leveraged, have failed to rationalize their costs, and are becoming prey to smaller, better-focused local competitors (Galloway 2008).

Whether the Australian scenario plays out in the United States is a subject of debate (and anxiety) among leaders of the U.S. radiology community. A significant practice consolidation in radiology will depend partly on whether cost containment continues to focus on imaging facility owners outside of hospitals—as it mainly has to date—or on the incomes of radiologists, as is scheduled to occur to a lesser extent during 2010–2014. If significant future cuts in professional payment result from future cost containment initiatives, the stage could be set for the consolidation of the highly fragmented professional side of radiology into larger entities.

In this event, consolidators will need capital, management systems for administration and billing, systems for consultative interchange with those who order exams, and PACS to store, move, and manage the images and associated reports. Capital and/or borrowing capacity also will be required to support the expected mergers and acquisitions, as well as to continuously renew the IT and scanning equipment.

The threat of corporatization is motivating independent radiology groups to rethink how they practice. Many groups have decided that sleeping with the enemy—the self-referring physicians—is better than losing their business outright. These radiology groups are electronically transporting and interpreting whatever imaging exams the doctors' offices are producing—CT scans, for example—in order to preserve the relationship with these physicians and continue to receive their referrals for MRI, PET, and other examinations. Small groups of radiologists are increasingly banding together via teleradiology to develop their own night call pools, rather than turning to the increasingly predatory teleradiology companies, as a means of protecting their contractual relationships with hospitals. Similarly, they are developing electronic regional networks with tertiary care hospitals to offer subspecialized services, as needed, rather than contracting out to teleradiology companies offering similar services.

Another possibility is that hospitals could become the corporate agents in rolling up radiology practices. Hospitals were the main beneficiaries of the DRA payment cuts to competing outpatient imaging centers. The further planned reductions in nonhospital outpatient technical payments might strengthen the role of hospitals as consolidators and shift power from entrepreneurial operators to hospital managements and their tightly linked or employed radiology groups. A movement to bundle radiology professional fees into the hospital diagnostic related group (DRG) payment, a possible consequence of future health care reform, would further increase hospitals' leverage over the profession while creating serious political and economic complications for independent radiology groups.[17]

The movement to screen orders for imaging studies for medical necessity—whether by RBMs, or by computerized decision support systems (both discussed in Chapter 5)—will both shrink the demand for studies of marginal benefit and raise the administrative expenses for supporting order flows. This will work to the disadvantage of smaller imaging actors—groups or companies—which may find the additional administrative costs too onerous, further tilting the playing field toward larger, better-organized competitors. Larger radiology groups or hospital imaging operators also will benefit disproportionately from superior capital access to adopt the intelligent order entry software.

The odds and the times favor consolidation of radiology practice into larger economic units in future years. Larger groups may find it easier to compete in a tightening radiology labor market by offering young recruits both flexible scheduling and a more complex and diverse clinical practice. Hospitals seem to enjoy many economic advantages in their relationship to radiology but historically have not demonstrated management competence in organizing or supporting physician practice. Nonetheless, whether or not hospitals play the role of radiology practice consolidator, Medicare payment policy seems to be on an inexorable course toward forcing radiology and hospital payment into tighter linkage as well as placing radiologists' incomes into more direct competition with those of other hospital-dependent disciplines.

Having said all this, it seems unlikely that a country with over 300 million people and with such huge geographic diversity as the United States will ever see the extent of consolidation in radiology practice experienced in Australia. As Americans seem to do, we are likely to develop new radiological practice arrangements in a uniquely chaotic and entrepreneurial manner. Radiologists are American medicine's most successful physician entrepreneurs. This entrepreneurial history confers on them a natural advantage in conditions of economic uncertainty. Radiologists' entrepreneurial skill will find new tests in a challenging and rapidly evolving economic environment.

---

[17] Specifically, this type of bundling would compel radiologists to negotiate their share of the global "bundled" payment with the hospital's medical directorate, finance office, or the hospital/physician organization (P/HO) joint venture. It would require radiologists to demonstrate how use of their services reduces hospitalization, unnecessary procedures, or readmissions. Bundling would place radiologists in explicit economic competition with other hospital consultants, as well as with post–acute care providers, within a fixed budget, a markedly different economic arrangement than contemporary fee-for-service.

## Summary

Innovations in information technology have affected the organization and management of radiology practice as profoundly as the introduction of any new scanning technology. Radiologists have been digital pioneers not only in the management of clinical information but also in the development of the supporting software to enable modern medical practice.[18] Radiology was the first clinical discipline to at least partially abolish the physical constraints of distance in medical practice.

In one important respect, radiologists may have arrived first at a central dilemma of twenty-first-century medicine: is medicine merely about interpreting data or is it something more complex? Teleradiology has led to the rapid expansion of remote reading of imaging studies. The next decade will see remarkable growth in the technical capacity to generate richer and more diverse real-time data feeds from patients with all types of medical indications from literally anywhere in the world. These remote presence tools will not apply merely to the *sick* — as we use that word today — but also to the asymptomatic well who might be at some risk of illness.

When this occurs, radiologists will not be able to remain isolated from the rest of medicine. They cannot simply act as purveyors of digital knowledge. Rather, they will increasingly become part of a team of counselors, advocates, and strategists helping us to live healthier lives. Radiologists must be full participants in clinical teams, using new and unique tools to assess risks, preempt illness, and intervene with precision in serious disease. Emerging digital technologies will enable our physicians to be better prepared, more accurate and precise in their estimate of what ails us, and better able to advise us on what we need to do about it.

Do radiologists need to be physically present or touch the patient or even be in the same room as their clinical team members to play this role? Not necessarily. But it is from the real-time interchange of intellectually curious, questioning caregivers that the best medicine emerges.

## References

Brennan PF, Starren JB. Consumer health informatics and telehealth. In: Shortliffe EH, ed. *Biomedical Informatics: Computer Applications in Health Care and Biomedicine*. 3rd ed. New York: Springer Science+Business Media; 2006:511–536.

Burkland J. Historical review of mergers and acquisitions in diagnostic imaging. *Radiol Bus J*. December 2008. http://imagingbiz.com/articles/rbj_view/historical-review-of-mergers-and-acquisitions-in-diagnostic-imaging/. Accessed December 14, 2009.

Cerf V, Kahn R. A protocol for packet network intercommunication. *IEEE Trans Commun*. 1974;22:637–648.

Clark DD. The design philosophy of the DARPA Internet protocols. *Comput Commun Rev*. 1988;18:106–114.

Friedman T. *The World Is Flat: A Brief History of the 21st Century*. New York: Farrar, Straus and Giroux, 2005.

Galloway H. Corporatization of radiology in Australia. *J Am Coll Radiol*. 2008;8:86–91.

---

[18] Radiologists have also been aggressive early adopters and users of speech recognition technology to aid in the preparation of their reports. The most advanced automated dictation applications in medicine can be found in radiology.

Greenes RA, Brinkley JF. Imaging systems in radiology. In: Shortliffe EH, ed. *Biomedical Informatics: Computer Applications in Health Care and Biomedicine.* 3rd ed. New York: Springer Science+Business Media; 2006:626–659.

Hammond WE, Cimino JJ. Standards in biomedical informatic. In: Shorliffe EH, ed. *Biomedical Informatics: Computer Applications in Health Care and Biomedicine.* 3rd ed. New York: Springer Science+Business Media; 2006:297–299.

Kahn CE, Carrino JA, Flynn MJ, et al. DICOM and radiology: past, present and future. *J Am Coll Radiol.* 2007;4:652–657.

Kaye AH, Forman HP, Kapoor R, et al. A survey of radiology practices' use of after-hours radiology services. *J Am Coll Radiol.* 2008;5:748–758.

Monaghan DA, Kassak KM, Ghormrawi HM. Determinants of radiologists' productivity in private group practices in California. *J Am Coll Radiol.* 2006;3:108–114.

Moser JW, Hastreiter DM. 2007 survey of radiologists: source of income and impact of the Deficit Reduction Act of 2005. *J Am Coll Radiol.* 2009;6:408–416.

Pianykh OS. *Digital Imaging and Communications in Medicine: A Practical Introduction and Survival Guide.* Berlin and Heidelberg: Springer Verlag, 2008.

Reinhardt U. The rise and fall of the physician practice management industry. *Health Aff.* 2000;19:42–55.

Robertson K. Sutter zaps pact with radiologists. Talks with radiological associates fail. *Sacramento Business Journal,* November 13, 2009, p. 31.

Teleradiology global market expected to grow at double digit rates in the next five years. TechNavio Reports. http://www.medicexchange.com/Teleradiology/teleradiology-global-market-expected-to-grow-at-double-digit-rates-in-the-next-five-years-technavio-reports.html. Accessed December 14, 2009.

White JP. The fifty largest radiology practices. *Radiol Bus J.* 2009;2:24–29.

Wiley G. FRA and Florida Hospital: a cautionary tale unfolds. *Radiol Bus J.* December 2008. http://imagingbiz.com/articles/rbj_view/fra-and-florida-hospital-a-cautionary-tale-unfolds/. Accessed December 14, 2009.

# 7

# Red in Tooth and Claw—Moral Hazard and the Struggle for Control of Imaging Services

*Bernice Mirowicz sat on the chilly, slick paper covering the examining table, periodically tugging at the hem of the skimpy gown to retain a modicum of modesty. It's hopeless, she thought. If I pull in one place, it just gapes in another. She could feel the draft of the air conditioner blowing through the gown's opening at her back. Why did I come here? I must be crazy. What's a little knee pain?*

*Actually, Bernice was not suffering from mental problems. Rather, she was a typical boomer, 58 years old and more interested in her health, functioning, and longevity than a member of any generation that had come before. She had led a healthy, active life. So, over the past several weeks, when she began having twinges in her knee during her aerobics classes, she'd gone online to get some insight into the problem. What she saw on the Web made her anxious: torn cartilage, degenerative arthritis, tibial stress fractures ... even metastatic cancer. She'd resolved to seek medical attention before whatever it was grew any worse.*

*Now, however, she was having second thoughts. The orthopedist was running late. She was nervous and regretted that she had pressured her primary care physician into giving her this referral. She had already made a cash copayment to the office assistant when she'd checked in. What in the world am I doing here? It's not like I'm going to be running any marathons.*

*Bernice's reverie was cut short as the examining room door flew open. The orthopedist strode into the room, perfunctorily asking how she was doing but not waiting for a reply before turning to wash at the sink. As he dried his hands on a paper towel, he introduced himself as Dr. Askew and asked what had brought her to see him.*

---

The title of this chapter is a reference to a line in a poem by Alfred Lord Tennyson—"In Memorium A.H.H." but commonly misattributed to Charles Darwin.

*"My knee. I—"*

*"Which one?"* he interrupted.

*"Th—the right one,"* Bernice stuttered. The orthopedist was a big man, wrapped in a knee-length white coat that he wore fully buttoned like armor. His blocky features exuded self-confidence.

*"Let's take a look at it,"* he said and bent to the task. He poked at various places around the knee joint, pulled on Bernice's flexed lower leg, and firmly twisted her limb from side to side. Bernice winced. She had questions to ask, but her initial attempts were met largely with nods, so she gave up and focused on answering the doctor's occasional queries about whether his manipulations were causing her any pain.

*"Mrs ... Mirkowitz,"* he said, standing and glancing quickly at the chart in his hand. *"Given that you haven't described any acute injury, I think you may have some arthritis in your knee ... perhaps a meniscal tear ... but I really can't tell much just from a physical exam. I'm going to recommend that you have an MRI."*

*"But ..."* started Bernice.

*"It's a very simple test, really. Not painful. My office assistant will set up an appointment for you to come back to the office within the next week."*

*"But doctor, an MRI. Do I really need an MRI? It's so expensive."*

*"Really? Well, that's what I recommend. Something serious may be going on, but I just can't tell without the imaging. We have MRI equipment right here in the office, and your insurance will pay for it. I wish I had more time to explain, but I've got other patients waiting. Please see Sylvia out front to make an appointment, and I'll speak with you again after I've reviewed the results,"* Dr. Askew said as he stood in the half-opened door, then turned and left. The visit had taken just over six minutes.

Bernice dressed. She stopped by the desk and once again offered her insurance card to the office assistant as she made the appointment for her MRI. While she waited for Sylvia to complete a preauthorization request to her health insurer, she nervously perused the circulars promoting the office's arthroscopy and rehabilitation services, which were neatly laid out on the counter in front of her. For a brief moment, she felt as though she were staring down the length of a dark tunnel.

*Do I really need the MRI?* She wondered. *And after that ... what happens to me?*

Medicine is fraught with risks. Managing those risks is one of society's most complex challenges. Not only is there the risk of illness itself, but also the risk of consequences from improper management of the illness. That risk includes a loss of income or the capacity to care for our families or, in some cases, even the loss of our lives. Risk also may be created by intervening in the illness when intervention might not improve the condition, but rather cause complications requiring further intervention.

And finally, there is the economic risk. As all of us know, medical care is very expensive—expensive enough that, absent sufficient insurance, a major illness can bankrupt even a family with substantial savings. To manage that risk, modern societies create both public and private health insurance. Insurance spreads the financial risk of illness and creates reserves for cushioning its economic effects on businesses and families. Given that the U.S. health care system is $2.5 trillion in size, the amount of societal economic risk related to medical use is enormous.

It gets worse. Having insurance creates a novel form of economic risk called *moral hazard*. Moral hazard arises from the fact that insurance causes us to be less vigilant about managing our risk in an economically responsible fashion. In the case of medical care, we become less concerned about the cost because someone else is paying for it. Moral hazard from the patient's perspective is compounded by a sub-species of moral hazard affecting physicians. The *principal-agent* moral hazard of Dr. Askew is the unscripted supporting character in Mrs. Mirowicz's angst-ridden physician visit.

The physician's moral hazard was succinctly described in Nobel laureate Kenneth Arrow's seminal 1963 paper on risk in medicine entitled "Uncertainty and the Welfare Economics of Medical Care" (Arrow 1963). Arrow notes that physicians must fight the temptation to enrich themselves by exploiting the asymmetry of knowledge between them and those they treat:

> By certifying to the necessity of a given treatment or the lack thereof, the physician acts as a controlling agent on behalf of the insurance companies. Needless to say, it is a far from perfect check; physicians themselves are not under any control, and it may be convenient for them or pleasing to their patients to prescribe more expensive medication, private nurses, more frequent treatments, or other marginal variations of care, *especially when they will financially benefit from doing so.* (Emphasis added) (Arrow, 1963, p. 946)

Arrow goes on to state that physicians' ethical standards play a crucial role in mitigating both the patients' and society's risk of excessive or inappropriate treatment:

> the social obligation for best practice is part of the commodity the physician sells, even though it is a part that is not subject to thorough inspection by the buyer ... the physician cannot act, or at least appear to act, as if he is maximizing his income at every moment of time. As a signal to the buyer that his intentions [are] to act as thoroughly in the buyer's behalf as possible, the physician avoids the obvious stigmata of profit maximizing. (Arrow, 1963, p. 947)

Precisely because we do not understand the nature of our medical risks, we delegate to physicians as our agents the task of evaluating and managing those risks for us. However, in practice, there is tension between physicians' professional responsibility to their patients and their desire to generate revenue from providing services. In one recent survey, fully 25% of physicians felt that monetary influences affected the care they provided to patients (which suggests, unfortunately, that the other 75% might be blissfully unaware of any conflict or else minimize its effects).[1]

## Medical Imaging and Moral Hazard

Thousands of variants of Bernice Mirowicz's encounter with Dr. Askew play out across the country every day. That encounter is a prime example of why imaging technology finds itself in the societal spotlight. Dr. Askew is a trusted agent of Mrs. Mirowicz's search for answers to her concerns. His imaging suite provides him a powerful tool for resolving her clinical uncertainty but also a powerful lever for

[1]   http://www.hschange.com/CONTENT/89/.

increasing his own income. Imaging has become a potent source of moral hazard for both patients and physicians.

High-technology imaging like CT, MRI, and PET was once the nearly exclusive purview of hospitals and the radiologists who worked in them. The equipment was so costly and so complex to operate that only hospitals could afford the devices and only radiologists knew how to use them properly. As advanced imaging technologies matured, however, miniaturization and simplification broadened their appeal in the outpatient setting. Such specialists as cardiologists, gastroenterologists, orthopedists, and neurologists—and, more recently, primary care physicians—are increasingly incorporating modalities like CT, MRI, and PET into their office practices, enabling them to refer their patients to their own imaging facilities (a practice commonly known as *self-referral*; (Pham et al. 2004). Revenues attained from billing the technical fee for high-technology imaging represent the leading edge of new income sources for these specialties (GAO 2008a).

In other words, technological advances have created a new big-ticket moral hazard—the hazard of economically motivated imaging studies. The democratization of imaging has ignited a titanic economic struggle for control of imaging between the aforementioned medical and surgical specialists, on the one hand, and their consultant radiologists and the hospitals, on the other. The stakes are high. As mentioned in Chapter 5, medical imaging has become a more than $170 billion industry.

### It's a Jungle Out There

*The Old Testament enjoins* and they shall beat their swords into plowshares, and their spears into pruning hooks: nations shall not lift up sword against nation, neither shall they learn war any more.

*Isaiah 2.4 KJV*

It hasn't worked out that way for medical imaging. The struggle for control over imaging technology has occurred largely out of public view. Nonetheless, it has occasioned bitter conflict over specialty certification, hospital privileges, a growing literature of economic studies, and a raft of new federal and state laws. An entire sub-species of health care legal practice and a rapidly growing moral hazard mitigation industry called *radiology benefits management* have developed around this issue.

Nonradiologists who control the testing of their patients and have acquired imaging modalities for their office practices have been at the center of the storm. Radiologists are dependent on other specialists for referrals for imaging.[2] As the incumbent specialists who have historically controlled the use of imaging technology, radiologists, not surprisingly, have been the most outspoken opponents of the diffusion of imaging into the practice spheres of other physicians and of what they perceive to be financially motivated imaging.

---

[2]  With only a few exceptions, like screening mammography or image-guided interventional procedures, radiologists must receive a consultation request for an imaging exam from a physician directly caring for the patient to receive payment for their services from insurers.

However, the development of interventional radiology has placed radiologists in a somewhat awkward position and has injected moral hazard into their traditionally purely consultative role. Interventional radiologists are increasingly competing with cardiologists and surgical subspecialists by establishing their own clinics and accepting both patients referring themselves and referrals from primary care physicians for the comprehensive care of patients. To practice their subspecialty effectively, interventional radiologists may refer patients to diagnostic radiologist in another practices, to other members of their own group, or acquire their own equipment and self-refer. Either of the latter two actions place them at risk for the same moral hazard as other self-referring physicians. Thus, as radiology has evolved from a purely diagnostic discipline to an interventional one (see Chapter 3), it has exposed itself to the same societal concerns about economically motivated care.

Even diagnostic radiologists may not be completely immune to accusations of financially motivated imaging. Although radiologists cannot directly refer patients for their services, they do have the capacity to induce additional referrals for imaging studies by recommending additional follow-up studies to resolve uncertainties to their referring clinicians. Referring physicians argue that although the radiologist's recommendations are nonbinding, they are compelling because ignoring them might increase their risk of being sued if patients experience a significant undiscovered condition. Thus, indirectly, radiologists have the capacity to induce additional referrals (called *auto-referral* to distinguish the practice from self-referral).

It's not just the imaging costs—substantial though they are—that worry policymakers. There is also the concern that what really motivates physicians to acquire high-technology imaging is their ability to control the downstream provision of other lucrative services, such as surgery or radiation therapy. As can be inferred from the example of Bernice Mirowicz, this concern ultimately threatens to undermine traditional public trust—the belief that physicians are acting purely on behalf of their patients.

The quaint 1960s concern about the mere appearances of physician disinterest that Arrow wrote about seems as far removed from today's high-technology medical industry as a faded rerun of *Marcus Welby*. Dr. Welby has left the building.

## Radiologists' Historical Control Over Imaging Technology

Key to the growth of radiology's preeminence in imaging was the partnership with and close integration into the hospital. At the dawn of high-technology imaging, radiology was a hospital-based specialty and benefited from a symbiotic, if not entirely conflict-free, relationship with the hospital. Hospitals provided both the capital base and the management framework for the acquisition of expensive new imaging devices, as well as a controlled framework for clinical practice. All but the smallest hospitals were able to generate the cash flows necessary to acquire high-technology imaging devices. Hospitals were also able to access tax-exempt financing markets or leasing opportunities. Those hospitals that could not generate cash or obtain credit were able to bring in mobile operators who made the technology investment for them. Radiologists benefited from the expanded capabilities of their departments and consequent growth in their professional franchises.

Cultural factors may also have played a role. Radiologists typically have been "gearheads," culturally attuned to welcome technical innovations. By constantly experimenting with these new technologies, in partnership with imaging equipment manufacturers, radiologists were able to both refine and extend their uses. Major multipurpose imaging innovations, like CT, MRI, and PET, have fit well into radiologists' historical generalist practice model of broad-based knowledge, high-volume referral of patients from a variety of sources, and efficient use of capital investment. As a result of all of these factors, radiologists had natural advantages in their adoption of high-technology imaging relative to other specialists (Brant-Zawadzki and Enzmann 2005).

Because new high-technology medical procedures were generally well paid, and because the number of applications of imaging were increasing, radiologists prospered. Radiologists have consistently ranked among the top five physician specialties in terms of income for over a decade. During the period of radiology's ascendancy, many medical and surgical specialists witnessed a decline in the real dollar (adjusted for inflation) payments for the services they most frequently provided. Despite spending a larger fraction of their time in clinical service, medical and surgical specialists' incomes diminished by 2.1% and 8.2%, respectively.[3] As these adverse economic changes occurred across many specialties, one can imagine affected physicians, radiologists' traditional customers (i.e. referral sources), thinking "How hard could it be to perform advanced imaging examinations?"

Imaging device companies like GE, Siemens, and Philips[4] have long sold equipment to nonradiologists for their office practices. Indeed, even before the advent of high technology imaging modalities, roughly half of all outpatient imaging work was performed by nonradiologists. Self-referral at this time was almost entirely confined to conventional film-based X-ray studies and, later, ultrasonography. The newer digital technologies, like CT and MRI, were largely restricted to hospitals because their size and expense prohibited most outpatient practices from acquiring them and because, as discussed in Chapter 5, many states regulated their dissemination by requiring a certificate of public need.

The device manufacturers recognized that focusing purely on the hospital market in selling high-technology imaging was limiting. The first step in the diversification away from the hospital customer base was to equip and support high-technology imaging in freestanding independent diagnostic and treatment facilities (IDTFs). The IDTFs began to appear in the early 1980s. Their development accelerated as MRI joined CT as a broadly accepted imaging modality.

Radiologists often participated in the development of IDTFs, both as consultants and, in many cases, as economic partners. Radiology groups took advantage of the IDTF movement to diversify geographically, following population growth patterns

---

3  Center for Studying Health System Change. Losing ground; physician income, 1995–2003 at http://www.hschange.com. http://www.hschange.com/CONTENT/851/SP3.htm?words=Losing+Ground. Accessed April 10, 2010.

4  There has been considerable consolidation in the medical device industry in recent years. There are smaller vendors, but by far, these are the "Big 3."

into the suburbs and the growing edge of the physician communities that relied upon radiologists for imaging diagnosis. Radiology's clinical franchise expanded aggressively as imaging became less hospital-dependent.

Nonradiologist physicians also became involved in the ownership of freestanding imaging centers. Their ability to supply patient referrals for imaging from their practices (rather than sending them to the hospital) often ensured the financial success of these ventures and made them attractive partners. The resulting explosive growth in imaging center volume drew the attention of Congress to the moral hazard that existed in such arrangements.

In 1992, federal legislation (the Stark II legislation mentioned in Chapter 5) restricted Medicare payment for high-technology imaging in freestanding centers in which physicians or their families held a financial interest. Significantly, as discussed later in this chapter, the law placed no limits on locating advanced imaging devices in physicians' offices. Equipment manufacturers recognized that this loophole created a large and potentially receptive untapped market. They responded with ingenuity. They developed less expensive instruments, often with less robust capabilities, and devices directed to imaging specific body parts to suit particular specialists' interests.[5] They manufactured imaging devices that were both more automated and more intuitive to use and required less training of supporting personnel. The engineering changes discussed above made it possible for small groups in a single imaging-intensive specialty, such as orthopedics or cardiology, or even individual practitioners, to acquire high-technology imaging devices.

To emphasize the benefits to physicians, the manufacturers developed marketing approaches that drove home to physicians the economic advantages of imaging technology ownership. They held financial seminars and presented physicians *pro formas* demonstrating the potential profitability of imaging. The manufacturers also made it much easier to acquire imaging devices by eliminating front-end cash outlays and bundling maintenance and other services into the annual payments. One brochure published by a manufacturer stated that physicians would be surprised at how easy it was to own a CT or MRI scanner; the *pro forma* indicated that with even 2 scans a day, physicians would break even in five years; with 10 scans per day, they would enjoy a $2.2 million profit over the same period. A *Wall Street Journal* investigative piece in 2005 described how a physician group could add an additional $122,000 per year to its practice's revenues by self-referring just 2 imaging studies a day under some scenarios—$610,000 if a group referred 10 a day (Armstrong 2005).

Thus, a combination of influences—cultural, organizational, financial, and technological—have resulted in the current state of unrest over which physician specialists will control the various technologies and perform imaging studies. Few dispassionate observers would worry about this struggle if it were not for two related sets of concerns: one is the large body of evidence that ownership of imaging technologies leads physicians to perform more imaging, and the other is evidence that the quality of imaging studies varies enormously, depending on who provides the care.

---

[5] As an example, the earliest single-purpose MRI scanners were designed for orthopedists to image only extremities.

## Concerns about the Cost of Care

One could view the struggle over imaging as simply an internecine struggle among physicians for control over a well-paid medical service. However, the rapid growth in high-technology imaging has enormous implications for patient care and costs to society. The main reason this struggle has risen into the public policy realm is concern over costs. There is a substantial body of research detailing how financial incentives promote inappropriate testing and generate increased costs without providing compensatory benefit to patients (Report to the Congress, Medical Payment Advisory Commission, 2009). This research focuses on the economic consequences of the moral hazard inherent in the democratized ownership of imaging technology.

But is moral hazard in imaging different than moral hazard in any medical service with regard to Arrow's classic scenario? As Arrow pointed out, medicine is rife with potential conflicts of interest that play out in practice every day. Consider a general surgeon evaluating a patient for elective surgery or a dermatologist considering whether he needs to freeze a precancerous growth. Both profit by performing the procedure whether it is needed or not. Most of us assume that physicians handle such conflicts fairly on the patient's behalf.

Where imaging differs is that imaging requires so much more capital investment and operational support than other forms of medical services. The motivations for acquiring imaging equipment are heavily weighted toward financial considerations. The considerable investment in and operating costs of high-technology imaging, as well as the lucrative payment for imaging procedures, are more potent influences on physicians' behavior than the many other opportunities for conflict encountered in daily practice. In other words, even though the conflict arising from owning imaging technologies is qualitatively similar to the conflicts commonly encountered in conventional medical practice, the amount of money involved matters greatly.

The concerns about the high utilization and costs of imaging, as well as the several reasons that the use of imaging is increasing so rapidly, were discussed at length in Chapter 5. What concerns policymakers most of all is the moral hazard—that the interests of insured patients (who want more care and are insulated from the financial consequences of expensive imaging examinations) and physicians (who can generate considerable additional practice income) conspire to encourage the performance of marginally important or unnecessary imaging exams. A patient's insistence that a problem be evaluated often causes a physician to order an imaging examination that he or she might not otherwise have ordered (whether the physician's financial incentive existed or not). The repetitive acquiescence to such requests ultimately becomes ingrained in the patterns of daily practice.

A sampling of some of the more prominent research into how physician ownership affects imaging utilization and costs supports this contention. Among the earliest studies addressing the financial impact of self-referred imaging was one conducted by the Florida Cost-Containment Board (Mitchell and Scott 1992). The study was facilitated by a legislative requirement that all freestanding facilities in Florida report their ownership interests. Astoundingly for the time, the report revealed that 40% of all Florida physicians had ownership interests in a freestanding (i.e., nonhospital) medical facility. Imaging facilities were the most popular investments for physicians in the state. In those days, prior to the institution of a federal fee schedule, physician-owned facilities charged higher fees and had higher utilization than hospital radiology departments. Particularly damaging politically was that physician-owned facilities were much less likely to provide access to the poor or underserved than hospital-sponsored facilities, despite the contentions of their proprietors.

In another study in Florida, the General Accounting Office (GAO) of the federal government published a follow-up study based on Florida Medicare claims data (GAO Report 1994). They found that 48% of Medicare referrals for imaging were generated through self-referral. For seven different imaging services, there was 2.5 times greater utilization by self-referral than when physicians referred their patients to radiologists.

Hillman[6] and colleagues developed a computer algorithm to define episodes of care for a number of conditions. The authors then interrogated two large national insurance claims databases to determine whether imaging occurred during an episode and who performed the imaging. The outcome in one study using a private insurer's database was that self referring physicians ordered imaging studies four times as much as with traditional radiologist referral, where referring physicians had no ownership stake (Hillman et al. 1990). Another publication by these authors employing a Medicare claims database reported 1.7–7.7 times the utilization, depending on the patients' clinical presentation (Hillman et al. 1992). A recent evaluation replicating the methodology of these studies but updated to include modern high-technology imaging like CT and MRI again showed uniformly increased utilization associated with self-referral (Gazelle et al. 2007). Self-referring physicians had 1.2–3.2 times greater utilization for similar types of patients for six presenting conditions, including coronary or cardiac disease, abdominal malignancy, and stroke.

The implication of these large studies is that the excess examinations performed via self-referral were neither necessary nor beneficial.[7] However, a methodological failure of all of these studies is that while the research shows large differences in utilization and costs between physicians who self-refer for medical imaging and physicians who refer their patients to radiologists, the research does not directly address whether the excess imaging was inappropriate. In other words, the evidence of economic abuse, while compelling, is largely circumstantial.

The only study of any scale to address appropriateness investigated services provided as part of the Workers' Compensation program in California (Swedlow et al. 1992). The authors evaluated the 1990–1991 claims for a variety of health care services. The only imaging service studied was MRI scans. According to the authors, self-referral led to a 38% rate of inappropriate requests for MRI, as opposed to 28% for physicians who referred their patients to radiologists. While these data show a large differential in ordering patterns affected by ownership, they raise larger questions than merely the propriety of self-referral. They call into question the appropriateness of a sizable fraction of radiological studies ordered through the traditional "disinterested" channels.

---

[6] One of the authors of this book.

[7] Those advocating self-referral deny that this is the case. They say that since outcomes are difficult to measure, some unmeasured benefit might have accrued to patients receiving the examinations.

The works of Mitchell and Scott, Hillman et al., and the GAO were persuasive in encouraging 29 states and the federal government to enact legislation restricting physicians from billing for examinations referred to freestanding imaging centers in which they had an ownership interest. Principal among these was the federal fraud and abuse Stark II legislation, named for Congressman Fortney (Pete) Stark (D-Cal), which imposed a substantial barrier to physicians referring their patients to freestanding imaging centers in which they had an financial interest.

However, there was an important exception built into this federal law, known as the *in-office ancillary services exception* (IOASE). The intention of the in-office exception was to allow physicians to continue to use simpler technologies like plain X-ray exams and ultrasonography in their offices—defined as the building in which they provide their traditional services—even as the broader scope of the law reduced self-referral for high-technology imaging provided in imaging centers.

What the Stark legislation didn't envision was the refinement of CT, MRI, and PET into office-based technologies. Since the initial passage of this legislation, it has been in physicians' offices that self-referred high-technology imaging has flowered. One can argue persuasively that there is nothing ancillary about a PET scanner in an oncologist's office or a CT scanner in a cardiologist's office since it provides such a large fraction of the physician's income. Technological advances have made a mockery of the original intent of the Stark laws, which was to protect patients from moral hazard–generated imaging.

There is a substantial body of work documenting the growing trend toward office-based self-referred imaging, largely conducted by ACR staff researchers and radiologists at Jefferson Medical College in Philadelphia. These can hardly be considered disinterested researchers. Nonetheless, the source of their data (CMS/Medicare) and the consistency of their results across a broad range of imaging technologies provide persuasive evidence that self-referred medical imaging is inflationary.

One example of this genre of research addressed the impact of noninvasive diagnostic testing for vascular disease using CT and MR angiography[8] on the rate of catheter-based angiography. Among radiologists, there was a notable substitution effect during the 2000–2004 dissemination of these new procedures. Radiologists' performance of catheter angiography fell 31%. At the same time, the rate of use of catheter angiography attributable to cardiologists and surgeons increased 70%, despite the availability of new, less invasive procedures (Levin et al. 2007).

Another example: Levin and colleagues charted Medicare payments for radionuclide imaging[9] of the heart. Cardiac nuclear imaging is both among the fastest-growing physician services in the Medicare program and, along with CT scanning, one of the procedures that generate the greatest exposure to ionizing radiation

---

[8] Both CT angiography and MR angiography require only an intravenous injection of contrast material (dye). Catheter angiography involves inserting a catheter into the femoral artery and, under X-ray guidance, directing the catheter to the vessels of interest before injecting the contrast material. The procedure requires extended observation to be sure that there is no postprocedural bleeding.

[9] Nuclear medicine testing for which a small amount of a radioactive substance is injected into a vein; a special "camera" is located over the chest to image the blood flow to the heart muscle, looking for areas of decreased flow that might be caused by atherosclerosis of the coronary arteries.

(Mettler et al. 2009). Between 1998 and 2002, the researchers found large increases in this procedure by cardiologists, which were most pronounced in cardiologists' offices. The rate of increase was more than six times greater than for radiologists' offices, indicating that the acceleration in billings for this test was probably attributable not only to a new application, but also to the compelling economic incentive to self-refer. Moreover, the increased use of myocardial perfusion studies did not replace other noninvasive tests like echocardiography (which is used for similar clinical indications) or more invasive catheter-based tests. Cardiologists performed both of these tests at an increasing rate during the same period, demonstrating the cascade effect of accelerated follow-up testing discussed in Chapter 5 (Levin et al. 2005).

Corroboration of the concern about whether a sizable fraction of self-referred cardiac nuclear studies are necessary arrived in 2009. A group of cardiologists worked with United Healthcare—the country's largest private payer—to evaluate the appropriateness of use of myocardial perfusion imaging (MPI) for 6351 patients at six sites. Using published appropriateness criteria and an automated computer algorithm, the investigators found that more than 14% of the exams were frankly inappropriate and nearly 30% were inappropriate or of questionable value (Hendel et al. 2009).

Research on the utilization of high-technology imaging in California revealed a 400% increase in PET scanning and lesser but still substantial increases in MRI and CT during the 2000–2004 period (Mitchell 2008). The author attributes much of the greater utilization to physicians' incorporation of these modalities into their office practices. As one example, another study found that cardiologists tripled the number of CT scanners installed in their offices during 2006–2008 (Barlow 2008).

Demonstrating its continuing concern that self-referred imaging provides a potential venue for abuse, the Office of the Inspector General (OIG) of the Department of Health and Human Services reported in 2008 a study of "connected services"—referrals where there is a connection between the physician ordering a service and the facility performing it—related to MRI exams performed in 2005 (Report of the OIG 2008). They found far higher utilization associated with connected services than when there was no financial relationship between the ordering physician and the MRI facility. The entities billing for the connected services were much more often nonradiologist physician groups than IDTFs or radiologists. Orthopedists and neurologists were responsible for ordering the largest number of connected examinations. Connected services tended to be billed as a technical component only, suggesting that most of the examinations were outsourced to radiologists for the professional interpretation.

## Moral Hazard in Imaging—The Teenage Years

As discussed in Chapter 5, the technical fee for supervising and performing the examination is the primary attractor for owning imaging modalities. As discussed earlier, the technical fee for high-tech imaging tends to be at three to five times the professional fee for the interpretation.[10] Moreover, once an imaging facility is established,

---

[10] The technical fee reimburses the provider for the high fixed costs of leasing or owning the equipment, by far the greatest expense related to performance of CT, MR, or PET studies.

the studies themselves are generally performed by technologists and other ancillary personnel, so little direct attention from the owning physicians is required.

As regulatory scrutiny of and legal restrictions on physicians' ownership of imaging services mounted during the 1990s, innovative legal advisers responded with new ownership structures intended to preserve physicians' opportunities to profit from self-referral. Federal law prohibits all quid pro quo arrangements for medical referrals under its antikickback policies. This means that physicians cannot receive any incentive to refer Medicare patients to a facility or be paid for their role as referrer on a per case or percentage basis.

To circumvent this regulation, some imaging facilities instituted what came to be known as *block time* and *per click* leasing arrangements. The former involves leasing a block of time on the scanner to physicians who are not part of the ownership interests. The facility charges the referring physician a fee that is less than what he or she can charge the insurer for the number of examinations that can be performed during the block time but sufficient for the facility to make a profit. The physician is highly motivated to be sure that his or her block of time is filled.

A variant of the block time approach, per click, is designed similarly from a financial perspective, but there is even less risk to the referring physician. The physician leases only when he or she actually has a patient to refer to the scanner. Researchers in the California study cited above found that block time and per click arrangements had become prevalent modes of CT, MRI, and PET utilization in that state. Thirty-three percent of MRI scans performed in the state in 2004 were by self-referral; 61% of these exams were billed by physicians who did not actually own or lease on a full-time basis any MRI equipment and therefore had to be billing through block time or per click arrangements with other entities. Twenty-two percent of all CT scans were self-referred, and 64% of these were billed via block time or per click mechanisms (Mitchell 2007).

Both block leasing and per click arrangements allowed physicians to gain additional income with little personal effort while being shielded from the capital risk associated with acquiring, maintaining, and operating the equipment. Centers that signed up enough users reduced their slack time and also profited from the practice while encouraging additional referrals from satisfied users.

Another strategy has been to profit from the difference between the global fee for imaging studies and the "market rate" for radiology interpretation. Because most self-referring physicians are untrained in imaging interpretation and fear the malpractice liability implications of reading their own imaging exams, many physician groups or imaging facilities outsource the interpretive service. The imaging operator charges the insurer the global fee[11] for the imaging service and then contracts out the interpretation to the lowest-bidding radiology group. By doing so, the operator profits not only from the technical component but also from keeping the difference between the insurer's reimbursement for the professional component and the operator's payment to the radiologist. Thus, radiologists have become potent enablers of self-referral.

---

[11] The global fee accounts for both performing and interpreting the examination; that is, it bundles the technical and professional fees.

During the past 20 years high-technology medical imaging has become the most profitable clinical service in hospital portfolios. During the past decade, this profit center has been threatened by the incursion of imaging in physicians' offices and freestanding imaging facilities, often built conveniently across the street from the hospital. Hospitals have been compelled by market exigencies to form joint venture imaging services with physicians, using the rationale that part of the imaging pie is better than no pie at all (The Advisory Board Company 2008).

In most of these arrangements, hospitals and physicians shared the investment returns, while the hospital or an imaging subsidiary functioned as general partner and source of the vast majority of the actual cash investment (the hospital also owned the credit risk). Such arrangements have, until recently, enjoyed some protection from regulatory concerns about whether these partnerships are simply a front to circumvent the Stark legislation, wherein the physician limited partners use the hospital as an agency through which their self-referrals are passed.

The practices detailed above confirm that financial incentives are a potent motivation for physicians to acquire and operate imaging modalities. Computed tomography is an especially attractive proposition. It has broad application and is both less expensive and easier to acquire and operate than MRI. Research focusing on 2001–2006 Medicare data shows that nonradiologists' share of CT scanning increased from 16% to 28% during the period, with the largest share of scans accruing to primary care physicians. Overall, nonradiologists' CT scan volumes increased 263% during the period versus 85% for radiologists (Levin et al. 2008). Despite the technological sophistication required to properly operate MRI technology and interpret the exams, this technology is following a similar pattern. Nonradiologists' billings to Medicare for MRI increased 254% (versus 83% for radiologists) between 2000 and 2005, and their market share climbed from 11% to 20% (Levin and Rao 2008).

Overall, radiologists accounted for about 52% of Medicare fee schedule billings for imaging in 1997 and 48.3% in 2002. In other words, radiologists lost market share in Medicare imaging services in that five year interval to other specialists. By contrast, cardiologists picked up three share points (from 19.8% to 22.8%). In 2006, right on the cusp of the DRA Medicare technical fee reductions, a MedPac analysis showed a continuation of the trend, with radiologists dipping to 43% of all imaging services billings and cardiologists' share growing to 25% (Medicare Payment Advisory Commission 2008). While this was troubling to radiologists, their workload actually grew, since overall Medicare imaging billings increased 78% during the time period.

No one is arguing that all imaging by nonradiologists is financially motivated. However, the sharp differences in the rate of increase in imaging billings on behalf of nonradiologist physicians raise the question of whether physicians have succumbed to principal-agent moral hazard and validate policymakers' concerns about inappropriate growth in imaging costs.

## Concerns Over the Quality of Care

A key factor inhibiting the use of market forces to control economically abusive imaging (often advocated by self-referring physicians) is not merely the patient's limited financial stake in imaging costs, but also his or her limited ability to discern the price–quality relationship—the core of the moral hazard problem.

Enforcing medical quality has historically fallen to voluntary professional self-regulation, in combination with government activities of various types. The medical profession has historically relied upon several mechanisms for ensuring quality medical care: medical licensure, regulated by individual states; accreditation of facilities by specialty organizations;[12] credentialing of a physician's ability to perform certain examinations and procedures by hospitals and other institutions; and board examinations leading to physician specialty certification.[13]

For the most part, the concerns over the quality of imaging relate to differences in training between radiologists and other specialists and the facilities they operate (see Chapter 1). Radiologists contend that while other specialists may receive some limited training in the imaging modalities used by their specialties, there is little testing of competence beyond the most rudimentary technical aspects of imaging and little education about the risks associated with imaging examinations. The concern is that non-radiologists have insufficient experience in performing and interpreting imaging studies to ensure that patients are not injured and that image quality is optimal. Several nonradiological medical specialty societies have developed so-called *rogue boards*—board examinations not approved by the American Board of Medical Specialties (ABMS)—to certify competency in specific imaging examinations relevant to their specialty. However, the ABMS, which represents all medical and surgical subspecialties, disputes rogue boards' contentions that they are effectively evaluating physicians' imaging capabilities. Their real purpose, the ABMS argues, is to provide political leverage in hospital credentialing battles with radiologists and to market their imaging services to patients.

## The Contribution of Training to the Quality of Imaging

The debate over the importance of training in imaging is not new. In a 1909 address to the New York State Medical Society, radiologist Eugene Caldwell said:

> The almost eradicable impression of radiographs as a picture or photograph which anyone can properly examine, interpret, and criticize has been a great hindrance to the progress of roentgenology … laymen and medical men alike are apt to regard it as a view and not suspect how incompletely and even how dangerous their overconfident interpretations might be" (cited in Berk 1995, p. 1321).

Research into the quality of imaging care provided by different medical specialties has been difficult to perform because many specialists refuse to participate in this type of research. Only a few studies, mostly using small samples of imaging examinations, address the issue of imaging quality.

---

[12] As an example, the ACR accredits individual facilities for a host of imaging modalities. While it offers accreditation to nonradiologists' practices, few actually seek accreditation on the grounds that the deck is stacked against them and the charge for nonmembers is too high. The Intersocietal Accreditation Commission accredits facilities for many of the same imaging modalities as ACR.

[13] The American Board of Medical Specialties (ABMS) is an organization of 24 member boards, including the American Board of Radiology (ABR). The ABMS must approve the content of the training and examinations of its members.

A study performed on behalf of a Connecticut insurer reviewed how the privileging of facilities[14] to receive insurers' payments affected the utilization of imaging and associated costs. Seventy-eight percent of inspected nonradiologists' imaging facilities showed important quality and safety deficiencies versus 0% for radiologists (Moskowitz et al. 2000). Restricting insurance payments to flagged facilities led to a precipitous drop in imaging utilization by nonradiologists, presumably because they either could not meet quality standards or did not wish to spend the time and money to do so.

This result confirmed the findings of an earlier study performed on behalf of Massachusetts Blue Cross and Blue Shield, which demonstrated that a much higher fraction of self-referring physicians' imaging examinations were uninterpretable compared to those of radiologists (Verrilli et al. 1998). Another insurer studied the quality of imaging facilities in several western states. The serious deficiency rate was 16% for orthopedists, 36% for urologists, 43% for family practitioners, and 48% for chiropractors (Levin et al. 2004). Many of the discovered problems related to failure to adhere to safety standards. Quality lapses were found in only 1% of radiologists' facilities.

The state of New Jersey instituted a quality program for plain radiography in 2001. The program was mandated for all facilities in the state performing X-ray examinations. During the first five years of the program, average radiation exposures decreased and the quality of the imaging improved, largely as a result of poor-quality providers ceasing to provide imaging services. Thirteen percent of nonradiologist physicians, 34% of chiropractors, and 33% of podiatrists stopped billing for plain radiography (Timmins et al. 2007).

More recently, the Blue Care Network of Michigan contracted with the firm RadMetrics to assess the quality of 3794 imaging studies performed by 100 nonradiologist providers in southeastern Michigan—primary care physicians, medical and surgical specialists, podiatrists, and independent testing facilities. Thirty-one percent of the exams, valued by RadMetrics at $2.6 million in global billings, had serious quality defects. Nearly 400 exams had defects that would potentially lead to missing important abnormalities. Among these were not including the region of concern in the imaged portions of the body, imaging with outdated or even incorrect equipment, and the production of artifacts that obscured potential areas of concern. Roughly 20% of the exams were billed incorrectly. Among the errors was the absence of an appropriate order from a referring physician, a request for payment for an inappropriate indication, and performing only a limited exam but billing for a comprehensive one. Physicians who were untrained in imaging commonly billed for interpretations. In an oral presentation of their findings to a gathering of radiologists, the authors concluded, "There are two standards of care today. One applies to radiologists and the other applies to the 74%[15] [of imaging] done outside your field of view."[16]

---

[14] A process by which an insurer determines that the quality of a facility is good enough to provide care to its beneficiaries and receive payments for its services.

[15] The source of the authors' estimate of 74% of imaging being performed by nonradiologists is unclear.

[16] Chesbrough RM, Hornick KJ. Quality and overutilization metrics of 100 outpatient radiology providers in Southeast Michigan. Presented at the 2009 annual meeting of the Radiological Society of North America, Chicago, December 2009.

With regard to interpretation capabilities, where training differences might be expected to be the most demonstrable, research again has suffered from small sample sizes. One study involving the interpretation of chest X-rays employed a commonly used metric, the area under the receiver operating characteristic (ROC)[17] curve (Potchen et al. 2000). The areas under the curves generated for both practicing radiologists and radiology residents were significantly greater than those of the non-radiologist interpreters, indicating higher interpretive performance. Johns Hopkins researchers used the same measure to compare the performance of radiology staff and residents with that of their emergency physician counterparts interpreting a variety of emergency room imaging examinations. Both radiology staff and residents performed significantly better than the emergency room physicians and trainees (Eng et al. 2000).

In a study of interventional radiology, Webster and colleagues (2004) evaluated 142 patients undergoing intradiscal electrothermal therapy for low back pain.[18] Patients of self-referring physicians required more narcotics, greater numbers of patients were eventually referred for more invasive back surgery because of treatment failure, and patients suffered a higher rate of absenteeism from work than patients who had been referred to radiologists. These differences may be explained as either a result of self-referring physicians treating patients who were less likely to benefit from intradiscal electrothermal therapy or the radiologists being more skilled in performing the procedure. While the researchers did not measure the radiation exposure, this is of particular concern for interventional procedures, which can take a lot of time. Techniques to reduce exposure[19] are essential to avoiding acute radiation burns to the skin and minimizing the greater long-term risk of developing cancer.

In general, the institutions responsible for overseeing the quality of care in medicine have been neutral on the issue of who should perform medical imaging examinations. State licensing boards do not restrict what aspects of medicine physicians may practice based on their training or board certification. In essence, the position of state licensing boards has been that physicians may practice any aspect of medicine and perform any procedure they wish to the extent that their patients will submit to their advice. In principle, were it not for the difficulty in obtaining malpractice coverage or hospital privileges, psychiatrists might legally perform brain surgery and orthopedists might treat borderline personality disorders.

Hospital credentialing committees have the authority to dictate which physicians provide imaging services inside the hospital. However, those decisions are frequently influenced by political or economic concerns, often by the hospital's desire not to drive away business. Cardiologists and surgeons are responsible for much of

[17] The ROC curve is a visual method for comparing imaging performance that incorporates both sensitivity (the true positive rate) and specificity (the true negative rate). The area under the ROC curve is the overall measure of performance.
[18] A percutaneous method to treat degenerated spinal discs that may be touching nerves and causing pain.
[19] As an example, using X-ray imaging guidance only intermittently as needed, instead of continuously. However, this requires greater experience and skill on the part of the practitioner.

hospitals' profits. Hospital administrators have been known to pressure credential-ing committees to confer imaging privileges to satisfy the desires of physicians who admit the greatest number of patients and bring in the most revenues to the hospital. Under any circumstances, credentialing committees have no say in what services physicians choose to provide in their offices.

## Policy Approaches to Address the Concerns about Financially Motivated Imaging

Given the foregoing, why don't government agencies and private payers intervene more aggressively than they have? The answers are difficult and relate to the politics of paying for health care.

Conservative policy gurus might argue that what we currently are witnessing with self-referral for imaging is a temporary aberration. The "invisible hand" of market forces will eventually ameliorate any abuses, if there was simply more dis-closure of the conflicts. However, there is little in health care that reflects a fairly operating market. Customers (patients) pay only a small fraction of the costs of care (moral hazard again), and there is much greater asymmetry of information between buyer (the patient) and seller (the doctor) than for most products and services we purchase (witness the interaction between Mrs. Mirowitz and Dr. Askew).

Moreover, genuine markets require that customers have a true choice among pro-viders and that there is unfettered competition on the basis of price and quality. It is hard to argue that such competition presently exists for imaging. The self-referral mechanism takes advantage of the fact that physicians control, either directly or indirectly, 85% of health care spending (The Advisory Board Company 2008). The magnitude of the financial risks involved in purchasing or leasing imaging equip-ment and the desire to make a profit militate against self-referring physicians send-ing their patients anywhere but to their own facilities—even if there is better quality and lower cost just down the street. In such circumstances, the invisible hand is not simply hard to see; it does not exist.

Similarly, one might question the effectiveness of further regulation in managing the situation. The self-referral mechanisms detailed above and their almost innu-merable variants demonstrate the American capacity for identifying and exploiting loopholes in regulation and raise doubts over whether the regulatory approach can deal with such a complex problem as self-referral (Hillman et al. 2007).

A third possibility is that payers and the employers that pay for their coverage might step in, as they have attempted to do in employing RBM's. Many readers may have the impression that the health insurance companies hold all the cards. In fact, something more resembling an uneasy balance of power exists between payer and provider. Insurance companies must have comprehensive, geographically inclusive networks of physicians who will treat the employees covered by their plans; other-wise, they cannot sell their coverage to employers. Physicians need insurers to pay for their services or their practices fail. Thus, neither insurer nor provider can sur-vive without the other. Neither can afford to unduly anger the other.

When the financial stakes of imaging were small, governments and insurers could afford to ignore the mounting evidence that financially motivated imaging was infla-tionary and avoid direct confrontations with providers. As detailed in an Chapter 5, this is no longer the case. A number of policy options have been suggested from various quarters to deal specifically with financially motivated imaging. While this section will mostly focus on the activities of the federal government (the single largest payer for health care in the United States), unique strategies are being employed by some states and private payers, including:

- Requiring physicians to disclose to patients when they have a financial interest in a facility to which they are referring the patient.
- Closing the Stark II loophole that allows in-office ownership of imaging modalities for high technology like CT, MRI, and PET.
- Prohibiting the worst abuses of in-office ownership, like block leasing and per click arrangements and hospital–physician relationships that are shields for self-referral.
- Revitalizing or strengthening state Certificate of Need (CoN) laws.
- Requiring accreditation and the use of appropriateness criteria in order to make imaging less attractive to financially motivated providers.
- Decreasing the financial attractiveness of performing imaging by instituting direct pay cuts or altering the payment system.

*Financial Disclosure*    Early on, it was suggested that physicians who had a financial interest in an imaging technology could simply inform patients whom they were sending for imaging studies that a potential conflict of interest existed. This strategy comports well with the market forces thesis, since informed patients can factor the physician's economic interests into their decision about whether to follow through on his or her referral recommendations. Financial disclosure is a popular manifestation of what we now call consumerism—empowering patients to decide what health care they need. The idea made some sense, since it already was a mandate of the AMA Council on Ethical and Judicial Affairs.[20]

A number of states have incorporated the practice into regulation. The problem is that such laws are largely unenforceable. In practice, few physicians disclose their conflicts of interest (Rodwin 1989). Even when physicians attempt to give patients information about their ownership interests, patients may be uninterested, either because they trust their physicians to advise them on what they think best or because they fail to grasp the implications of the conflict.

Despite the general failure of disclosure laws to reduce abuse, in 2008 Charles Grassley introduced a new disclosure law in the U.S. Senate, The Sunshine in Medical Imaging Act. Provisions from this bill have been incorporated into the recently signed Patient Protection and Affordable Care Act of 2010. Specifically, physicians financially benefiting from a referral they make must disclose their ownership interest in facilities to patients in writing and provide them with a list of alternative imaging facilities where they could receive care. However, these provisions are unlikely to

---

[20] In 2008, the AMA Council on Ethics and Judicial Affairs reemphasized that informing patients of their financial involvements is a responsibility of physicians (KB O'Reilly. AMA meeting: doctors told to reveal financial stake in referrals. amednews.com, December 1, 2008. http://www.ama-assn.org/amednews/2008/12/01/prsf1201.htm. Accessed April 2, 2010. The AMA is a voluntary physician organization that has no enforcement powers.

have any meaningful effect on the practice of financially motivated imaging, since the powerful incentives to increase physician income remain in place.

*Closing Stark II Loopholes*  An obvious solution to the self-referral problem would be to tighten federal Stark II restrictions on self-referral by terminating the in-office ancillary services exception mentioned earlier in this chapter. Opponents of self-referral argue that the IOASE was never intended to protect office-based high-technology imaging and should be amended or abolished. In fact, one state, Maryland, did pass just such a law in 1993 (back before so much money was involved), which has withstood numerous challenges. The law specifically cited CT, MRI, and radiation therapy services as being outside the bounds of the IOASE. However, there was no initial enforcement of the law, and self-referral operations flourished until a suit by the ACR was upheld by Maryland state courts in 2005. Since that time, there has been a flurry of legal and legislative attacks on the legislation, which continue to put the law in jeopardy.

A number of other state radiology organizations have lobbied unsuccessfully for similar legislation in their states. The ACR has abetted these efforts and also has lobbied the federal government for years to try to close the federal loophole. Broad efforts to close the loophole in a single stroke have failed because of the resistance of a powerful political coalition. Symbolic of the tenacity of what has become a coordinated effort opposing the elimination of the IOASE was Resolution 235 of the 2004 American Medical Association (AMA) House of Delegates, which passed overwhelmingly over radiologists' objections. Sponsored by nine specialty societies, the resolution read in part:

> AMA should ... work collaboratively with state medical societies and specialty societies to actively oppose any and all federal and state legislative and regulatory efforts to repeal the in-office ancillary exception to physician self-referral laws, including as they apply to imaging services.

At the same time as the resolution was being developed, the American College of Cardiology (ACC) introduced a new consortium called Physicians for Patient-Centered Imaging (PPCI), now called the Physician Coalition for Patient-Centered Imaging (PCPI). The ACC argued in a press release sent by e-mail to thousands of physicians that the true motivation of the radiology community was franchise protection. The PCPI has portrayed radiologists as obstructing optimal patient care, which could only be ensured by giving patients access to facilities controlled by their own physicians.

Numerous professional societies joined the PCPI coalition, which also enjoyed the backing of the major imaging equipment manufacturers. "It's a political issue," said an officer of one leading manufacturer. "Our business is not about deciding who will make money but how to get [the technology] to patients" (Becker 2004).

The support garnered by the PPCI initiative was telling for the opponents of self-referral. Beyond the obvious reality that radiologists were greatly outnumbered, there lay this simple fact: Nearly every congressperson and senator had a cardiologist or another personal physician who had the legislator's ear in a most intimate locale—the examining room. Almost none of them had a personal radiologist. In an address to the 2007 annual meeting of the ACR, Congressman Pete Stark, the godfather of Medicare fraud and abuse legislation, evinced no stomach for a fight to broaden his eponymous legislation. Attacking the IOASE head on remains unlikely. Representatives Jackie Speier and Bruce Braley introduced legislation in 2009 that would have had this effect, but their provisions were not included in the Patient Protection and Affordable Care Act of 2010.

Radiologists and their allies also have pursued the regulatory route of advocating piecemeal elimination of the more egregious abuses of the Stark II law. With regard to the practice of awarding the interpretation of imaging examinations to the lowest-bidding radiologist, CMS developed an *anti-markup* provision which took effect January 2008. The provision limits the self-referring physician or IDTF to billing either the usual fee schedule payment or what the physician paid the radiologist for the interpretation, whichever is less. The expectation is that many professional services formerly charged by the self-referring physician will now be billed directly by the contracting radiologist.

With regard to block time and per click leasing arrangements, in 2007 the Illinois Attorney General filed suit against 20 Chicago area imaging facilities on the grounds that referring physicians were earning a profit by making referrals without actually providing medical services and were hence in violation of the antikickback laws (Japsen 2007).[21] Fourteen of the involved imaging centers were owned by a single entity, which settled with the state in 2009, paying Illinois fines totaling $1.2 million. The defendants admitted no wrongdoing but ended the offending practice (Japsen 2009). Similar suits followed in Florida and Louisiana.

Perhaps in response to states' concerns, CMS issued a final rule, effective January 2008, that abolished per click arrangements. The agency put off implementing the rule until October 2009 in response to involved practitioners' outcries over the decision. Currently, CMS considers block time leasing to be legal under Stark II but plans to continue to monitor these arrangements for abuse.

CMS also moved to limit the *under arrangements* joint ventures typified by some hospital–physician partnerships by broadening the definition of what is covered by the Stark II regulations. The move was intended to halt the abuses associated with physicians using the hospital as an agency through which to practice self-referral. Although the rule originally was scheduled for implementation in January 2008, it was delayed until October 2009 to allow these partnerships to undergo legal review and determine whether they met the terms of the regulation or needed to be modified or dissolved.

**State Certificate of Need Laws**   An alternative regulatory approach has been more vigorously to enforce existing state laws concerning who can own high technology imaging facilities and where the technologies can be located. Certificate of need (CoN) (sometimes called *certificate of public need* [COPN]) regulations require that a prospective owner of a technology request permission from the state and show a need based on a deficiency of access to a specific technology or for any service costing above a specific dollar limit.

[21] The facilities were profiting by selling time to referring physicians (per click) who were billing for the CT and MRI exams even though they had nothing to do with providing the services.

As discussed in Chapter 5, CoN laws vary greatly from state to state. In most states that do maintain active CoN laws, like Virginia, where both authors live, regulators have attempted to maintain some balance between open competition and the desire of hospitals to keep control of important revenue-generating imaging technologies. The Virginia Hospital and Healthcare Association has tacitly worked with the radiologists in the state to derail annual attempts by entrepreneurial physicians to diminish or circumvent the regulations.

More dramatically, in 2006, the West Virginia Health Care Authority issued a moratorium on the placement of CT scanners in physicians' offices. The action was stimulated by a request from the West Virginia Hospital Association based on the hospital administrators' concern that a further siphoning away of their imaging revenues would impact their ability to provide uncompensated care for West Virginia's uninsured. In 2007, the Health Care Authority announced that it would rescind the moratorium but was overruled by the governor, keeping the stay on further office-based expansion of CT capacity in effect (Messina 2007). It is not clear that reinstituting CoN coverage of imaging equipment will make much of a dent in financially motivated imaging because of the huge installed base of imaging equipment already in the marketplace.

*Quality Initiatives to Reduce Financially Motivated Imaging*   At the same time as it pursued the legislative and regulatory approaches, the ACR initiated a campaign to make self-referral more difficult by convincing policymakers and insurers that improving the quality of imaging could also reduce costs. The strategy was based partly on successful advocacy during the early 1990s dealing with breast imaging and leading to the passage of the Mammography Quality Standards Act (MQSA). The result was that many borderline mammography providers chose to discontinue offering mammography services. As a result, nearly all mammography is now performed by radiologists. Mammography, however, is different from most other imaging services. Unlike CT, MRI, or PET, which have applications to many organ systems and diseases, mammography is almost entirely directed at detecting only one condition: breast cancer. The group that benefits from mammography is well defined (almost entirely women over age 40). And mammography is far less lucrative than the high-technology modalities mentioned above.

Defining quality standards for all of advanced imaging—which may be applied to hundreds of conditions—is a more daunting task. For years, the ACR has worked with its members to develop guidelines for how advanced imaging examinations should best be performed, appropriateness criteria defining the best imaging exam for a particular clinical presentation, and accreditation programs delineating quality standards for facilities providing imaging services. The ACR recently updated and expanded its appropriateness criteria and began to promote an online version to insurers. At the same time, the ACR expanded the accreditation program to cover a larger number of technologies.[22] These actions have facilitated the use of ACR guidelines as a foundation for insurers' efforts to reduce cost through quality improvement.

---

[22] The Intersocietal Accreditation Commission addresses accreditation for many of the same imaging modalities as ACR.

In 2005, Highmark Blue Cross Blue Shield, which is the dominant private insurer in western Pennsylvania, instituted a policy that it would not pay for outpatient imaging except from a provider it had evaluated and determined was qualified to perform imaging studies. In order to be considered, facilities had to be owned or leased by the billing providers on a full-time basis (i.e., no block time or per click arrangements). A facility had to be open at least 40 hours per week and offer at least five different imaging modalities (a particularly costly requirement geared to excluding marginal imaging operations). Qualified facilities had to be accredited by the ACR or the Intersociety Accreditation Commission (IAC) and use licensed technologists. The effect has been to exclude from coverage by Highmark many marginal office-based imaging operations.

In 2007, the country's largest private health care insurer, United Healthcare, announced that it would require accreditation of all providers wishing payment for advanced imaging by October 2008. The action has been indefinitely delayed because of the pushback from many affected providers. Following United's lead, CMS has disseminated a rule requiring all facilities offering CT, MR, and PET to be accredited by 2012 to receive Medicare payment for imaging for its beneficiaries. Almost certainly, the accreditation requirement will drive out some marginal imaging providers and should improve imaging quality for patients. There are numerous outmoded pieces of equipment still in service that may not pass muster under an accreditation program.

However, as we have noted, the financial incentive to continue to provide in-office imaging is a potent one. Many nonradiologists who are providing imaging services may prove resilient and may work to comply with the new regulations. It remains to be seen whether the "quality approach" will prove effective in controlling the moral hazard of economically motivated imaging studies.

## A Nuclear Winter for Medical Imaging?

The most draconian approach to reducing the rate of increase of imaging expenditures—what one might term the *nuclear winter* payment option—is simply to pay much less generously for imaging services. One school of thought is that even though the payments for imaging have been established in the same manner as for any other medical service (the valuation method known as the *resource-based relative value system* [RBRVS] was discussed in detail in Chapter 5), the reason that so many doctors want to provide imaging is that imaging services are "over-valued" (Winter and Ray 2008).

Those who espouse this belief say that the payment rates set at the time of initial value determination for tests like CT and MRI might have been accurate then, or were no more overvalued than other big-ticket procedures were at the end of the halcyon era of charge-based payment. However, as advanced imaging technologies like CT and MR have improved, operating efficiencies have increased per case profits under technical fee schedules that remained essentially fixed. Because private and public health insurance insulates the ultimate user from these costs, the conventional market forces of price competition have neither reduced prices nor meaningfully restrained demand for imaging care.

Proponents of dramatic payment reductions for imaging argue that the growth rate of imaging utilization would lessen if there were less money to be made. The year 2007 provided a test of this theory. Two years earlier, Medicare rules governing the growth of Part B physician payments called for a 4.4% average reduction in professional fees paid to all doctors in 2006. Congress recognized that the reduction might cause physicians to withdraw from participation in the Medicare program[23] or else not accept any new Medicare patients. Congress struggled to find a way to avoid implementing the pay cut while still limiting the growth of the Medicare budget, as required by law.

## Baby, It's Cold Out There

Influenced by staff at CMS and an analysis by the congressionally chartered Medicare Payment Advisory Commission (MedPac), Congress enacted reductions in nonhospital imaging technical payments that they projected would save about $2.8 billion—more than half of what they needed to cover the Part B "savings" they needed to generate under law. The Deficit Reduction Act of 2005 required imaging providers to accept the lesser payment of the RBRVS-determined technical component for advanced imaging services (MR and CT) under the Medicare physician fee schedule or the Hospital Outpatient Prospective Payment System (HOPPS) payment rate assigned for the service. There was no reason, lawmakers argued, for physicians performing scans in their offices or entrepreneurs owning imaging centers to be paid more than hospitals for equivalent services.

In addition, DRA mandated a two-step reduction over consecutive years in how much providers could charge for scanning contiguous body parts by CT or MRI during the same scanning session. That is, instead of charging the entire technical fee for a CT scan of the abdomen and the entire technical fee for a CT scan of the pelvis captured in a single scanning session, as previously, there was a 25% reduction in the fee for the less expensive body part in January 2006 and a further reduction to 50% in 2007. The second reduction was delayed but reappeared in the Patient Protection and Affordable Care Act of 2010, and is scheduled to take effect in January, 2011. The rationale for this action was, lawmakers argued, that there were efficiencies in scanning adjacent body parts like not having to place an additional IV line, renotifying the patient of potential risks of the procedure, or stationing the patient on the scanner table a second time.

The DRA managed to infuriate all physicians who used imaging, both on emotional and technical grounds. The core concern, however, was purely economic. Why should imaging physicians bear such a disproportionate share of the reductions as opposed to sharing the pain with a broader cross section of physician colleagues? As can be imagined from the foregoing, the political alliances formed to fight the imaging cuts made for odd bedfellows.

Nonetheless, the temporary spirit of bonhommie among competing specialties was for naught. The political reality was that imaging presented a large, easy target that did not require line-by-line revision of the fee schedule, and the cuts affected

---

[23] Physicians may choose not to accept payment according to the Medicare fee schedule and bill patients directly for their services.

only a small minority of all physicians, who were, by the way, some of the most highly paid specialists in medicine. Congress opted to anger a few relatively wealthy physicians greatly rather than many physicians slightly.

Despite concerns about the DRA cuts reducing access to imaging care, the federal government saved a lot of money, breaking a multiyear trend of double-digit Medicare spending increases for advanced imaging in FY 2007, the first full year of DRA implementation (GAO Report 2008b). Despite capping only 20% of overall Medicare imaging paid under the fee schedule (the most expensive 20%), a GAO analysis for FY 2007 showed that total Medicare imaging spending fell 12.7%, a remarkable result against a background of nearly a decade of hefty increases. Tellingly, however, the advanced scanning volume rose four times the rate of overall imaging in 2007, suggesting that self-referring physicians markedly dialed up the volume of imaging tests to offset the cuts (GAO Report 2008b). This finding is consistent with earlier studies that found that rate cuts do spur increases in provider-controlled scanning volume.[24] This phenomenon is known in the health wonk world as the *behavioral offset*. The volume increases argue persuasively that access to imaging services had not meaningfully decreased.

Recent analysis of 2008 Medicare data showed a year-over-year increase of 2.8% in overall imaging spending on a 1.5% volume increase. Advanced imaging spending rebounded, growing 2.3%, on a little over a 1% volume increase. In other words, advanced imaging volumes and costs increased in the second year following the DRA cuts, but certainly had not regained the volume or cost growth trends prevailing before DRA (Moran Company 2009).

The ACR estimates that the actual reductions in payments to radiologists may have been two to three times greater than projected (RSNA News 2008). Examination of trends for office-based advanced scanning showed that radiologists' payments for MR fell by 30%, CT payments fell by 5.2%, and payments to other specialists for MR fell by 23.5%, while payments for CT for other specialists actually rose by 8.2% due to an 18% volume increase. This suggests that radiologists continued losing market share in advanced imaging because (as discussed previously) they have limited influence over the volume of services they provide compared to other physician specialists (Levin and Rao 2009).[25]

So, while in one sense—reducing the growth rate in imaging expenditures—the DRA might be viewed as a success. However, it actually seems to have resulted in greater imaging utilization among some physicians, because self-referring physicians increased their referrals to sustain their facilities and meet revenue targets.[26]

Most significantly, the 2010 health care reform legislation will result in a phased-in rebasing of equipment utilization rate from 50% to 75% over 2 years (62.5% in 2010). The legislation replaces a 2010 CMS ruling that would have set the ultimate utilization rate at 90% with a 4 year phase-in period through 2014.

---

[24] Offsetting a payment reduction for imaging was the principal result of a study by Hillman et al. when the United Mine Workers Union Health and Retirement Funds decreased payments for self-referred imaging in Appalachia (Hillman et al. 1995), and both the utilization of their beneficiaries and their overall imaging outlays increased.

[25] Since radiologists depend on referrals from other physicians, they do not have the capacity to offset.

[26] Geraldine McGinty, ACR Advisor to the AMA Relative Value Committee, oral communication, National Health Policy Forum, November 2008.

Health reform legislation will have the effect of further reducing the component of the technical payment attributed to compensating providers for purchasing and maintaining the equipment. The 2010 payment rules represent the second significant reduction in imaging technical payments in three years, targeting non-hospital imaging providers.

Finally, a rebalancing of professional fee payments among specialties will result in an expected 6% reduction for radiologists over the next four years. An initial evaluation by the ACR indicates that practices only billing the global fee (professional plus technical) in offices and outpatient centers may see 30%–40% decrements in their revenue once all reductions are fully implemented in 2012. The average practice—with both hospital and outpatient activities—is expected to see a 16% decrease.[27]

A concern of radiologists is that since some physicians have the capacity to offset price reductions with higher utilization—and seem to be doing just that—Medicare and private insurers might continue iteratively to impose further cuts in unit payment for imaging until imaging is no longer profitable for any provider. At some point, nonradiologist physicians might simply dissolve their imaging operations and move on to more promising entrepreneurial activities.

The result of a nuclear winter payment policy could be that radiologists and hospitals would be left with an enormous burden of examinations that would have become both undervalued and underpaid. In such circumstances, established radiologists might stop recruiting newly trained radiologists into their practices or might decide on early retirement for themselves. The combination of the two might indeed engender a crisis in patient access to medical imaging examinations. Reductions in imaging activity under this scenario might have the collateral result that imaging equipment manufacturers reallocate their R&D spending to focus technical innovation on other, more lucrative areas.

## Summary

The public is generally unaware of the conflicts among specialists over which physicians perform high-technology medical imaging examinations. However, because of the possible influence of moral hazard, patients should have reasonable concerns over whether the imaging examinations recommended to them are appropriate and necessary. Patients should recognize that while the benefits of modern imaging are undeniable, imaging examinations are not always appropriate or necessary and could cause them both economic and physical harm. The findings of imaging examinations can also set off a chain reaction of additional diagnostic and therapeutic care that might be neither appropriate nor beneficial. The biological effects of repeated exposure to diagnostic ionizing radiation accumulate over a lifetime and may pose a threat to health. Patients should question their physicians about the possible benefits and harms of any medical imaging exam and ask about any conflicts that might affect their physician's recommendation.

The dynamics underlying the conflicts between radiologists and other physicians, and the financial incentives that underlie them, make it virtually certain that the unseemly wrangling over who controls imaging technology will continue in the future (Fig. 7-1). As an example, many gastroenterologists currently base their

---

[27] Personal communication, Bibb Allen, MD, November 2009.

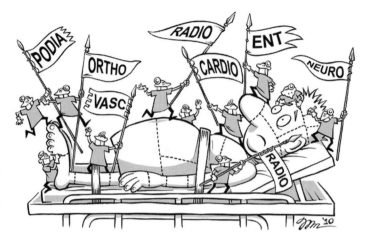

FIGURE 7-1

*The conflict among
specialists to provide
medical services.*

practices almost entirely on performing endoscopy examinations of the colon and are threatened by the ongoing emergence of CT colonography. Interventional radiologists and surgeons are aggressively competing over new catheter-based methods to treat aneurysms. As noted earlier, interventional radiologists are becoming much more aggressive in soliciting patients to seek their services as direct caregivers in direct competition with surgeons.

The battles among specialties over imaging might work out in several ways. One is the continuation of what is mostly going on now—each turf battle is fought hand-to-hand in each individual locale. However, the continuation of turf battles has the potential to damage the public's perception of medicine and contribute to a public perception that economic concerns trump concerns about the patient's welfare.

An alternative approach is collaboration. Collaboration might be abetted by the current trend of many hospitals returning to service line organizational structures for their major clinical programs. Service lines focus on specific medical problems (cancer, diabetes, etc.) that cross disciplinary boundaries. They seek to promote collaboration among specialties in the patient's interest. In such service lines, imaging experts are paired with their specialist colleagues to deliver care focused on specific organs and diseases. The development of organ-based multispecialty groups is spilling over into office practice. The most noticeable example is the proliferation of comprehensive breast care centers. Subspecialist breast imaging experts are colocated in an interactive environment with breast specialists trained in medical oncology, surgery, and pathology. Patients get one-stop shopping for their problem in a single location. And clinical protocols, not competitive forces driven by economic interests, determine which specialist does what.[28]

---

[28] This trend might be further reinforced if Medicare begins paying for care based upon episodes of illness, rather than a la carte (per visit, per hospital admission, per scan, etc.). The Patient Protection and Affordable Care Act of 2010 envisions a raft of experiments with more unified forms of health care payment that would reward interdisciplinary collaboration and lead to new Medicare payment approaches.

The fundamental concern of this chapter remains the injurious effects on patients of unnecessary imaging examinations motivated by financial gain. Legislative and regulatory efforts to control injurious financial incentives to perform marginal and unnecessary imaging have been inconsistently effective. Future reforms must consider how rationally to reduce incentives to perform unnecessary exams while avoiding any negative impact on patient access to high-quality and beneficial medical imaging. As the issue of how to deal with inappropriate imaging overlaps with so many other concerns about how society can afford to pay for the remarkable continuing advances in medical imaging, this book will address possible policy approaches in its final chapter.

## References

The Advisory Board Company. Physician-hospital alignment. Document #16984. Washington, DC: The Advisory Board Company, 2008.

Armstrong D. Own image: MRI and CT centers offer doctors way to profit on scans. *Wall Street Journal*, May 2, 2005:1A.

Arrow K. Uncertainty and the welfare economics of medical care. *Am Econ Rev.* 1963;53:941–973.

Barlow RD. CT installed base triples in cardiology practices. 2008. http://www.auntminnie.com/index.asp?Sec=sup&Sub=imc&Pag=dis&ItemID=84071&wf. Accessed April 2, 2010.

Becker C. Imaging imbroglio. Battle over self-referrals is pitting doc against doc. *Modern Healthcare*, December 6, 2004, p. 16.

Brant-Zawadzki M, Enzmann D. The disaggregation of radiology. *J Am Coll Radiol.* 2005;5:1181–1185.

Berk RN. Why Caldwell? *AJR.* 1995;164:1321–1322.

Christiansen CM. *The Innovator's Dilemma: When New Technologies Cause Great Firms to Fail.* Boston: Harvard Business School Press, 1997.

Council on Ethics and Judicial Affairs, American Medical Association. Conflicts of interest. Physician ownership of medical facilities. *JAMA.* 1992;267:2366–2369.

Eng J, Mysko WK, Weller GER, et al. Interpretation of emergency department radiographs: a comparison of emergency medicine physicians with radiologists, residents with faculty, and film with digital display. *AJR Am J Roentgenol.* 2000;175:1233–1238.

GAO Report to the Chairman, Subcommittee on Health, Committee on Ways and Means, House of Representatives. *Referrals to Physician-Owned Imaging Facilities Warrant HCFA's Scrutiny* (GAO/HEHS-95-2). Washington, DC: General Accounting Office, 1994.

GAO Report to Congressional Requesters. *Medicare Part B Imaging Services. Rapid Spending Growth and Shift to Physician Offices Indicate Need for CMS to Consider Additional Management Practices* (GAO-08-452). Washington, DC: Government Accountability Office, 2008a.

GAO Report to Congressional Requesters. *Medicare: Trends in Fees, Utilization, and Expenditures for Imaging Services before and after Implementation of the Deficit Reduction Act of 2005* (GAO-08-1102R). Washington, DC; Government Accountability Office, 2008b.

Gazelle GS, Halpern EF, Ryan HS, et al. Utilization of diagnostic medical imagining: comparison of radiologist referral versus same-specialty referral. *Radiology.* 2007;245(2):517–522.

Hendel RC, Cerqueira M, Douglas PS, et al. A multicenter assessment of the use of single-photon emission computed tomography myocardial perfusion imaging with appropriateness criteria. *J Am Coll Cardiol.* 2009;55:156–162.

Hillman BJ. Government health policy and the diffusion of new medical devices. *Health Serv Res.* 1986;21:681–711.

Hillman BJ. Trying to regulate imaging self-referral is like playing Whack-a-Mole. *AJR Am J Roentgenol.* 2007;189;267–268.

Hillman BJ, Joseph CA, Mabry MR, et al. Frequency and costs of diagnostic imaging in office practice—a comparison of self-referring and radiologist-referring physicians. *N Engl J Med.* 1990;323:1604–1608.

Hillman BJ, Olson GT, Colbert RW, et al. Physicians' responses to a payment policy denying reimbursement of non-Radiologists' professional charges for diagnostic imaging. *JAMA.* 1995;274:885–887.

Hillman BJ, Olson GT, Griffith PE, et al. Physicians' utilization and charges for outpatient diagnostic imagining in a Medicate population. *JAMA.* 1992;268:2050–2054.

Japsen B. Doctors took MRI kickbacks, suit says. State alleges fraud costs insurers, patients millions. *Chicago Tribune,* January 18, 2007:1.

Japsen B. MRI centers to settle illegal kickback case. *Chicago Tribune,* January 14, 2009:1.

Lee S, Saokar A, Dryer K, et al. Does radiologist recommendation for follow-up with the same imaging modality contribute substantially to high-cost imaging volume? *Radiology.* 2007;242:857–864.

Levin DC, Intenzo CM, Rao VM, et al. Comparison of recent utilization trends in radionuclide myocardial perfusion imaging among radiologists and cardiologists. *J Am Coll Radiol.* 2005;2:821–824.

Levin DC, Rao VM. Turf wars in radiology: updated evidence on the relationship between self-referral and the overutilization of imaging. *J Am Coll Radiol.* 2008;7:806–810.

Levin DC, Rao VM, Orrison WW Jr. Turf wars in radiology: the quality of imaging facilities operated by non-radiologist physicians and of the images they produce. *J Am Coll Radiol.* 2004;1:649–651.

Levin DC, Rao VM, Parker L, et al. The effect of the introduction of MR and CT angiography on the utilization of catheter angiography for peripheral arterial disease. *J Am Coll Radiol.* 2007;4:457–460.

Levin DC, Rao VJ, Parker L, et al. Ownership or leasing of CT scanners by non-radiologist physicians: a rapidly growing trend that raises concern about self-referral. *J Am Coll Radiol.* 2008;5:1206–1209.

Levin DC, Rao VJ, Parker L, et al. The disproportionate effects of the Deficit Deduction Act of 2005 on radiologists' private office MRI and CT practices compared to those of other physicians. *J Am Coll Radiol.* 2009;6:620–632.

Medicare Payment Advisory Commission. *Report to the Congress: Variation and innovation in Medicare.* Medicare Payment Advisory Commission Washington, DC: June 2003.

Medicare Payment Advisory Commission. *Data Book, Healthcare Spending and the Medicare Program.* Medicare Payment Advisory Commission Washington, DC: June, 2008.

Messina L. Manchin wants HCA to revisit CT scan decision. *Charleston Daily Mail.* December 10, 2007:1.

Mettler FA, Bhargavan M, Faulkner K. Radiologic and nuclear medicine studies in the United States and worldwide: frequency, radiation dose, and comparison with other radiation sources—1950–2007. *Radiology.* 2009;253:522–531.

Mitchell JM. The prevalence of physician self-referral arrangements after Stark II: evidence from advanced diagnostic imaging. *Health Aff.* 2008;26:W415–W424.

Mitchell JM, Scott E. Evidence of the prevalence and scope of physician joint ventures. *JAMA.* 1992;268:80–84.

Moran Company. *Trends in Imaging Services Billed to Part B Medicare Carriers and Paid Under the Physician Fee Schedule 1998–2008.* Moran Company Washington, DC: October 2009.

Moskowitz H, Sunshine J, Grossman D, et al. The effect of imaging guidelines on the number and quality of outpatient radiographic examinations. *Am J Roentgenol.* 2000;175:9–15.

Patti JP, Berlin JW, Blumberg AL, et al. ACR White Paper: the value added that radiologists provide to the health care enterprise. *J Am Coll Radiol.* 2008;5:1041–1053.

Pham HH, Devers KJ, May JH, et al. Financial pressures spur physician entrepreneurialism. *Health Aff.* 2004;23:70–81.

Potchen EJ, Cooper TG, Sierra AE, et al. Measuring performance in chest radiology. *Radiology.* 2000;217:456–459.

Report of the OIG. *Provider Relationships and the Use of Magnetic Resonance under the Medicare Physician Fee Schedule* (OEI-01–06-00261). Washington, DC: Office of the Inspector General, 2008.

Report to the Congress: Improving Incentives in the Medicare Program. Medical Payment Advisory Commission. Washington, DC, June, 2009:81–96. http://www.medpac.gov/documents/Jun09_EntireReport.pdf. Accessed April 5, 2010.

Rodwin MA. Physicians' conflicts of interest. The limitations of disclosure. *N Engl J Med.* 1989;321:1405–1408.

RSNA News. Practices still faltering despite temporary DRA relief. October 2008.

Salary Survey Results Questioned. RSNA News, November 2008. http://www.rsna.org/Publications/rsnanews/November-2008/salarysurvey_feature.cfm. Accessed December 13, 2009.

Sunshine JH, Lewis RS, Bhargavan M. Diagnostic radiologists' subspecialization and the new final board examination. *AJR Am J Roentgenol.* 2008;191:1293–1301.

Swedlow A, Johson G, Smithline N, et al. Increased costs and rates of use in the California workers' compensation system as a result of self-referral by physicians. *N Engl J Med.* 1992;327:1502–1506.

Timmins J, Orlando P, Lipoti J. The New Jersey radiographic quality assurance program at 5 years. *J Am Coll Radiol.* 2007;4:691–698.

Verrilli DK, Bloch SM, Rousseau J, et al. Design of a privileging program for diagnostic imaging: costs and implications for a large insurer in Massachusetts. *Radiology.* 1998;208:385–392.

Webster BS, Verma S, Pransky GS. Outcome of workers' compensation claimants with low back pain undergoing electrothermal therapy. *Spine.* 2004;29:435–441.

Wilson IB, Dukes K, Greenfield S, et al. The patients' role in the use of radiological testing for common office practice complaints. *Arch Intern Med.* 2001;161:256–263.

Winter A, Ray N. Paying accurately for imaging services in Medicare. *Health Aff.* 2008;27:1479–1490.

# 8

# Using Imaging to Screen for Life-Threatening Diseases—Its Promise and Its Problems

*Bernardo Martinez lit up a Winston and tuned in to his favorite salsa station on the car radio. It had been a stressful day at work, as most days were in the mortgage business since the housing crash. The double bacon cheeseburger his assistant had gotten him for lunch hadn't helped matters. He'd hurriedly wolfed it down at his desk while he worked out a thorny set of numbers on his computer. His heartburn still hadn't receded. It felt as though a clenched fist were tightening in his chest.*

*He tried to relax to the beat of music he'd loved since he was a child growing up in Little Havana. How things had changed! Hard work and a few loans had gotten him through college. Now he had a large home in a new development on the water, a wife and three kids, and a little money he could save each month after all the bills were paid. He had trouble getting to sleep at night. Bernardo felt a lot of pressure to maintain the life he'd built. What, he mused, would become of my family if something were to happen to me?*

*The song finished with a flourish and was replaced by a man's voice. Bernardo had been daydreaming during the music, but the urgency of the man's pitch made it seem that he might be saying something important. "I want to tell you about something I did several months ago," said the man. "It didn't just change my life. It saved it! I underwent a simple medical test ... a CT scan of my heart. It took only a few minutes of lying still in a quiet room. The radiologist spoke with me right after the scan. He showed me a picture of a narrowing in one of the blood vessels to my heart ... what he called 'a widow maker.' I had it taken care of, and I can tell you I feel twenty years younger. To think I'd been walking around like that...." The commercial continued, but Bernardo was only half listening now. That could be me, he thought. He took note of the name of the imaging center and vowed to call them when he got home. He knew that his health insurance wouldn't cover it—the commercial had said so—but what he'd heard had been compelling. He'd spend the money. Bernardo opened the windows of his car. He crushed out his cigarette and took a deep breath of fresh air.*

Depending on where you live, you too may have heard radio commercials like this one or other messages promoting what purports to be a great medical advance—using modern imaging technology like CT or MRI to screen for life-threatening conditions like atherosclerosis of the coronary arteries to the heart or cancer. The commercials would have you believe that even though you feel fine, these conditions are silently and insidiously propelling you toward your imminent demise,[1] but that a "simple, noninvasive test" (words commonly used in these commercials) can catch the disease early and save your life. The not so subtle message is that you might be a ticking time bomb. You should hurry in to the advertised imaging facility. You might not have a minute to spare.

Screening for serious disease is not a new idea. Though not without periodic controversy, mammography screening for breast cancer, colonoscopy for colon cancer, and nonimaging screening tests like PAP smears for cervical cancer have been propelled by highly successful social marketing campaigns. The best evidence is that these tests reduce the mortality rate for their respective diseases. Perhaps as a direct result, the public is highly receptive to the idea of screening for disease. A 2004 survey (Schwartz et al. 2004) revealed that 87% of Americans believed that screening for disease was almost always a good idea. Nearly as many, 74%, believed that screening for cancer saved lives. An amazing 98% of adults who had actually undergone a screening exam and initially got an incorrect result (usually a false-positive result when they did not actually have the disease) said they were nonetheless glad that they had done it.

Public opinion aside, however, there are few other situations in which the current scientific evidence favoring imaging screening in otherwise healthy individuals is as compelling as it is for mammography. In particular, the value of other, newer imaging screening tests—such as whole body CT scanning and CT screening for coronary artery disease (the idea that so appealed to Bernardo)—remains unproven. Indeed, as this chapter will discuss, screening tests involving imaging of any sort can have both positive and negative consequences that can impact the individuals undergoing screening and society at large.

## The Outcomes of Screening Examinations

To begin, let's consider what the term *imaging screening* actually means. Imaging screening is the application of an imaging technology to:

> the systematic testing of individuals who are asymptomatic with respect to some target disease. The purpose of screening is to prevent, interrupt, or delay the development of advanced disease in the subset [of individuals] with a preclinical form of the target disease through early detection and treatment. (Hillman et al. 2004, p. 862)

That means that for imaging screening to be effective in large populations, two important conditions must hold: First, the preclinical phase of the disease—when disease or predisease is present but is not causing symptoms—must be long enough

---

[1] There is some truth to this. Death is the first "symptom" for roughly a third of heart attack patients.

that regular screening will catch a large number of cases before they have progressed; second, the test must be sensitive enough to detect the preclinical form of the disease before symptoms have developed.

In addition, good screening tests should appeal to patients and providers so that the test will be widely available and people will wish to undergo it. This means that the test should cause little pain or discomfort, be reliably reproducible both across a broad geographic range and over time, and especially, be affordable, since screening tests often are not covered by insurance. Most importantly, there must be an important and measurable health benefit that is derived from the screening. Ideally, this means that there exists a treatment that is more effective when disease is found early than when the condition becomes symptomatic.

This last qualification is often debated. Insurers usually take the position that if no treatment exists to improve the condition of individuals identified by the exam, then there is no reason to use the test. Caregivers respond that the knowledge provided by the exam is valuable in itself, since it can guide patients in deciding how to live their lives. One example is the recent development of PET imaging using amyloid plaque-specific radionuclides to diagnose and chart the progression of Alzheimer's disease. Although there is little available to treat the fundamental problem, a patient and his or her family can use the test outcome to make decisions about the need for and expense of future care.

An important word in our definition of imaging screening is *asymptomatic*, because this means that the imaging test is being applied to healthy people. This is distinctly different from using imaging to diagnose disease in someone who is experiencing health problems, because imaging screening has the potential to make patients out of people who believed that they were healthy until they were tested. In some cases, such as for the character in the radio commercial, this works out quite nicely. For others, problems can develop.

To see how this occurs, let's consider an analogy. Woody Hayes, the legendary football coach of Ohio State University, renowned for his disdain for the passing game, famously said, "There are three things that can happen when you pass, and two of them ain't good" (http://buckeyefansonly.com/woody). The same is true for imaging screening, except that there are not three but four possible outcomes (Table 8-1).

Consider the risks and benefits of each possible outcome of an imaging screening. One possibility is that the test will be negative and the patient will be truly healthy. Doctors refer to this outcome as a *true-negative* test result. There can be no quibble over this one; it is the best and least complicated possible outcome. The test verifies that the person is healthy. Screening has been such a positive experience that he or she likely will want to be screened again at the recommended interval.[2] The patient may even increase his or her use of other valuable health-promoting behaviors, like eating more healthfully and exercising regularly.

---

[2]  Historically, for mammography, the recommendation has been annual screening after age 40. As we discuss later in this chapter, controversial 2010 recommendations of the U.S. Preventative Services Task Force now suggest every-other-year screening beginning at age 50. Other experts dispute these recommendations.

TABLE 8-1　*The Possible Test and Health Outcomes of Imaging Screening Tests*

| Status of Test and Individual | True Negative | True Positive | False Negative | False Positive |
|---|---|---|---|---|
| Definition of Status | Test is negative. Individual is healthy. | Test is positive. Individual has the condition. | Test is negative. Individual has the condition. | Test is positive. Individual is healthy. |
| Possible Outcomes | Less anxiety and improved sense of well-being. | Reduced chance of death; and/or better health; or no change in illness or time of death. | Delay in treatment may reduce the chance of a cure. | Increased anxiety; more testing and/or inappropriate treatment. |

Beyond the true negative result, things grow more complicated. As with any medical testing, imaging screening may provide different types of incorrect results. Both *false-negative* and *false-positive* test results can occur. A false-negative test is one that is interpreted as showing no disease, but the individual actually has the condition for which the test is intended. This is clearly an unfortunate result, since the individual will incorrectly believe himself or herself to be healthy and may ignore early signs and symptoms. What may have been early, curable disease at the time of the screening examination, or even when the patient first begins to have symptoms, may become incurable in the time that elapses before a correct diagnosis is made. In some cases, interpretive mistakes are responsible; in others, a false-negative diagnosis simply reflects a limitation of what the test is capable of detecting. Regardless of the true cause, medical liability lawyers make their livings off such cases, calling them *failure to diagnose.*

In the case of a false-positive result, the test indicates that the person has the target disease, but the person is actually healthy. This is not a benign circumstance. The individual will almost certainly receive additional imaging testing, perhaps an invasive diagnostic procedure (a biopsy or catheterization, for example), or even incorrect treatment, before it is determined that a mistake has been made. The actually healthy individual will be treated as a patient with a serious health problem. He or she may incur substantial harm and experience significant anxiety, and both the person and society will pay unnecessary costs.

### "The Only Normal Patient Is One Who Has Not Yet Undergone a Complete Workup"

A cautionary real-life example of how a false-positive imaging screening result can turn a healthy individual into a patient is a radiologist and friend, Bill Casarella (Casarella 2002). Dr. Casarella had arrived at the age at which the American Cancer

Society recommends that all men and women should be screened for colon cancer. Eschewing the conventionally accepted colonoscopy, Dr. Casarella opted for a relatively new imaging screening test for colon cancer called *virtual colonoscopy* (also known as *CT colonography* [CTC]). This test will be discussed in greater detail later in this chapter. Briefly, the procedure involves inserting a tube into the rectum and filling the colon with air to smooth out the normal folds of the colon and improve the ability to see small polyps[3] and cancers. A CT scan is performed using very thin slices (to improve the visualization of small abnormalities), which a radiologist can then view conventionally as cross sections of the body or have the computer reconstruct into a three-dimensional image so that he or she can "fly through" the colon virtually. In recent clinical trials, CTC has been shown to have accuracy in finding colonic polyps comparable to that of conventional colonoscopy[4] (Pickhardt et al. 2003; Johnson et al. 2008).

However, CTC has an additional capability beyond that proffered by colonoscopy. The images allow the interpreting radiologist to see not only the abnormalities inside the colon, but also the surrounding organs in the abdomen. To the uninitiated, this may seem like a good thing. Indeed, in some cases it does identify important, treatable extracolonic abnormalities. But for Dr. Casarella, this capacity led to considerable unnecessary distress.

Dr. Casarella's colon was entirely normal, but at the margins of the images of his colon, the radiologist detected a lump on the kidney, several liver masses, and some nodules at the base of the lungs. Without any doubt, his situation was exacerbated by his being a prominent physician in his medical center. As a group, doctors receive excessive medical care. Because Dr. Casarella's colleagues were concerned about him, he received as follow-on testing an abdominal CT scan with intravenous contrast material, a high-resolution CT scan of the lungs, a CT-guided liver biopsy, a PET scan, and video-guided thoracoscopy and wedge resection of the lung nodules.[5]

All of this caused extraordinary anxiety to Dr. Casarella and his family (who believed he had metastatic cancer). It also led to a two-week hospitalization, five weeks of considerable pain from the thoracoscopy (which resulted in a partial lung collapse), bed rest and rehabilitation, and medical expenses (mostly paid by insurance) in excess of $50,000. In the end, the renal mass turned out to be a benign cyst, and the liver and lung lesions were residual inflammations (termed *granulomas*) from a long-ago bout with a common fungal infection called *histoplasmosis*.[6] While not all false-positive screening results produce such an extraordinary cascade of events, clearly there is the potential for devastation. Dr. Casarella, who felt fine at the time

---

3   Most colon cancers begin as benign polyps that protrude into the colon from the most superficial layer of the colon wall, called the *mucosa*. It usually takes many years for a polyp to become a cancer—one of the reasons colon cancer screening is so effective.

4   For colonoscopy, a scope hooked to a video camera is placed into the rectum and manipulated around the entire colon to directly see polyps or cancers.

5   A surgical procedure using a scope to ensure that the lung nodules were properly resected.

6   Histoplasmosis is most commonly encountered in the Midwest. It often heals by leaving small nodules in such organs as the lungs, liver, and spleen. Many of these nodules contain calcium and do not present a diagnostic problem. When they are noncalcified, they may be confused with cancer.

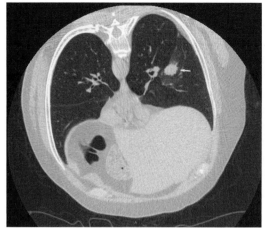

he was screened, declared, "The only normal patient is one who has not yet under-gone a complete workup" (Casarella 2002).

Finally, a *true-positive* result occurs when the test is positive and the individual, in fact, has the condition for which he or she is being screened. There are several possible outcomes in this situation. The most salubrious is that the disease will be found early, at a treatable stage. This may allow for less intensive treatment, less dis-comfort, and a shorter convalescence. The individual is cured and goes on to lead a long, healthy life. Some of you undoubtedly know a relative, a friend, or a friend of a friend who responded to a commercial, paid out of pocket for a screening examina-tion, and serendipitously had his or her cancer found early (Fig. 8-1). "The surgeon got it all," this person tells you. "The CT scan saved my life!"

## The Problem of Pseudodisease

Here, the plot thickens. In some cases, screening did save the person's life. But there is another possibility: the screening examination detected a lesion that, even if it had not been found, would never have harmed the patient. Screening experts refer to these types of abnormalities as *overdiagnosis* or *pseudodisease*. Consider, as an example of overdiagnosis, an atherosclerotic lesion found by a newly developed imaging screening test called coronary CT angiography (CCTA).[7] This was the test advertised in the opening vignette in this chapter that so appealed to Bernardo. The "widow maker" may actually have been the death-dealing lesion described, or it may simply have represented pseudodisease. In fact, most men and women over the age of 50 have at least some coronary atherosclerosis, but for many, this disease is

---

[7] This exam requires the injection of contrast medium and then immediately scanning with very thin slices through the heart to see actual atherosclerotic foci, called *plaques*, and how they might be narrowing the coronary arteries. Coronary CT angiography serves the same function as coronary catheterization but without the need for an invasive procedure. As a result, some authorities have suggested that the test could be used as a screening examina-tion. At this time, the impact of CCTA screening has not been thoroughly evaluated.

not life-threatening. The problem is that the mere identification of atherosclerosis is often sufficient to initiate a cascade of tests. When the screening test depicts pseudodisease, all of what follows generates societal costs but provides no measurable benefit for patients.

How is it possible to have a condition that is truly pathological when the relevant cells are examined under a microscope but that doesn't affect the patient in his or her lifetime? The answer is that many potentially serious human diseases, like atherosclerosis and cancer, vary enormously in their aggressiveness. It is well known, for example, that as one ages, the likelihood of developing certain cancers—such as prostate, breast, and thyroid cancer—increases dramatically. However, the patient doesn't necessarily die of these cancers. As the saying goes, "She didn't die *of* the cancer, she died *with* the cancer."

From the perspective of designing imaging screening programs for large populations, the identification of pseudodisease on imaging screening examinations will have no impact on how many people die of the disease. To say it another way, finding pseudodisease does not reduce the death rate (also known as the *mortality rate*) from the illness—the number of deaths caused by the disease per thousand members of the screening-eligible population per year.

Unfortunately, at this stage of its development, imaging screening technology cannot successfully differentiate aggressive, life-threatening disease from pseudodisease. Right now, we only know the aggressiveness of an abnormality once the disease has become clinically apparent (aggressive disease) or when the abnormality is found incidentally on autopsy (pseudodisease). Because even small tumors can metastasize early, the present tendency is to treat every finding as though it is life-threatening. However, even frequent screening might not change the death rate for patients with these aggressive tumors because we lack treatments that work any better against early, screening-identified disease than they do against disease that is diagnosed after symptoms appear. Once again, screening has no capacity to reduce the death rate for these unfortunate patients.

A good example would be if Bernardo has a screening CT scan and the radiologist finds an early pancreatic cancer. Many pancreatic cancers are highly aggressive but frequently exhibit no or only very vague symptoms. Treatment is futile for most patients. As a result, because the cancer has been found earlier than it would if no screening had occurred, Bernardo lives for a longer period knowing that he has a death-dealing illness but dies at exactly the same time as if he were not screened. For many people, this screening result would lead to a diminished quality of their remaining life.

The foregoing discussion validates the contention stated at the beginning of this chapter. Proven imaging screening has the potential to save many from the ravages of incurable disease, but there is also great potential to induce harm by applying unproven imaging screening technology to the general population of asymptomatic Americans. As one screening authority, Bill Black, has put it, "If you screen the general population, you can wreak havoc on the general population" (Spurgeon and Burton 2000). More recently, in light of renewed concerns over the human and monetary costs of false-positive diagnoses and pseudodisease, Dr. Otis Brawley, Chief Medical Officer of the American Cancer Society, caused controversy by saying, "We don't want people to panic, but I'm admitting that American medicine has overpromised when it comes to screening. The advantages of screening have been exaggerated" (Kolata 2009).

## Gauging the Costs and Benefits of New Imaging Screening Tests

To be acceptable to the general public and to public and private health insurers, imaging screening must improve the health of those who are screened at a price that patients, insurers, and society can afford. Cost is a necessary consideration because imaging screening has the potential to add tens or even hundreds of billions of dollars to our already very high national health care expenditures. Since, ultimately, we all pay for what we spend on health care through taxes and our and our employers' contributions to health insurance programs, we want to be certain that if we spend such a large amount, society is getting good value for the money. This section will review the benefits and harms of screening and describe how benefits and costs are evaluated.

As noted above, a reduction in the number of deaths caused by the disease is usually the desired goal. At the very least, screening must result in an important reduction in illness or an improvement in the patient's quality of life.[8] Even if we can demonstrate a benefit to screening, however, we also need to weigh that benefit against the potential harm caused. Popular advertising of imaging screening tends to overstate the benefits of imaging screening while glossing over or even ignoring the risks of potential harm. Nonetheless, these risks are real and must be considered in any estimation of the value of population-based screening. One must subtract from the identified benefit any loss of health or duration or quality of life that occurs as the result of screening to arrive at a "net benefit" for the screening test.

The most obvious risks of harm are ones we've already discussed in detail: false-positive and false-negative diagnoses and the identification of pseudodisease. Other commonly encountered risks of imaging screening examinations include adverse reactions to contrast material and harm that might result from long-term accumulation of radiation. These risks and others were described in detail in Chapter 4.

One reason imaging screening is so popular is that it gives us the impression that we have greater control over our health and lives. We are grateful for this opportunity, particularly if someone else is paying the bill. However, to receive value for the money we invest, we must understand the risks and benefits of a given imaging screening exam. Screening for serious diseases in large populations is almost always a very expensive endeavor, requiring considerable financial and human resources. In fact, despite what we often hear from advocacy foundations, some professionals, and politicians who are personally invested in a particular disease or test, screening large populations usually is more expensive for society than waiting until people get sick and then treating them. But that's not the whole point. We believe as a society that good health has value and that we're willing to pay for that value … but only so much.

---

[8] An example is bone density screening in postmenopausal women, intended to identify osteoporosis or "weak bones." Even here, however, the goal is to reduce fractures, which in the elderly have a strong correlation with the likelihood of earlier death.

Several factors drive cost. The first is the size of the population that might be offered the new imaging test. The better the general population can be *stratified* (i.e., put into categories of risk), such that only higher-risk individuals receive the screening examination, the lower the costs to society. The ultimate stratification would be one in which we could identify inexpensively before we provide the imaging test those who have any chance of developing the target disease. Only those people would receive the test, saving society the cost of testing the unaffected population. Unfortunately, we do not yet possess accurate methods for doing this for any major application of imaging screening. Instead, we do the best we can, using age, family history, a little genetic testing, and potential environmental factors to determine who will be tested.

As one obvious example, unless an asymptomatic woman under 40 carries a specific genetic code identifying her as being at high risk for breast cancer (such as an aberrant BRCA gene), breast imaging experts would not normally recommend that she have screening mammography. Another good example is using chest CT scanning to screen for lung cancer. As detailed below, this is a highly controversial clinical practice. However, there are several large clinical trials testing whether CT screening lowers the death rate from lung cancer. In these trials, both advanced age and a long, intense smoking history are required for individuals to enter the trial. Including others at lower risk would both unfairly lower the potential benefit of screening and unreasonably raise the societal cost.

The accuracy of an imaging screening test is one of the most important factors that determines what it will cost society to perform population-based screening. The test must be sensitive enough (i.e., have a high true-positive rate) to identify accurately the patients who actually have the disease while not generating so many false-positive results that the cost and risk of follow-on testing become overwhelming.

In fact, the biggest driver of costs for most screening tests is usually not the cost of the test itself but all the follow-on diagnostic and treatment costs for individuals who test positively. These costs are both expected and acceptable so long as the identification of positive cases significantly reduces the death rate. When these follow-on costs are mainly devoted to false-positive tests and pseudodisease, or when there is no treatment available that results in greater longevity or improved health, the follow-on procedures can be not only injurious to patients but also wasteful of scarce resources.

Once the net benefit of an imaging screening test is established and its costs are known, health services researchers and policy experts are able to estimate the value of the test by conducting a cost-effectiveness analysis. The goal of this exercise is to determine whether the value of the new screening test can be compared to that of other medical interventions in practice. The outcome of conducting a cost-effectiveness analysis is a ratio—the cost divided by the benefit—usually expressed in terms of the number of dollars that would have to be spent to add a year of life[9] beyond what would be expected if the screening test were not employed. The result can be used by

---

[9]  This is often written as $/LYS, where LYS is life years saved. Recognizing that a year of life with a serious illness is often not experienced the same way as a healthy year, methods have been developed to discount the value of an illness-affected year. When this is entered into the analysis, the ratio becomes $/QALY, or cost per quality-adjusted life year saved.

payers, regulators, and legislators in making decisions about whether insurers, and particularly the federal government through its Medicare and Medicaid programs, should pay for an imaging screening test.

## Screening Is a Political Minefield

So, how much money is too much to spend to add, on average, a year of life to each individual in a screening population? Ultimately, that's a societal decision. Traditionally, health policy mavens have talked about a maximum threshold of $50,000 per year of life saved, but there has been some reconsideration of this number in recent years. Indeed, there may be no specific amount that can be cited, because in some ways, this is the ultimate value judgment: an estimate of the value of a human life.

As we've learned recently with the controversy over mammography screening, for politicians and policymakers, these discussions are an ethical and political minefield. The adoption of a new imaging screening test into medical practice and its payment by insurers is ultimately a political process. As with all political processes, vested interests impinge on policy decision making and almost always muddy the influence of scientifically acquired data. Even so, the character of our times is raising the bar on what information and what level of value are needed to impel the acceptance of a new imaging screening test. The continuing and constant rise in the fraction of our gross domestic product occupied by health care, and particularly the remarkable increase in the use and cost of medical imaging, make it likely than any new imaging screening test will be subject to considerable scrutiny from both a benefit and a cost perspective.

## Examples of Imaging Screening Technologies

As many as 50 applications of imaging screening examinations for specific diseases have been suggested in the medical literature (Hillman et al. 2005). Most fail on one or more of the requirements for successful screening detailed in the previous section or have been too little investigated to determine whether population-based screening can be done cost-effectively.

This section will address both a widely accepted imaging screening technology (mammography for breast cancer) and other technologies that are in various stages of clinical investigation. We will also explore whole body CT scanning, which has been popularly marketed but shows little evidence of effectiveness and has the potential for considerable harm.

*Mammography Screening for Breast Cancer*    Breast cancer is the most commonly encountered cancer and the second leading cause of cancer death among women. In 2007, approximately 41,000 women died of breast cancer in the United States and roughly 465,000 worldwide. The breast cancer mortality rate has been declining in developed countries since 1990, largely due to both the increased availability of and compliance with mammographic breast cancer screening and better access to improving therapies.

(a) 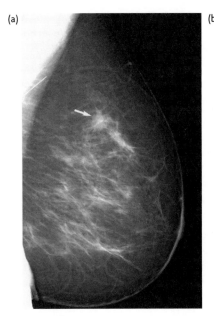 (b)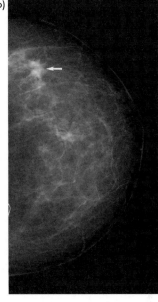

FIGURE 8-2

*A 50-year-old asymptomatic woman found on mammography to have a subcentimeter breast cancer (arrow), seen on (a) the mediolateral (ML) projection; (b) the lesion is confirmed by its visualization (arrow) on the caudocranial (CC) projection. (Courtesy of Michael Cohen, MD, the University of Virginia.)*

There are now multiple imaging modalities available for breast cancer screening—including X-ray mammography, ultrasonography, and MRI—but the standard screening test for women with an average risk of developing breast cancer remains mammography. Mammography is essentially like any X-ray examination, except that the equipment is adapted to the special characteristics of breast tissue.

The effectiveness of mammography (Fig. 8-2) in reducing the death rate from breast cancer is hardly debated,[10] thanks to a number of large randomized and practice-based clinical trials. The clinical studies have been conducted over the past 40 or so years. Even allowing that both the mammographic techniques and the average expertise of interpreting radiologists have improved over time, the results are both consistent and meaningful. Depending on the randomized trial, women who received mammography had roughly 20%–30% lower death rates than women who did not (Duffy et al. 2002). Practice-based research has validated the outcomes of the randomized trials. Indeed, because of the methodological rules employed in randomized clinical trials, it appears that the effect of mammography in reducing breast cancer–related death may actually have been understated in the randomized trials when viewed from the perspective of broader clinical practice (Feig 2002).

One problem with mammography is that there is considerable variability among radiologists in how well they interpret the images (Beam et al. 1996; Sickles et al. 2002). More experienced radiologists and those specializing in breast imaging tend to perform better than radiologists who interpret mammograms as part of a more general radiology practice (Taplin et al. 2008).

[10] Gotzsche and Olsen (2000) revived the debate over the value of mammography in a letter to the *Lancet*, based on their contention that a number of the supporting clinical trials were biased; however, few agree with their position.

Another problem is that mammography produces a significant number of both false-positive results and pseudodisease. The former derives from the fact that finding cancers against a complex background of normal glandular structures is a very difficult visual task. The false-positive results may go on to biopsy and produce short-term anxiety until the situation is clarified (Smith et al. 2003). The pseudodisease is related to a phenomenon we discussed earlier—the enormous variability in how quickly breast cancer grows. Mammography uncovers a sizable number of tumors that grow so slowly that they will not affect the woman in her lifetime. Pseudodisease will be surgically removed, but its excision will not positively affect the health of the patient.

The concern about false-positive diagnoses and pseudodisease has led directly to a very public disagreement over what is the best screening regimen. The ACR and the ACS recommend annual mammography screening for women with average risk factors beginning at age 40. This has been the standard regimen—broadly accepted by women and their physicians—for the past decade. In November 2009, a U.S. Preventative Services Task Force (USPSTF)[11] panel determined that women between ages 40 and 50 did not necessarily require mammograms and that screening biannually after age 50 would be sufficient.[12] The basis for their recommendation was that, in the panel's view, relatively few women develop breast cancer in their 40s and that annual screening was resulting in too many follow-up studies and biopsies. In the panel's opinion, the excess findings were causing unnecessary anxiety among patients called back for additional tests and biopsies.

The USPSTF recommendation was met by outrage from the ACR, the ACS, many breast imaging specialists and other breast physicians involved in breast cancer care, and women's health advocates.[13] Critics felt that the panel's conclusions were based more on saving costs than saving lives (Thrall 2010). Health and Human Services Secretary Kathleen Sebelius immediately distanced herself from the report, saying that "middle-aged women should keep on doing what they're doing, getting yearly testing."[14] Two days later, task force spokeswoman Dr. Diana Petitti clarified that the USPSTF was not against women having mammograms in their 40s. They simply felt that this should not be recommended as a matter of routine medical practice and that it was a decision to be made individually by a woman and her physician (Wang et al. 2009). It is too soon to tell whether women and their physicians will change course to follow the new recommendations. Initially, advocates were concerned that payers might force physicians' hands by denying payment for the more frequent, hence more expensive, ACS- and ACR-endorsed regimens. However, the recently passed 2010 health care reform legislation specifically prohibits insurers from denying coverage for breast cancer screening exams based on the USPSTF recommendations.

---

[11] The USPSTF is an activity of the Agency of Healthcare Research and Quality (AHRQ) in the Department of Health and Human Services (DHHS).

[12] http://www.ahrq.gov/clinic/uspstf/uspsbrca.htm.

[13] http://www.acr.org/HomePageCategories/News/ACRNewsCenter/USPSTFDetails.aspx.

[14] *ABC World News*, November 18, 2009.

A new mammography technology, digital mammography, is poised to replace conventional film-based mammography because of several key attributes. Digital mammography uses projectional radiography[15] just like film mammography. The only difference is that the technique employs an electronic image receptor to display the mammogram on a video screen in place of film. Using an electronic receptor offers several advantages. The image can be "windowed and leveled" (i.e., the darkness and contrast of the image can be manipulated) in an almost infinite number of combinations to make it optimal for the interpreting radiologist. Digital mammograms can also be sent over the Web for distant consultation as needed. More than one individual (say, the radiologist and the physician caring for the woman) can view the mammogram at distant sites at the same time. And electronic storage is potentially eternal, with little or no image degradation. A recent 50,000-woman clinical trial comparing the accuracy of radiologists' interpretations of film and digital mammograms showed digital mammography to be superior to film for younger and perimenopausal women and women who had dense breasts (Pisano et al. 2005).[16] Radiologists diagnosed the film and digital mammograms equally well for all other women.

Newer screening modalities like breast ultrasonography and MRI (Fig. 8-3) have shown promising results in sizable clinical trials (Lehman et al. 2007; Berg et al. 2008). Magnetic resonance imaging, in particular, doubtless finds cancers missed by other methods, but it is more expensive. Moreover, the exquisite sensitivity of MRI means finding more cancers that matter to the health of the patient but also identifying and working up more lesions that do not represent a true threat to health. A strong family history of breast cancer or a genetic test showing the woman to have the BRCA 1 or BRCA 2 genes that greatly increase the likelihood of her developing breast cancer argues for more frequent screening and/or screening by a more sensitive technique like MRI. The ACR and the Society of Breast Imaging recently

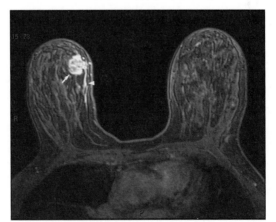

FIGURE 8-3

*Axial contrast-enhanced MRI scan of the breasts showing a 2 cm cancer in the right breast. The enhancement is primarily around the rim of the mass (arrow), where the vessels support rapidly growing tissue. The hypovascular center is necrotic (dead). A large vein (arrowhead) drains the tumor. (Courtesy of Michael Cohen, MD, Emory University.)*

---

[15] This refers to radiography that does not involve computerized image reconstruction, as in CT or MR.

[16] Breasts with more glandular tissue and less fat are radiographically more dense and may obscure breast cancers.

have issued new recommendations for how best to employ the various technologies under different screening scenarios (Lee et al. 2010).

There is no recommended upper limit of age for continued screening so long as the overall health and expected life span of the woman support her being treated for a breast cancer if one is identified (Smith et al. 2003).

*CT Colonography Screening for Colon Cancer*   Colon cancer is the third most common cancer and the second leading cause of cancer death in the United States. Unlike many other cancers, the natural history of colon cancer is fairly well understood. There is usually a long precancerous development phase (up to 10 years or more) in the form of a polyp (also called an *adenoma*), which grows from the superficial layers of the colon wall. Small polyps have little potential to become cancers, but as they grow greater than 1 centimeter, the risk increases considerably. There is good evidence that screening for colonic polyps reduces both the development of cancer and the death rate from colon cancer (Eddy et al. 1987; Selby et al. 1992). That colon cancer is so amenable to screening[17] helps to explain why there are so many tests that can be applied, including the stool guiac test (a chemical test looking for blood in the stool),[18] barium enema,[19] optical colonoscopy, and CTC.

Colonoscopy has been the gold standard (even if an imperfect one, since it misses 8%–11% of cancers in various studies) for screening for colon cancer. Unfortunately, despite the effectiveness of the test and considerable promotion of the value of screening (newscaster Katie Couric famously had a colonoscopy on her daytime news show to encourage viewers to get theirs), there has been poor public adherence to screening recommendations. This is largely because colonoscopy is uncomfortable, expensive, time-consuming, and, to many, embarrassing. The procedure requires rigorous preparation to cleanse the colon beginning the night before (many would say this is the worst part), remaining "npo" (nothing per mouth, meaning no eating or drinking) until the procedure is performed the next day, and a cocktail of drugs that usually puts the person to sleep (this is somewhat anomalously referred to as *conscious sedation*). As a result, most people lose a day from work. Clearly, there is a niche for a less complicated test that would address some of these problems and hopefully increase screening compliance.

Computed tomographic colonography has some of the virtues one would desire in this regard. It is considerably cheaper than colonoscopy, does not require anesthetic agents, and can be performed in minutes, allowing the individual to return to work the same day. Still, as currently performed, CTC requires a preprocedural colonic cleansing equivalent to that for colonoscopy. The patient must also remain npo until the CTC procedure is performed.

The radiologist pumps air or carbon dioxide through a tube into the rectum to expand the colon. Very-thin-slice CT scans cover the full extent of the colon in the

---

[17] Three major criteria for successful screening are satisfied: there is a long preclinical phase; we have tests that can find preclinical abnormalities; and removing polyps before they become cancer saves lives.

[18] Polyps and cancers have fragile surfaces that tend to bleed.

[19] Barium is a dense material that can be inserted into the colon, along with air, by a tube placed in the rectum. Polyps and cancers are seen as defects in the barium-coated colon.

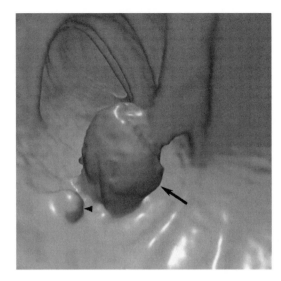

FIGURE 8-4

*Three-dimensional reconstruction of a CTC exam. A 1 cm polyp (arrow) on a stalk and another suspicious area—possibly a small, broad-based polyp (arrowhead)—lie adjacent to each other. (Courtesy of Drew Lambert, MD, the University of Virginia.) (See Color Figure 8-4 in the insert.)*

supine and prone positions so that polyps on all surfaces of the colon can be seen surrounded by gas. Radiologists view the images as axial (horizontal) slices through the abdomen and pelvis to search for abnormalities both within and outside the colon. They also have the computer reconstruct the images into a three-dimensional format, which they can view as a "fly-through" (Fig. 8-4). This Isaac Asimov-like fantastic voyage is like being in an airplane soaring through the colon. The three-dimensional search technique complements the painstaking two-dimensional search of the axial images to improve the detection of colonic polyps.

Colon perforation from the inflation tube is extremely rare. There is no need for intravenous contrast material. Concerns over the radiation dose are somewhat ameliorated by the fact that the exam is recommended only for those over 50 and only every 5 years in average-risk individuals. As a result, there is a very low risk of developing radiation-related cancers.

The early results of clinical studies showed both promise and disappointment. Computed tomography colonography did well at demonstrating very large polyps but less well with smaller polyps that many still consider to be important. More recently, three studies, each involving multiple sites, produced very different results (Pickhardt et al. 2003; Cotton et al. 2004; Johnson et al. 2003). It is not uncommon to see disparate results among different studies, especially when a technology is new and developing rapidly. In this case, many of the differences in results probably had to do with both differing CTC techniques and the generation of CT scanners that were employed.[20] The most recent studies—including a large multicenter clinical trial—showed true-positive rates comparable to those of colonoscopy (Kim et al. 2007; Johnson et al. 2008) with an acceptably low false-positive rate. In one study,

---

[20] New CT scanners have 4 to 64 detectors, allowing for scanning at higher speeds (to reduce motion) and producing thinner slices to better see small abnormalities.

patients indicated a clear preference for the new, imaging-based CTC procedure (Pickhardt et al. 2003).

Despite the apparent success of CTC in detecting polyps, there are problems that reduce the general acceptance of the procedure. To some extent, these revolve around the fact that CTC is strictly a diagnostic procedure, while colonoscopy is both diagnostic and therapeutic when polyps are found (when the colonoscopist finds a polyp, he or she inserts an instrument through the scope and removes it). Around 7%–10% of patients have polyps detected on CTC that will require colonoscopy, in addition, for their removal (Kim et al. 2007; Johnson et al. 2008). Ordinarily, this would mean a second, very discomforting colon-cleansing preparation prior to the colonoscopy. However, institutions, along with collaborating radiologist and gastroenterology practices, are increasingly working to arrange follow-up therapeutic colonoscopy on the same day as the positive CTC exam.

Nonetheless, it is unclear whether referring clinicians will be willing to simply follow 5- to 8-mm polyps, which are less accurately depicted by CTC, with subsequent repeat CTC or insist that they be removed by colonoscopy, as they mostly are today. In part at least, this decision may be related to turf issues over colon cancer screening and the fact that the colonoscopic removal of polyps is well paid. The success of CTC puts colonoscopy at risk, and colonoscopy is a substantial fraction of the work of many gastroenterologists. As a result, the rise of CTC has engendered considerable political conflict.

The positive results of the multicenter National CT Colonography Trial (NCTCT), a large, generalizable study validating the effectiveness of CTC (Johnson et al. 2008), led the ACS to recognize CTC as a front-line method of screening for colon cancer. The ACR and three gastroenterological societies joined the ACS in issuing joint guidelines recommending screening CTC for the first time. However, since removing polyps requires a separate clinical encounter involving colonoscopic removal of the offending lesion, payers have concerns about the potential of CTC to increase costs.

Currently, few insurers pay providers for performing CTC as a screening procedure.[21] In 2009, CMS declined to pay for CTC screening on its first evaluation for Medicare coverage, saying that the positive results of the major trials were not specifically designed for the Medicare age group (Dhruva et al. 2009). The American College of Radiology Imaging Network (ACRIN), which conducted the NCTCT, is reviewing the data with an eye to performing additional analyses to address CMS's concerns.

*CT Screening for Coronary Artery Disease*   Coronary artery disease kills more than 500,000 Americans annually and accounts for the single greatest disease expenditure in U.S. health care (Thompson and Stanford 2005). The principal disease process responsible for all of this illness and death is atherosclerosis. Atherosclerosis involves lipid (fat) deposition in the arterial wall and inflammation within the plaque deposits. A thin cap over a lipid core can rupture, leading to bleeding into the vessel

---

[21] Many payers have been reimbursing providers for CTC performed on patients who can not undergo colonoscopy or where colonoscopy was unsuccessful in seeing the entire colon.

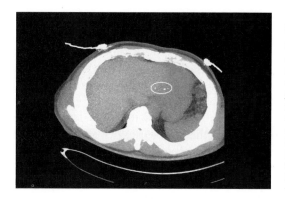

FIGURE 8-5

*Noncontrast CT calcium scoring exam of the heart in a patient with occasional chest pain. There are several small atherosclerotic calcifications in the expected course of the left coronary artery. (Courtesy of Patrick Norton, MD, the University of Virginia.)*

wall that facilitates clot formation resulting in an abrupt stoppage of blood flow to the heart muscle. This is known as *myocardial infarction* (heart attack). A screening test that would reduce mortality from this condition—the second leading killer of Americans behind cancer—would be an extraordinary benefit to the overall well-being of the population. Two imaging tests have been employed to conduct imaging screening for atherosclerosis: coronary artery calcium scoring and, more recently, CCTA.

The more established test is coronary calcium scoring (Fig. 8-5). As atherosclerotic foci (called *plaques*) age, they undergo an inflammatory reaction that can calcify. These calcifications can be seen on CT scans and the amount of calcification estimated. The idea behind the test is that the greater the amount of calcification, the higher the person's risk of having a coronary event. To some extent, this has been verified. People with a zero calcium score have little risk of a near-term coronary event (O'Rourke et al. 2000). Individuals with the highest scores have up to a six-fold increased likelihood of suffering a myocardial infarction (Shemesh et al. 2003). Intermediate-level scores hold up less well in predicting the risk of coronary events. This may be because a great deal of atherosclerosis is not calcified, so the test tends to underestimate the extent of disease (Thompson and Stanford 2005). The location of calcifications does not necessarily correlate with the actual locations of important narrowings and does not relate to weakened areas that may rupture.

Initially, a special technology was designed specifically to evaluate coronary artery calcifications, known as *electron beam CT* (EBCT). More recently, less expensive and more widely available multidetector CT (MDCT) has progressed to the point where its speed and resolution have been shown to be equivalent to those of EBCT for coronary calcium scoring (Daniell et al. 2005). From the perspective of a provider, the advantage to acquiring MDCT, rather than EBCT, for coronary calcium scoring is that MDCT is applicable more broadly to all CT applications throughout the body.

This said, there still is debate over the potential for coronary calcium scoring as a population-based screening test. There is some concern over the variability seen in the same patient with repeated testing over time. Scanning the same person at different sites can produce very different results. Most importantly, there is no solid research to confirm that population-based screening will do what it must do to be of value—significantly reduce serious illness or the number of deaths caused by coronary atherosclerosis.

The costs of population-based screening for coronary atherosclerotic disease would be even more astounding than for any cancer because atherosclerosis is so prevalent—indeed, ubiquitous—in our middle-aged and elderly populations. For many, this is a significant condition that will eventually cause problems or even death. For many others, it is an incidental abnormality (pseudodisease) that will be detected by the great sensitivity of CT and cause greater distress than if they had not undergone the screening exam. Given what would be a stupendous cost if insurers were to pay for coronary calcium screening to the general population, better data concerning the health impact of coronary calcium screening is essential.

A review article (Thompson and Stanford 2005) summarizing the consensus view of the utility of coronary calcium screening concluded that given the dearth of outcome data associated with screening and concerns over the cost of offering generalized screening with uncertain benefit, coronary calcium screening should be considered on a case-by-case basis in the following circumstances:

1  As an additional data point in individuals who have other important risk factors for coronary artery disease;
2. When evaluating low-risk individuals who present with atypical chest pain (note: this would not truly qualify as screening since these individuals are symptomatic);
3. For nonscreening applications, such as consideration of initiating or following patients on drug treatment regimens;
4. Many insurers pay for coronary calcium scoring but only in situations like those above for which physicians consider the test medically necessary.

Coronary calcium scoring is an *indirect test.* That is, the test does not directly visualize the specific lesions that will produce harm. A newer imaging test that actually does depict the narrowings in the coronary arteries is coronary CTA (CCTA) (Fig. 8-6). Coronary CTA involves the administration of contrast material, followed

FIGURE 8-6

*A CTA with a single stenosis of the left anterior descending artery (arrow) feeding the myocardium (heart muscle) of the left ventricle. (a) Two-dimensional cross-sectional view and (b) three-dimensional reconstruction. (Courtesy of Patrick Norton, MD, the University of Virginia) (See Color Figure 8-6b in the insert.)*

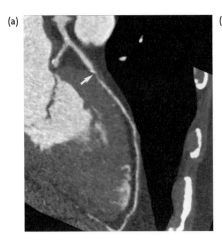
(a)

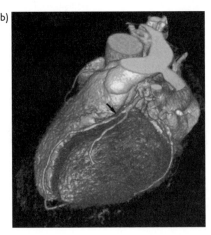
(b)

by very rapid (to "outrun" the motion of the heart and prevent blurring of the images) thin-slice CT scanning through the heart and adjacent major blood vessels, like the aorta and pulmonary arteries. The contrast material fills the coronary arteries, allowing the physician interpreting the study (usually a cardiologist or radiologist) to determine whether the coronary arteries are narrowed. Narrowings (called *stenoses*) of greater than 50% are considered clinically important and may require catheterization, during which the vessel can be further examined, and, if necessary, widened or stented.

As with most newly developed tests, there are numerous small and single institutional studies that indicate positive prospects for CCTA (e.g., Min et al. 2008). No major multicenter trials have been reported to indicate how the test would perform in a broad screening application. However, there is sufficient consistency in the research to suggest that CCTA is both sensitive (finds a high fraction of stenoses) and specific (accurately excludes serious disease in normal individuals) (Miller et al. 2008).

There are three critical issues that confront the acceptance of CCTA as a screening test. One we have already discussed in the context of the other possible imaging screening tests: there will be a large number of individuals who will have extensive atherosclerosis but who will not be clinically affected by their condition. These people will be at risk for unnecessary downstream imaging and overtreatment. A second concern is that CCTA may not be identifying the individuals at greatest risk of an acute cardiac event. There is mounting evidence that many, if not most, heart attacks are the result not simply of narrowed blood vessels but of an inflamed, weakened coronary artery wall (i.e., vulnerable plaque). Bleeding into the artery wall acutely blocks off blood flow to the heart muscle, which dies for lack of oxygen. Currently, there are no proven tests to detect these arterial wall abnormalities. Third, CCTA delivers high radiation doses to the thorax. Using CCTA regularly to examine normal individuals bears the risk of precipitating additional cancers (see Chapter 4). Coronary CTA is not recommended as a population-based screening test even for high-risk individuals (Kramer 2008).

Although some insurers are paying for CCTA examinations for specific clinical indications, no organization has yet supported population-based screening, nor does health insurance cover the procedure.

*CT Lung Cancer Screening*   Among both men and women, more deaths are caused by lung cancer than by any other malignancy—roughly 30% of all cancer deaths in the United States. One of the reasons lung cancer is so deadly is that it tends to grow silently for a variable period of time, so that when symptoms finally bring a patient to medical attention, the tumor has already spread (metastasized). Once metastases have occurred, the cancer can no longer be treated by surgical removal, and it is much less likely that the patient will survive. Hence, a method of screening that would accurately identify more disease in the asymptomatic phase might help reduce the death rate from this deadly disease.

Chest X-ray has been discarded as too insensitive for the efficient detection of early lung cancer. With improvements in CT—especially the introduction over the

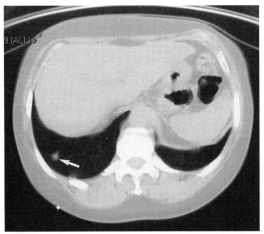

FIGURE 8-7

*A CT scan of the chest in a 71-year-old man who had smoked two packs of cigarettes a day for over 40 years. The arrow points to a stage I lung cancer found on a CT screening exam. (Courtesy of Mathew Bassignani, MD, the University of Virginia.)*

past several years of multidetector scanners[22]—there has developed great interest in employing annual chest CT to detect lung cancer in the at-risk population of middle-aged, long-term cigarette smokers.

With the exception of the risks of repeated irradiation,[23] there is limited procedure-related harm to individuals from CT screening for lung cancer, since contrast material is not routinely administered. Some studies suggested that screening CT identifies a large fraction of lung cancers in the earliest stage (Fig. 8-7) and has the potential for great improvements in long-term survival (Henschke et al. 1999, 2006; Kaneko et al. 2000). These studies fueled excitement over the possibility of population-based CT screening for middle-aged and elderly individuals with a long smoking history.

However, there have also been contradictory studies (Gohagen et al. 2005; Swensen et al. 2005; Bach et al. 2007) finding no mortality advantage in using CT to screen for lung cancer. Cost-effectiveness calculations have thus varied wildly, from just a few thousand dollars to hundreds of thousands of dollars per year of life saved.

The main reason for such disagreement is that all of the published results are based on *observational* studies. This means that all participants in the study have received screening CT. There is no *control*, or comparison, group of participants, who has not received screening CT that would make it clearer whether regularly performed screening CT actually reduces the death rate. Critics of the positive observational

[22] Multidetector CT scanners, as their name implies, have more than one digital "plate" to receive the X-rays that have passed through the patient's body. With more detectors comes the capability of producing more slices simultaneously through the body. The result is faster scanning with the capability of generating thinner slices in the same or less time as older single-detector scanners. This means that multidetector scanners can produce better images of smaller abnormalities. Manufacturers now commonly produce and sell 16- and 64-detector scanners, and 254-slice scanners are available.

[23] Computed tomography scans generate 70 times the radiation of a chest X-ray, but this is of less concern for carcinogenesis in the target middle-aged and older age groups.

studies point to biases in observational research that can explain the strikingly positive results (Black and Baron 2007). These critics say that only randomized clinical trials (RCTs) with experimental and control groups—the conventional gold standard of clinical research—can truly determine whether there is a benefit in reducing the death rate. Such trials are underway in both the United States and Europe. The various trial results are scheduled to be reported between 2011 and 2015.

There is some debate as to how much CT screening would have to reduce the death rate to be considered effective. Based on a statistical extrapolation of their observational data, the International Early Lung Cancer Action Project (I-ELCAP) researchers believe that 80%–90% of lung cancer deaths could be avoided. The largest RCT, the National Lung Screening Trial (NLST), has repeatedly screened 50,000 subjects with either CT or chest X-ray to determine if the death rate has been decreased by at least 20%. The debate is not merely of academic interest. If CT lung cancer screening proves effective, it might save tens of thousands of lives annually. At the same time, regularly screening U.S. smokers would be very expensive, adding tens of billions of dollars annually to the health care budget and perhaps taking resources away from other important uses. As some smoking cessation advocacy groups have pointed out, it also begs the question of whether scarce dollars spent on screening could better be spent getting smokers to quit smoking.

The main reason CT screening would be so expensive is that the remarkable spatial resolution of multidetector CT enables radiologists to see very small nodules (lumps) in the lungs. Such nodules are extremely common. In one large case series, 74% of the 1520 people enrolled had lung nodules (Swensen et al. 2005), yet only a small fraction of the nodules discovered by CT was actually cancer. Most of the rest were meaningless inflammatory nodules from a previous infection like histoplasmosis or tuberculosis. Nonetheless, many of these benign nodules will compel further workup (mostly repetitive CT and PET scans over as much as two years) and produce great anxiety among patients. A small number would even go on to biopsy or removal (remember the story of Dr. Casarella). By far the greatest generator of costs in lung cancer screening relates to these false-positive diagnoses.

The ACS and the American College of Chest Physicians continue to recommend against CT screening for lung cancer pending the results of RCTs, whereas the USPSTF and the ACR do not make specific recommendations either for or against the practice. There is little, if any, insurance payment for CT lung cancer screening. While some individuals who are anxious about their smoking history have been willing to pay for CT screening themselves, this trend has not caught on among the large number of current and former cigarette smokers, perhaps because of the significant recurring cost of annual screening recommended by screening advocates.

*Whole Body CT Screening*  Despite the huge amount of publicity about whole body CT screening in the past decade, there has been little research on the effectiveness of this modality in reducing death rates. In fact, a large part of the problem is that, unlike all the other accepted and proposed imaging screening tests, with whole body CT screening there is no specific target condition. Facilities that offer whole body scanning tend to offer coronary calcium scoring for atherosclerosis, CTC for colon cancer, and a general cancer screen in addition.

Depending on the imaging center, a whole body scan includes anything from just the chest, abdomen, and pelvis to the full Monty—from the top of the skull to the tips of the toes. Most facilities conducting whole body scanning do not inject contrast material, so contrast allergy poses a problem only in the minority of facilities where the use of contrast media is part of the protocol. Radiation exposure is a concern for whole body scanning. There is potential for a long-term accumulated radiation dose, since the examination is being touted by some as appropriate for adults of all ages. This means that younger individuals who received repeated exams over several years could potentially accumulate enough radiation and have enough time for radiation-related cancers to develop. The use of the newer multidetector scanners exposes patients to higher radiation doses, which further increases the risk of radiation-induced cancers over time.

To an extent even greater than for other imaging screening exams, whole body screening raises concerns for both false-negative and false-positive diagnoses. The ability to accurately detect abnormalities inside organs depends heavily on the use of contrast material. With or without contrast material administration, false-positive diagnoses and pseudodisease are extremely common. Some centers have reported that they find abnormalities in more than 90% of the people they screen. The great majority of these findings are not significant threats to health. Indeed, they are overwhelmingly likely to be simple anatomical variations that either mimic disease or are what clinicians call *incidentalomas*—abnormalities like cysts of the kidneys or liver, benign tumors of the adrenal glands, or liver hemangiomas—which are extremely common but will not adversely affect health. Regardless, the identification of these abnormalities often provokes further testing (usually at the screening center that identified the original finding) and, in rare instances, inappropriate treatment. The false-positive diagnoses associated with whole body CT scanning pose by far the most significant risk to individuals choosing to undergo this procedure.

One might reasonably ask, "What's the harm? It's a free country." If people wish to spend their discretionary income on a whole body CT screening exam and assume the risks of an incorrect diagnosis, that's their concern. As with most things in health care, it's not so simple. While the initial screening exam itself is paid for by the individual receiving the service, the follow-on studies generated by the large number of false-positive findings are usually paid for by the individual's health insurance or by government programs like Medicare. The positive screening finding—whether it identifies a life-threatening condition, a false positive, an incidentaloma, or pseudo-disease—creates a situation of "medical necessity." As a result, all of whatever diagnosis and treatment that occurs afterward is paid for by either governmental or private insurance. Once discovered, the screening finding may also serve as a benchmark for a "preexisting condition" which may adversely affect someone's ability to obtain health insurance, or increase their premiums. In other words, ultimately, we all pay a portion of the cost of false-positive outcomes of whole body CT screening in the form of higher taxes or insurance premiums.

The large number of individuals who would have to be studied and the related enormous expense of an RCT of whole body CT screening ensure that such a trial will likely never occur. When a clinical trial is impossible, an alternative approach is to perform a *decision analysis*. In conducting a decision analysis, researchers employ the best available information and expert opinion to develop a sample of virtual patients. The decision analysis models what fraction of patients will show disease and what might happen to them in terms of diagnosis, treatment, and outcome, depending on whether or not they receive the screening test. One such cost-effectiveness analysis for whole body screening addressed six common cancers, coronary artery disease, and abdominal aortic aneurysm.[24] The finding was that whole body CT screening was not cost-effective, with a probable cost of $149,500 per year of life saved[25] (Beinfeld et al. 2005).

No major organization supports the concept of CT whole body screening. The ACR has made the following statement:

> The ACR, at this time, does not believe there is sufficient evidence to justify recommending total body CT screening for patients with no symptoms or a family history suggesting disease. To date, there is no evidence that total body CT screening is cost effective or effective in prolonging life. In addition, the ACR is concerned that this procedure will lead to the discovery of numerous findings that will not ultimately affect patients' health but will result in unnecessary follow-up examinations and treatments and significant wasted expense.[26]

## The Business of Imaging Screening

Although the cost-effectiveness of screening provides the backdrop for payment and policy decisions, it is the business of imaging screening that has drawn commercial, consumer, and most media attention.

At first glance, imaging screening seems to be a very good business. The public believes in screening (Schwartz et al. 2004), and the kinds of diseases new imaging technologies like CT are good at detecting are the most common killers in developed societies—cancer and cardiovascular disease. Almost everyone has heard a compelling anecdote of how imaging screening has saved a life and, at least subconsciously, has considered whether some deadly process is insidiously developing within his or her own body. Many people may have read in the lay press about the much ballyhooed successes of various screening procedures in observational studies. These results have been avidly promoted by imaging screening facilities with little regard for the scientific deficiencies of the studies.

Entrepreneurs—physicians and nonphysicians alike—flooded into the imaging screening center business in the early 1990s. The early market leaders developed facilities devoted primarily to imaging screening, often backed by supportive equipment

[24] An abdominal aortic aneurysm is a widening of the body's biggest vessel as it courses through the belly. The bigger the aneurysm gets, the more likely it is to contain clot that could break off and be carried to the kidneys, other organs, and legs or rupture and cause almost instant death.

[25] Any cost-effectiveness analysis requires many assumptions that can vary greatly. A good cost-effectiveness analysis, therefore, requires that numerous calculations be performed, producing both a "most likely" result and a range of other possible expenditures that might occur if other assumptions prove more accurate.

[26] http://ww.acr.org/s_acr/doc.esp?trackID=&SID=1&DID=16014&CID=2192&VID=2& RTID=0&CIDQS=&Taxonomy=False&Specialsearch=False.

manufacturers, who felt that this might provide the next boost for an already rap-idly growing industry. Mostly located in larger cities, these entrepreneurial facil-ities heavily marketed the benefits of screening and offered "special discounts" for organizations like church groups and civic organizations. There soon developed a glut of facilities that began to undercut each other on price, particularly in areas like southern California and Florida, where competition to provide imaging screen-ing services was most intense (Kolata 2005). The marketing arguments for imaging screening typically focused on just a small set of issues:

"It's like an annual physical exam, but much more precise."

"When someone is willing to pay, should anyone be able to deny that person valu-able information about his or her own body?"

"It's like screening mammography, which has saved countless lives."[27]

Typically, the bread-and-butter screening service was *unenhanced* (no contrast medium) whole body CT screening. Many operations featured an immediate con-sultation with the radiologist to go over the preliminary imaging results.[28] Patrons often received a CD of their images to take home for their own future viewing or for consultation with their physician (or to share with their friends). The intent was to provide a more personal, customer-friendly experience than often occurs in hospital outpatient imaging facilities or even radiologists' private offices.

Initially, imaging facilities dedicated to screening were a going concern. They appealed to the worried well, particularly the boomer generation, whose members have both a greater preoccupation with their health and more money to spend on health and longevity than preceding generations (Goldsmith 2008). Imaging screen-ing procedures were uncritically popularized in the media. Oprah underwent a whole body screening CT, invited the well-known radiologist-entrepreneur owner of the facility[29] onto her television show, and told her millions of fans how wonder-ful it was to know that one was truly well. Investors flocked to rapidly growing chains.

And then, all of sudden, the party was over. To understand why, consider the instructive example of radiologist Michael Brant-Zawadzki, who related how his initially lucrative business in imaging screening went into precipitous decline and cratered in less than three years.

Dr. Brant-Zawadzki, known to many as BZ, was part of an 18-person radiol-ogy group in Orange County, California. There, he witnessed firsthand the birth of the concept of *high-touch*, consumer-oriented imaging screening as practiced by Harvey Eisenberg, another Orange County radiologist who is generally recognized as a pioneer in this field.

BZ became convinced not only of the potential benefits to health of CT screening (Brant-Zawadzki 2002) but also of its viability as a business. In the waning years of the twentieth century, his group opened a screening center in Southern California

---

[27] We hope we have adequately explained in preceding sections why each screening applica-tion is different.

[28] Radiologists vary enormously in the amount of time it takes them to fully review a set of CT images, so, most often, a full and final report would be sent to the patient at a later time.

[29] Dr. Harvey Eisenberg, introduced below.

and saw their professional revenues increase by over 10% in the first year of operations. Emboldened, BZ gathered what he described as "friends and family" investors to finance four screening centers in New York City, where he saw a nearly virgin market for imaging screening services. The first center opened under the rubric of CT Screening International (CTSI) in May 2001. As BZ described it, the events of 9/11, just four months later, may have had the most salient adverse effect on his business.

However, he also recognized that there were important problems with both his marketing assumptions and the business model that contributed to his venture's rapid demise. With regard to the former, he believes that the public and, more importantly, other physicians were not yet ready for the *concierge* model of health care delivery now gaining popularity among the well-off in some areas of the country. CTSI had not made the connections they needed with primary care physicians nor given them any reason to refer their patients. With respect to the business model, BZ felt that radiologists—who have been well compensated for their traditional activities—failed to perceive the potential of imaging screening. He also believed that any number of facilities failed because they couldn't interest radiologists in a high-touch patient care model, wherein radiologists meet and talk with clients following each examination.

As one examines the large number of similar failures, fundamental flaws in the basic business model are revealed. Fewer people were willing to pay out of pocket (in those heady early days, as much as $2000 a scan) than the entrepreneurs had imagined. Even more importantly, once patients had undergone scanning and learned that they were healthy (perhaps after several anxiety-provoking diagnostic tests to follow up on the screening findings), there were few repeat customers. As has been noted on several occasions in this chapter, screening should occur at regular intervals to pick up newly developed (*incident*) disease. The fact that there were (and still are) no authoritative recommendations on what might be an appropriate interval for repeating an unproven screening test did little to encourage customers to return.

Slowly, media skepticism increased, drawing public attention to the potential for abuse (Kolata 2005). The FDA published a warning about the risks of radiation associated with CT screening on its public Web site [http://www.fda.gov/cdrh/ct] and insurers, perhaps worried more about the downstream costs than the possible health effects, supported the government's concerns.

Perhaps most importantly, traditional purveyors of imaging—mainly hospitals and radiologists, but also other specialists with imaging equipment in their offices—began to take on some of the newer focused imaging screening procedures, particularly chest CT for lung cancer and coronary calcium screening for coronary artery disease. These entrenched providers, with their well-established networks of physician referrals and their greater resource base, usually proved to be too much competition for less well-known screening newcomers.

In addition, because of their physician-to-physician relationships, established imaging providers were in a better position to provide the follow-on imaging tests that resulted from the initial screening exams. While patients can refer themselves to some providers for a self-pay screening test, insurers require a referring physician in order to pay for "medically necessary" follow-on imaging tests. Many radiologists offering screening tests will not accept individuals who refer themselves, requiring an order from their referring physician. In part, this may be because of concern that the screening test is not indicated, but the radiologist also may be concerned that, in the absence of a referring physician, he or she will be taking on legal responsibility for the care of the patient if abnormalities are discovered. Few diagnostic radiologists seek or are equipped to accept direct patient care responsibilities.

## Ethics, Politics, and Money

In addition to the issues cited in the preceding section, there are a number of ethical and economic concerns related to the diffusion of unproven imaging screening tests. The most significant, perhaps, is the one already discussed: while individuals who choose to undergo screening may or may not benefit from it, the costs they generate in the diagnosis of screening findings are shared by us all. The situation is exacerbated by a small number of unscrupulous providers who recommend to referring physicians that patients with positive screening findings undergo unnecessary testing for incidentalomas and other marginal indications—a process known as *churning*—to increase revenue.

Radiologists already are stressed by the work of interpreting diagnostic imaging studies. An increase in examinations related to unproven screening methods might overwhelm radiologists and shift their work from helping to diagnose patients with symptomatic disease to purposes of lesser societal value. Of even greater social concern is that if only those who can afford to pay out of pocket for screening examinations receive them, there will be an even greater disparity in health care access and utilization between rich and poor than already exists today. Because of the subsidization of follow-on studies in positive cases, in essence the poor might actually be supporting unnecessary care for the wealthy, as well as experiencing lengthening delays in receiving treatment themselves.

These equity considerations receive little attention because, although they are important, more practical considerations of personal preferences, politics, and money generally carry the day in deciding whether individual screening exams are performed and, ultimately, whether screening programs are covered by payers.

Research into the value of screening is also susceptible to infringements by political and financial concerns. As a prime example, consider the case of CT screening for lung cancer. Earlier in this chapter, we reviewed the case for lung cancer screening, indicating that this is an application that remains in dispute. In fact, the argument between those who favor the immediate institution of a national screening program and those who wish to wait for the outcome of RCTs to decide whether broad-based screening is cost-effective has been highly politicized. On one side are the I-ELCAP researchers who generated the positive observational results detailed earlier. They are joined by the medical device industry and some advocacy groups—notably the Lung Cancer Alliance (LCA)—which see CT screening as potentially lifesaving.

The I-ELCAP researchers have repeatedly called for government and private health insurers to pay for CT screening immediately, based on their observational study results. They have called RCTs like the National Lung Screening Trial unethical given their positive interpretations of their own results (Goldberg 2007a). The other side is largely represented by the researchers involved in the RCTs—most notably the NLST[30] in the United States—the government agency funding the trial (the National Cancer Institute, [NCI]), and government and private insurers leery of the expected costs of a population-based screening program. Their argument is that the I-ELCAP observation of prolonged survival is explainable by the biases of observational screening studies and that no benefit of screening in lowering the death rate has been shown.

The debate has grown nasty at times. Reputations are on the line, and big money is involved. There have been claims of conflict of interest on both sides that call into question the validity of the other's research. The Lung Cancer Alliance (LCA) discovered that one of the two lead researchers (known as the *principal investigator* [PI] of the NLST,[31] radiologist Denise Aberle, had, at around the time of the initiation of the trial (2003), provided in a Louisiana state court scientific evidence on CT screening as a witness for the American Tobacco Company (now part of Reynolds American, Inc.) (Armstrong 2007). Her university (UCLA) was paid for her testimony. This was inflammatory to the LCA because many smokers were suing the tobacco companies for the cost of lifetime CT screening as partial compensation for their tobacco-related injuries.

The LCA first sought to have NIH terminate the NLST on the basis of what they perceived to be a serious conflict of interest that might affect the veracity of the trial. When this met resistance at the highest levels, the LCA leadership suggested that the NLST data accrued through 2007 be combined with NLST data and the data of two foreign trials. The NCI investigated the possibility but eventually opposed this action. The methods of the trials were sufficiently different that any result would be questionable. Indeed, biostatistician Dr. Donald Berry, a member of the panel appointed by the NCI to study the question, said it was like "pooling apples, oranges, lemons, and limes" (Goldberg 2008b).

Perhaps contributing to the panel's decision was that, at about the same time, the I-ELCAP researchers also were implicated in conflicts of interest. An investigation by *The Cancer Letter* revealed that the I-ELCAP research had been partially supported by a foundation funded by the tobacco industry (Goldberg 2007b).

Superficially, the interest of the cigarette manufacturers might seem counterintuitive. However, tobacco companies might well benefit from the adoption of CT lung cancer screening. A reliable screening test that would identify curable cancers might encourage hard-core cigarette smokers to risk continuing their habit. At the very least, insurer payment for screening CT scans might limit the liability of the tobacco companies from smokers asking the courts to make the tobacco companies pay for these exams.

*The Cancer Letter* also found conflicts related to the I-ELCAP researchers' relationships with the medical device industry (Goldberg 2008a). Two lead researchers had failed to disclose to journals publishing the research information concerning

---

[30] One of the authors of this book, Dr. Hillman, was principal investigator of ACRIN, an organization partnering with NCI in the design and conduct of the NLST.

[31] The NLST is actually a collaboration of two research entities. Dr. Aberle directs the efforts of ACRIN. The other PI is Dr. Christine Berg, an NIH employee who heads the Lung Screening Study (LSS).

patents they held related to CT screening and had received licensing revenues from the industry (Goldberg 2008a). Failing to disclose financial relationships that might influence their research was viewed by many as an infraction of research ethics and led ACS Chief Medical Officer Otis Brawley to indicate that a thorough audit of I-ELCAP data would be necessary before its published results could be taken seriously. "If you're using blood money, you need to tell people you're using blood money," said Brawley (Goldberg 2008c, p. 2). The ACS provided I-ELCAP more than $100,000 in grants from 2004 to 2007, money it probably would not have given had it known of the tobacco industry grants (Harris 2008).

The accusations of conflicts of interest on both sides spurred a broader investigation of conflicts affecting federally funded research undertaken by Representative John Dingell, chairman of the House Energy and Commerce Committee, and Representative Bart Stupak, chairman of the House Subcommittee on Oversight and Investigations.

It is not just at the elevated levels of government and industry that conflicts over new imaging screening tests occur. Indeed, the most vigorous battles are fought among physician specialists, hand to hand on the ground, where clinical services are provided. Imaging screening has attracted a good deal of attention from numerous medical specialties.

For example, many gastroenterologists—the specialists who primarily perform colonoscopy—feel threatened that CTC screening could greatly reduce the performance of their bread-and-butter procedure, colonoscopy. As a response, small gastroenterologist practices are coalescing into mega-groups to acquire CT scanners for their office practices so that they can perform CTC. Similarly, as described above, cardiologists are buying CT scanners to perform a host of cardiac procedures, including CT screening examinations.

There are important societal implications here. The financial imperative to fill the capacity of the scanners might encourage self-referring physicians to recommend unproven screening examinations to their patients as a vehicle for generating downstream therapeutic procedures. As mentioned earlier, research on regional variations in the use of health care services has found a strong correlation between the number of scanners in a locale and the number of examinations performed.

## The Future of Imaging Screening

The goal of this chapter has been to educate readers on what imaging screening is, how it works, why proven screening is beneficial, and why readers should be careful in deciding to undergo an unproven screening examination.

Several technical advances could make imaging screening work more efficiently and produce more accurate and meaningful results. It is wasteful to screen the entire population when only a portion of the population is susceptible to the target disease. Identifying more accurately who is at greater risk of a given illness would help reduce the costs of both the screening examination and the number of false-positive diagnoses. It would ensure that fewer individuals would be harmed by the screening process and greatly reduce the wasted follow-on medical expense.

For example, molecular medicine might spur great increases in screening efficiency by improving risk stratification. Imagine, for example, a simple, inexpensive blood or urine test that could determine whether a patient's genetic code puts her at risk for developing, say, breast cancer.[32] Imagine, moreover, that this molecular test was very good at expressing the actual risk, enabling physicians to tailor the optimal screening approach for her as an individual—including determining which test would best demonstrate her cancer if it existed, how frequently she should be screened, or even if she needed any imaging screening at all. The issue of how imaging fits into the new world of molecular medicine will be explored in greater detail in Chapter 9.

The other major scientific advance that could promote more effective screening would be tests that could measure the biological aggressiveness of the abnormalities found on screening. As noted several times in this chapter, the greatest harm and cost associated with imaging screening programs derive from the fact that imaging "sees too much." Imaging screening identifies many more insignificant findings than ones for which treatment would really benefit patients. Tests that could rapidly and accurately differentiate benign from malignant growths, as well as slow-growing abnormalities that are actually pseudodisease, would help narrow treatment choices, relieve patients' anxiety, and greatly diminish screening-related costs.

Some candidate technologies are emerging that might help in this regard. As one example, the PET imaging compound, 18-FLT ([F-18]-3″-fluoro-3′-deoxy-L-thymidine), has been shown in a number of small single-institutional trials to be taken into cancer cells more than into normal cells. Thymidine is a building block of DNA, so 18-FLT is a measure of how quickly cells are proliferating. Future trials will indicate whether 18-FLT can serve as a measure of a cancer's aggressiveness, for which tumors 18-FLT PET can be accurately applied, and what relationship exists between using the test and improving patients' health outcomes.

For the present, however, we have little that is really effective in helping us to distinguish clinically significant from insignificant findings revealed by imaging screening. Tests that would help us determine which abnormalities need to be treated and which could be left alone would be a tremendous advance in making imaging screening better for patients and more cost-effective for society.

Improving the science behind imaging screening is the one thing that would do the most to address a much broader question: even if we had a good new imaging screening test, how would we pay for it? A new screening test for a widespread deadly condition would add billions of dollars of cost. Regardless of what benefits we'd enjoy, this might mean that to implement the new test, we'd have to forego some other valuable medical service or transfer moneys originally intended for education, road building/repair, high speed rail, or other services. This thorny problem is addressed in the concluding chapter.

At present, the prices charged for unproven imaging screening examinations poorly reflect their costs. In the absence of insurance coverage, the prices are set by providers based on what they believe will be attractive to individuals seeking the examination or to serve broader organizational goals, like capturing individuals with

---

[32] This is not as simple as identifying a single gene, like BRCA. Most cancers develop as the result of a not fully understood complex of multigenetic activity and interaction with environmental influences, such as diet, infections, and other stressors.

positive findings for follow-on imaging studies and treatment. As a result, individuals seeking screening may pay highly variable amounts for the same procedure.

There still remains the question of how to deal with individuals who choose to undergo unproven imaging screening tests and how their actions can adversely affect others who do not. We have noted in this chapter that individuals choosing to be screened by unproven tests must pay the initial cost of the test itself. A large fraction of these individuals will have positive findings. These findings generate further imaging and nonimaging testing, which, because "medical necessity" is triggered, is paid for by private and government insurance programs, regardless of whether the findings represent a truly dangerous and treatable condition, a false-positive diagnosis, or pseudodisease. This leads to a skewed distribution of medical resources that adds considerable cost to society and threatens access to needed care.

One solution would be for insurers not to pay for the downstream costs of unproven screening tests until a positive diagnosis is made and the patient must undergo treatment. Putting the individual choosing to undergo unproven screening at financial risk would be a fairer solution than what occurs today. Or, as P.J. O'Rourke wrote, "There is only one basic human right, the right to do as you damn well please. And with it comes the only basic human duty, the duty to take the consequences."[33]

Authoritative organizations like the ACR and the ACS can help reduce the burden of costs associated with unproven imaging screening tests by providing better information to guide public actions (Black and Baron 2007). As examples, one group of screening experts has advised the ACR to develop a "screening scorecard" that would be regularly updated and would inform the public of the scientific and insurance payment status for a host of popular imaging screening examinations (Hillman et al. 2005). The organization also was advised to develop an "informed consent" document that radiologists could use to detail the risks and benefits to individuals before they undergo imaging screening. Fully informed individuals might make very different choices about whether to undergo imaging screening, to the benefit of us all.

Future imaging screening has considerable potential to improve health, particularly as molecular medicine begins to provide tools for radiologists to shift from screening large, undifferentiated populations to monitoring disease in individuals who have a demonstrably higher risk. The prudent use of imaging screening tests requires that the public better recognize both the personal and societal downsides of imaging screening. Finally, public dialogue must address the issue of how we will pay for all of the extraordinary advances in imaging screening technologies that could potentially improve the public's health in the future.

## References

Armstrong D. Critics question objectivity of government lung-scan study. *The Wall Street Journal,* October 8, 2007:B1. http://online.wsj.com/article/SB119179920110451468.html?mod=googlenews_wsj. Accessed April 3, 2010.

Bach PB, Jett JR, Pastorino U, et al. Computed tomography screening and lung cancer outcomes. *JAMA.* 2007;297:953–961.

[33] http://www.cato.org/speeches/sp-orourke.html.

Beam C, Sullivan D, Layde P. Effect of human variability on independent double reading in screening mammography. *Acad Radiol.* 1996;3:891–897.

Beinfeld MT, Wittenberg E, Gazelle GS. Cost-effectiveness of whole body CT screening. *Radiology.* 2005;234:415–422.

Berg W, Blume J, Cormack J, et al. Combined screening with ultrasound and mammography compared to mammography alone: results of the first year in ACRIN 6666. *JAMA.* 2008;299:2151–2163.

Black WC, Baron JA. CT Screening for lung cancer: spiraling into confusion? *JAMA.* 2007;297:995–997.

Brant-Zawadzki M. CT screening: why I do it. *AJR Am J Roentgenol.* 2002;179:319–326.

Casarella WJ. A patient's viewpoint on a current controversy. *Radiology.* 2002;224:927.

Cotton PB, Durkalski VL, Pineau BC, et al. Computed tomographic colonography—a multi-center comparison with standard colonoscopy for detection of colorectal neoplasia. *JAMA.* 2004;291:1713–1719.

Daniell AL, Wong ND, Friedmena JD, et al. Concordance of coronary calcium estimates between MDCT and electron beam tomography. *AJR Am J Roentgenol.* 2005;185:1542–1545.

Dhruva SS, Phurrough SE, Salive ME, et al. CMS's landmark decision on CT colonography—examining the relevant data. *N Engl J Med.* 2009;360:2699–2701.

Duffy SW, Tabar L, Smith RA. The mammography screening trials: commentary on the recent work by Olsen and Gotzsche. *CA Cancer J Clin.* 2002;535:68–71.

Eddy DM, Nugent TW, Eddy JF, et al. Screening for colon cancer in a high risk population: results of a mathematical model. *Gastroenterology.* 1987;92:682–692.

Feig SA. Effect of service screening mammography on population mortality from breast carcinoma. *Cancer.* 2002;95:451–457.

Gohagen JK, Marcus PM, Fagerstrom RM, et al. Final results of the Lung Screening Study: a randomized feasibility study of spiral CT versus chest X-ray screening for lung cancer. *Lung Cancer.* 2005;47:9–15.

Goldberg P. Study finds no benefit from CT screening; advocacy group alleges "delaying tactic." *Cancer Letter.* 2007a;33(March 9):1–4.

Goldberg P. House committee begins investigation of NCI's National Lung Screening Trial. *Cancer Letter.* 2007b(October 26);33:1–7.

Goldberg P. I-ELCAP leaders named as inventors on 27 patents: journals probe disclosures. *Cancer Letter.* 2008a;34(January 18):1–8.

Goldberg P. Panel recommends against pooling results on NLST, European studies and I-ELCAP. *Cancer Letter.* 2008b;34(September 26):1–7.

Goldberg P. ACS Chief Medical Officer Brawley urges audit of I-ELCAP lung screening data. *Cancer Letter.* 2008c;34(September 26):1–3.

Goldsmith J. *The Long Baby Boom: An Optimistic Vision for a Graying Generation.* Baltimore: Johns Hopkins University Press, 2008.

Gotszche PC, Olsen O. Is screening for breast cancer with mammography justifiable? *Lancet.* 2000;355:129–134.

Harris G. Cigarette company paid for lung cancer study. *New York Times,* March 26, 2008. http://www.nytimes.com/2008/03/26/health/research/26lung.html?_r=1&sq=gardiner %20harris%20&st=nyt&scp=2&pagewanted=print&oref=slogin. Accessed April 3, 2010.

Henschke CI, McCauley DI, Yankelevitz DL, et al. Early Lung Cancer Action Project: overall design and findings from baseline screening. *Lancet.* 1999;354:99–105.

Henschke C, Yankelevitz D, Libby DM, et al. Survival of patients with stage I lung cancer detected on CT screening. *N Engl J Med.* 2006;355:1763–1771.

Hillman BJ, Amis ES, Weinreb JC, et al. The future of imaging screening—proceedings of the fourth annual ACR Forum. *J Am Coll Radiol.* 2005;2:43–50.

Hillman BJ, Black WC, D'Orsi C, et al. The appropriateness of employing imaging screening technologies—report of the methods committee of the ACR Task Force on Screening Technologies. *J Am Coll Radiol.* 2004;1:861–865.

Johnson CD, Chen MH, Toledano P, et al. Accuracy of CT colonography for detection of large adenomas and cancers. *N Engl J Med.* 2008;358:1207–1217.

Johnson CD, Harmsen WS, Wilson LA, et al. Prospective blinded evaluation of computed tomographic colonography for screen detection of colorectal polyps. *Gastroenterology.* 2003;125:311–319.

Kaneko M, Kusumoto M, Kobayashi T, et al. CT screening for lung cancer in Japan. *Cancer.* 2000;89(suppl):2485–2488.

Kim DH, Pickhardt PJ, Taylor AJ. CT colonography versus colonoscopy for the detection of advanced neoplasia. *N Engl J Med.* 2007;357:1403–1412.

Kolata G. Rapid rise and fall of body-scanning clinics. *New York Times*, January 23, 2005. http://www.nytimes.com/2005/01/23/health/23scans.html?pagewanted=print&position. Accessed April 3, 2010.

Kolata G. Cancer Society, in shift, has concerns on screening. *New York Times*, October 20, 2009:A1.

Kramer CM. Should all high-risk patients be screened with computed tomography angiography? *Circulation.* 2008;117:1333–1339.

Lee CH, Dershaw DD, Kopans D, et al. Breast cancer screening with imaging: recommendations from the Society of Breast Imaging and the ACR on the use of mammography, breast MRI, breast ultrasound, and other technologies for the detection of clinically occult breast cancer. *J Am Coll Radiol.* 2010;7:18–27.

Lehman C, Gatsonis C, Kuhl C, et al. MRI evaluation of the contralateral breast in women recently diagnosed with breast cancer. *N Engl J Med.* 2007;356:1295–1303.

Miller JM, Rochitte CE, Dewey M, et al. Diagnostic performance of coronary angiography by 64-row CT. *N Engl J Med.* 2008;359:2324–2336.

Min JK, Kang N, Shaw LJ, et al. Costs and clinical outcomes after coronary multidetector CT angiography in patients without known coronary artery disease: comparison to myocardial perfusion SPECT. *Radiology.* 2008;249:62–70.

O'Rourke RA, Brundage BH, Froelicher VF, et al. American College of Cardiology/American Heart Association expert consensus document on electron beam computed tomography for the diagnosis and prognosis of coronary artery disease. *Circulation.* 2000;102:126–140.

Pickhardt PJ, Choi JR, Hwang I, et al. Computed tomographic virtual colonoscopy for colorectal neoplasia in asymptomatic adults *N Engl J Med.* 2003;349:2191–2200.

Pisano E, Gatsonis C, Hendrick RE, et al. Diagnostic performance of digital versus film mammography for breast cancer screening. *N Engl J Med.* 2005;353:1773–1783.

Schwartz LM, Woloshin S, Floyd FJ, et al. Enthusiasm for screening in the United States. *JAMA.* 2004;291:71–78.

Selby JV, Friedman GD, Quesenberry CP, et al. A case control study of screening sigmoidoscopy and mortality from colon cancer. *N Engl J Med.* 1992;326:653–657.

Shemesh J, Apter S, Itzchak Y, et al. Coronary calcification compared in patients with acute versus in those with chronic coronary events by using double sector spiral CT. *Radiology.* 2003;226:483–488.

Sickles EA, Wolverton DE, Deke KE. Performance parameters for screening and diagnostic mammography: specialists and general radiologists. *Radiology.* 2002;224:861–869.

Smith RA, Saslow D, Sawyer KA, et al. American Cancer Society guidelines for breast cancer screening: update 2003. *CA Cancer J Clin.* 2003;53:141–169.

Spurgeon D, Burton TM. For the very cautious a physical exam now includes a CAT scan. *Wall Street J.* March 23, 2000:A1.

Swensen SJ, Jett JR, Hartman TE. CT screening for lung cancer: five-year prospective experience. *Radiology.* 2005;235:259–265.

Taplin S, Abraham L, Barlow WE, et al. Mammography facilities characteristics associated with interpretive accuracy of screening mammography. *J Natl Cancer Inst.* 2008;100:876–887.

Thompson BH, Stanford W. Update on using coronary calcium screening by computed tomography to measure risk for coronary heart disease. *Int J Cardiovasc Imag.* 2005;21:39–53.

Thrall JH. U.S. Preventative Services Task Force recommendations for screening mammography: evidence-based medicine or the death of science? *J Am Coll Radiol.* 2010;10:2–4.

Wang S, Rockoff JD, Martinez B. Group issues clarification on mammography advice. *Wall Street J.* November 20, 2009:A1.

# 9

# The Future of Medical Imaging

*The year is 2036. A seemingly healthy 46-year-old woman named Lucinda Hanson enters an octagonal room for her annual imaging screening examination. A technologist sits behind a computer console directing the study. A fellow technologist in the adjacent scanner room hooks a vaporizer mask over Lucinda's nose and mouth. Lucinda lies recumbent, fully conscious, in a sophisticated advanced imaging device known as the Omniscient. The Omniscient employs a completely safe radiant energy, discovered in 2027 during testing of advanced positron-based target sensing technology by the Defense Advanced Research Projects Agency.*

*The lead technologist directs his colleague to administer a completely safe, odorless, gaseous molecular contrast agent and then conducts a scan that assesses genomic risk. The agent passes into the bloodstream and attaches to specific genetic sequences in the nucleus of cells inside Lucinda's body, identifying a known genetic lesion that predisposes her to the highly aggressive pancreatic cancer #236R (by this time, there are 335 known genetic variants of cancers arising from the pancreas). In less than 15 minutes, the risk assessment phase of the scan has been completed. The initial gas is rapidly metabolized and excreted from Lucinda's body by respiration.*

*The technologist calls for a second gas. A molecular agent contained in this gas specifically targets the surface receptors of metabolically hyperactive cells of pancreatic cancer 236R. This second scanning phase detects a submillimeter-size lesion in the tail of the pancreas. A software program highlights the abnormality in lavender and sets off a beeping sound as reinforcement. The scanner—assisted by advanced computer-aided detection (CAD) technology—has found a site of active cancer. The technologist instructs the Omniscient to emit a series of radiofrequency pulses directed to the pancreas. The pancreatic lesion turns brilliantly red on the screen, confirming the tumor's highly aggressive nature. The scan has revealed that the pancreatic lesion is indeed the rapidly progressive 236R. Fortunately, it has been found early. The subsequent whole body scan finds no other hot spots, showing with 98% reliability that there are no metastases.*

*At the direction of the technologist, the Omniscient transmits a new and unique set of energy pulses precisely focused on the abnormality. The pulses cleave the contrast agent's molecules attached to the cancer cells, transforming the contrast agent into a highly effective therapeutic molecule (such agents, which are both diagnostic and therapeutic, are referred to as* theranostics*). The molecule triggers apoptosis, the internal cellular programming that destroys the tagged cells. Because the agent is selectively attached to tumor cells, the surrounding normal pancreatic tissue is completely unharmed. Lucinda is cured of a disease that, 30 years earlier, lurked undetected for years and, when finally discovered, was almost invariably fatal. She drove herself home immediately following the procedure.*

This scenario is science fiction. There may never be an Omniscient. But one can see numerous strains of technological development today that might produce elements of such a device tomorrow. Numerous innovations in imaging diagnosis and therapy could provide faster, safer, less discomforting, and more valuable contributions to clinical care than anything presently available. Future medical imaging methods likely will involve the marriage of sensitive image acquisition devices (like CT and MRI) and biological agents targeted to specific cellular and subcellular abnormalities. Computer software programs will fuse anatomical and physiological images for improved diagnosis, as well as identify potentially troublesome findings for the radiologist to examine more closely.[1] There may be combined technologies that both diagnose and treat disease. Five-dimensional imaging—comprising length, width, depth, time, and function—will span the spectrum from the subcellular to the organismal.

To be successful, these new imaging methods must possess a number of important qualities. At a minimum, any nascent imaging technology must provide new and valuable clinical information. This means that the technology must be applicable to one or more conditions that affect a large number of individuals. These disease conditions must be important ones, causing a significant amount of illness or death. And using the technology should, in some empirically definable way, lead to better health outcomes.

However, while biological and clinical rationales for a new technology are essential, they are not sufficient to ensure acceptance into clinical practice. A complex of hard-to-predict environmental factors must align favorably to enable a promising technology to overcome financial, regulatory, payment, and cultural barriers. The barriers have grown taller as society's tolerance for the accelerating costs of imaging has worn thin.

This chapter will discuss what influences are driving imaging innovation and what new capabilities may emerge. The chapter will also consider some promising candidate technologies now being evaluated in animal models, clinical trials, and limited clinical practice. Finally, it will identify the factors that may support or impede the acceptance of new imaging technologies.

---

[1] There already exist examples of such fusion technologies, like PET-CT and PET-MRI scanners.

## Trends in Medicine Guide Imaging Innovation

In a 2007 presentation to the Radiological Society of North America, the then director of the NIH, radiologist Elias Zerhouni, addressed medical and societal trends that he believed would necessarily direct imaging innovation in the future (Zerhouni 2008).

Zerhouni explained how new research emphases and altered provider behavior would be necessary to achieve better care at less cost. Specifically, he talked about *P4 medicine*. Future health care, he said, would have to be predictive, personalized, preemptive, and participatory.[2] Ideally, advances in imaging could help actualize each of these characteristics of future health care:

*Predictive*   There are important differences among all of us in our susceptibility to important diseases. These differences are based on both genetic factors and environmental influences to which we are exposed, like an injury, exposure to a virus or an environmental toxin. As an example of how genetics and the environment interact differently among us, we all recognize that smoking cigarettes is harmful. However, the vast majority of smokers do not develop clinical emphysema or die of lung cancer. The same is true of heart disease. High serum cholesterol levels have been shown to be an important risk factor for future serious cardiac events like heart attacks and heart failure. But again, there is no certainty that the individual will ever be clinically affected.

Health care would be both more effective and less costly if we knew in advance which patients truly needed more intensive prevention (pharmaceutical or behavioral) or early treatment. The potential virtues of predictive imaging are extraordinary. Imaging tests can be performed noninvasively and repeatedly over time to accurately inform the patient's physician of changes in the risk of disease. If we pair this knowledge with earlier and more effective personalized therapies (see below), the patient would have a better health outcome, with less discomfort and less potential for harm related to treatment. The efficiencies of reducing missteps would lead to lower costs. In this model of care, imaging will employ panels of *biomarkers*, which identify and track biological processes.

*Personalized*   *Personalized medicine* has gained currency in the parlance of both medical researchers and health policy workers. The term implies that the best treatment for any given disease will vary from person to person and that medicine's job will be to tailor treatment to the unique characteristics of that person and his or her disease. The reason for this is that individuals differ meaningfully in measurable ways in their predisposition to diseases with genetic roots. They also differ in their immunocompetence (i.e., their inherited capacity to defend themselves against diseases) and in their capacity to metabolize drugs.

In addition, there are important genetic differences among conditions currently considered a single disease that may vary at the level of the individual person. What

---

[2]   For his RSNA address, Zerhouni modified the ideas of the originator of the term *P4 medicine*, biologist Leroy Scott. Scott's original formula was predictive, preventive, personalized, and participatory (http://www.systemsbiology.org).

we call diseases today are really families of different diseases, with different prognoses and requiring different treatments. Better recognizing these differences could positively influence the outcomes of care. As an example, breast cancer is at least several (if not many) diseases, based on genetic differences in cancer cells. As discussed earlier, some breast cancers will not progress rapidly enough to affect women during their lifetimes. As detailed in Chapter 8, such cancers are termed *pseudodisease*. Other cancers are highly aggressive, causing death in a short period. Hence, different diseases have different biologies and clinical courses, progress differently individual to individual, and respond differently to specific treatments.

What if medical imaging could illuminate these differences—that is, could predict the biological behavior of the disease in a specific person? The central tenet of personalized medicine is that a person's genetic and environmental individuality should inform considerations of his or her care. Imaging as a precursor to individualized treatment on any reasonable scale is a very long-term goal, but its potential to improve care and make treatment more efficient could be extraordinary.

*Preemptive*   It is an axiom of medical care that finding disease earlier in its course is better than discovering disease after it has become established or spread. This is certainly the case for many conditions, such as identifying colonic polyps before they develop into cancers. Ideally, then, wouldn't it be best to identify a much larger fraction of serious disease in healthy-seeming individuals before they manifest symptoms? This seems to make such good sense that the American public overwhelmingly believes that screening[3] for disease is always a good thing (Schwartz et al. 2004).

We explain in Chapter 8 why the public's expectations of imaging screening are unrealistic given the current state of imaging technology. However, future advances in imaging could alter today's problematic balance of cost, risk, and benefit both for individuals and for society as a whole. Indeed, the ability of imaging research (and related research into point-of-care laboratory testing) to create more accurate and less expensive predictive tools will improve the effectiveness of imaging as a screening tool. The key problem with current imaging screening strategies is that they depend on very coarse indicators of who should be screened. Using some preliminary and inexpensive form of imaging (or perhaps more traditional in vivo diagnostic blood or urine tests) to help stratify populations into risk groups would greatly reduce the cost of screening programs by focusing the screening effort on those with the highest risks.

Ideally, physicians could reliably tell their patients where they fall along a continuum of risk—from needing no screening at all to needing frequent and intensive screening with the most sensitive technologies—and engage them based on their personal tolerance of risk. Even more significantly, results of imaging tests could be biomarkers for the aggressiveness of a found abnormality. An effective test for the biological aggressiveness of lesions found on screening would indicate whether an abnormality really required treatment or could be left alone. Reliable information on whether an abnormality was a threat to health or life could greatly reduce

---

3   The word *screening* means looking for disease in asymptomatic individuals.

follow-on testing and inappropriate treatments, which are the greatest generators of patient harm and cost associated with current imaging screening scenarios.

*Participatory*    Patients no longer compare the service they receive from one doctor or one hospital with the care they get at another. They evaluate their health care experiences with the same expectations that they bring to their favorite Starbuck's *barista*, or to Amazon.com or FedEx. Patients want to participate in their care in unprecedented ways. To the extent that future imaging can enhance the health care experience—making care faster, safer, less painful, cheaper, and more convenient for the patient,[4] with better outcomes—imaging innovations will find a receptive audience.

Almost all physicians experience daily the confluence of patients' elevated expectations and their access to extensive health-related information via the Internet. Patients' expectations for their own health and tolerance for risk vary. Patient demand may compel radiologists to provide patients with instant access to their images and radiological reports, shortcutting the traditional reporting chain of radiologist-to-referring physician-to-patient. Treatment decisions must thoughtfully incorporate these factors into shared decisionmaking about how their health risks are addressed. Even today, imaging facilities are increasingly sending patients home from an exam with a DVR of the scan to share with their physician or, if they wish, to engage a second opinion.

## Medical Imaging in Transition

To support P4 medicine, medical imaging is in transition from:

- Depicting gross anatomical abnormalities to detailing cellular and subcellular structures;
- Interrogating anatomy to evaluating metabolic activities like glucose metabolism, cell reproduction, and cell death;
- Imaging broad, nonspecific physiological processes to interrogating highly specific molecular targets along the molecular pathways of disease;
- Qualitative description to quantitative measurement.

This is not to say that all of the current gross anatomical imaging will disappear, but as medicine becomes more molecularly oriented, new roles for imaging will take priority. The opening anecdote about the Omniscient illustrates how P4 medicine and the new medical imaging might converge to accomplish the following objectives:

- Predict which individuals may be more susceptible to specific diseases;
- Detect disease earlier and in a more treatable state;
- Stage and map the extent of disease more accurately;
- Predict the disease's course based on biological aggressiveness and susceptibility to treatment;

---

4    Read Chapter 7 on moral hazard; cheaper for the patient does not necessarily mean less expensive for society or beneficial for the U.S. economy.

- Discern what might be the best treatment, and at what dose, before it is given;
- Determine the susceptibility of the patient to unusually toxic effects;
- Guide less invasive therapy;
- Monitor the patient's response to treatment early on to avoid unnecessary discomfort and harm and reduce the cost of ineffective therapy.

The goal is to improve care and health outcomes for patients. To achieve this goal at a cost society can afford, new imaging modalities must provide greater sensitivity to abnormalities than current methods, with fewer false-positive diagnoses and better discrimination of which abnormalities do and do not require further care. Imaging diagnoses and image-guided treatment must go beyond simply providing more information to improving the outcomes of care. Successful technologies should cause little or no discomfort, impose minimal inconvenience, and induce as few complications as therapeutically possible.

Finally, to be acceptable to an environment increasingly sensitive to the rising cost of health care, successful new imaging methods must reduce or moderate the rise in overall health care expenditures.[5] New imaging technologies should reduce clinical uncertainty more effectively and enable clinicians to rule out marginally effective care pathways. Their use should be grounded in solid empirical evidence of clinical effectiveness. Ideally, future imaging technologies—devices, biological agents, and treatment energies—should painlessly complete the continuum from risk assessment and early disease surveillance through definitive treatment during a single patient visit ... much like the Omniscient.

## Imaging's Emerging Toolbox

Unfortunately, there is no Omniscient on the near horizon. However, new imaging technologies are emerging that might combine to produce many of the Omniscient's key features. Given a welcoming environment, the next 20 years could see a second revolution in medical imaging that could overshadow the contributions of the past 4 remarkable decades.

Medical imaging already is very sophisticated. Merely continuing the steady increase in computing power, combined with more sophisticated image acquisition and display software, will ensure continuous improvement in what already are very powerful tools. However, new capabilities for diagnosis and therapy are emerging from both industry and academic research venues. The following section will provide a few examples of the hundreds of imaging innovations that might offer benefits in the future.

*Superparamagnetic Iron Oxide (SPIO) Nanoparticles and MRI to Stage Cancer*  Nanotechnology is an active arena for research in many fields, including medical imaging, because of the strength and versatility of such small particles (a nanometer is one-billionth of a meter—one thousandth of the diameter of a human hair). Nanoparticles useful in medicine tend to range in size from a few to 100 nanometers. To be employed in imaging, specific targeting molecules are

---

[5]  Imaging costs could be greater so long as total health care expenditures were lessened.

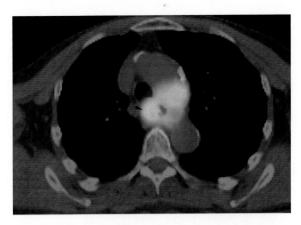

COLOR FIGURE 2-16

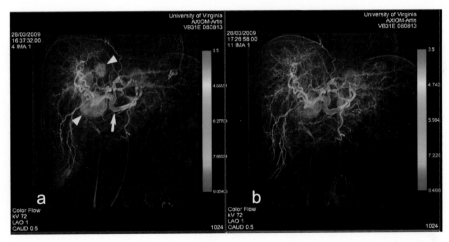

COLOR FIGURE 3-5

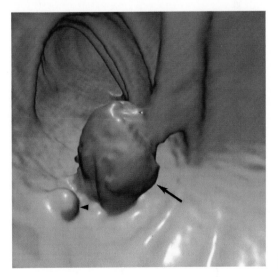

COLOR FIGURE 8-4

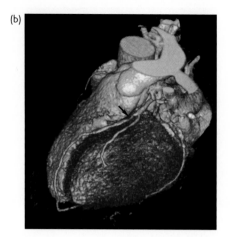

COLOR FIGURE 8-6b

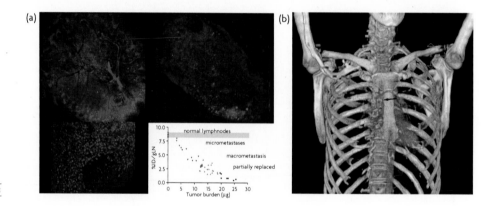

COLOR FIGURE 9-1

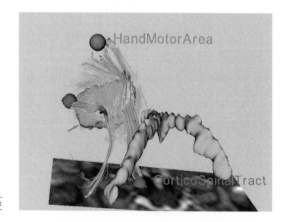

COLOR FIGURE 9-2

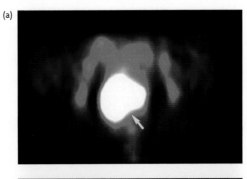

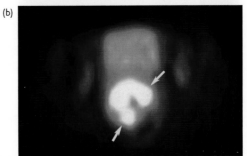

(b)

COLOR FIGURE 9-4

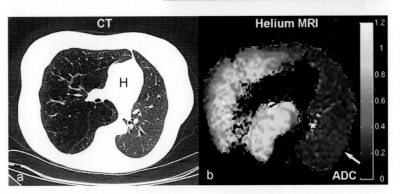

COLOR FIGURE 9-5

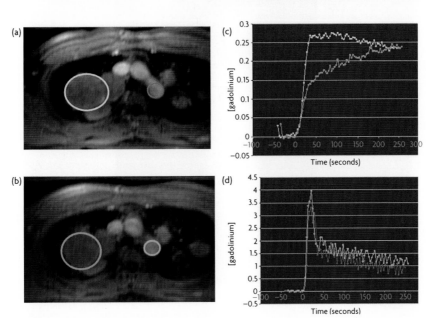

COLOR FIGURE 9-6

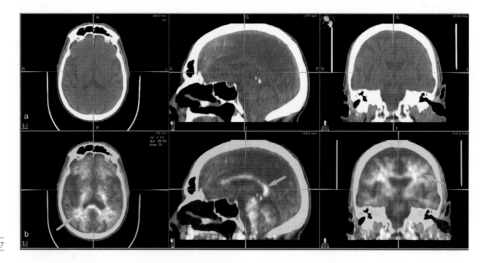

COLOR FIGURE 9-7

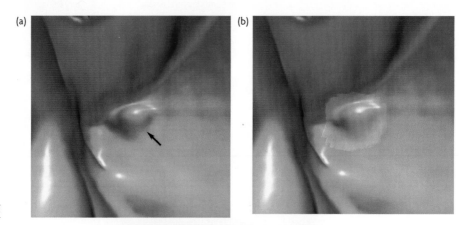

(a)

(b)

COLOR FIGURE 9-8

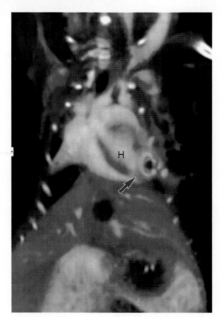

COLOR FIGURE 9-9

hooked to nanoparticles to act as targeted contrast agents, treatments, or theranostics combining both functions (Islam and Josephson 2009). One example of
a nanoparticulate targeted contrast agent is an iron-based MRI contrast agent to
evaluate patients for the spread (metastasis) of cancer to lymph nodes. For most
types of cancer, whether the primary tumor has metastasized to the lymph nodes
greatly affects the type of treatment patients receive and their likelihood of being
cured.

The current method of determining lymph node involvement by cancer is imaging by CT or MRI. For both radiological modalities, size is used as the criterion; if a
lymph node (oval in shape) is larger than 1 centimeter in its narrower diameter, it is
considered cancerous. Radiologists make this diagnosis knowing that it is a highly
inaccurate approach. Nodes smaller than 1 centimeter may be infested by cancer
cells. Bigger lymph nodes may merely have been enlarged by inflammatory cells and
contain no cancer cells at all. One multicenter trial pitting CT against MRI for staging cervical cancer showed very poor results for evaluating lymph nodes for both
methods based on size alone (Hricak et al. 2006).

The SPIO nanoparticles can be used to target macrophages in the lymph nodes,
which engulf (*phagocytize*) the SPIO particles (Fig. 9-1). Cancer cells do not. As a
result, the normal lymph nodes appear as a "void" or black region on MRI scans. In
other words, the SPIO nanoparticles are a "negative" contrast agent. Clinical studies have shown much better accuracy in determining whether there are lymph node
metastases using this approach compared to conventional CT and MRI scanning.
Because normal lymphatic flow is altered even with microscopic levels of metastases, the method can detect even subvisual levels of tumor involvement (Harringsani
et al. 2003).

### Advanced Preoperative Visualization of Brain Tumors

Imaging will become "the eyes
of the interventionalist." Imaging tools are becoming increasingly useful in reducing
complications and improving the outcomes of surgery. The increased integration of
imaging into both surgical planning and surgery itself is a major strain of technological development in imaging.

Advanced surgical visualization techniques have been developed to guide brain
tumor interventions. These techniques define the margins of the tumor (called

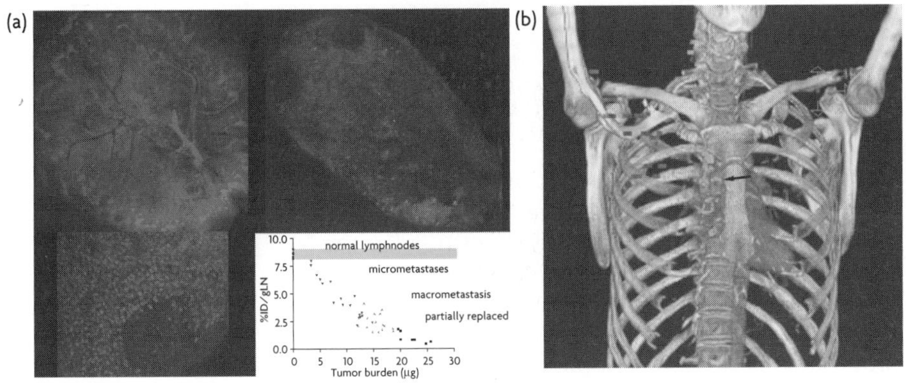

(a)   (b)

FIGURE 9-1

*(a) Surgically resected lymph nodes containing fluorescently labeled magnetic particles. The orange areas are where the nanoparticles have distributed following injection. The graph at the lower right shows the relationship between nanoparticle uptake in nodes (vertical axis) and the amount of tumor in lymph nodes. (b) A plot of the lymph nodes on a three-dimensional representation of the thorax show where cancer-affected nodes are localized as a means of planning surgical treatment. The color coding reflects different nodal status. For example, the cluster of green nodes in the central thorax (arrow) represents nodes partially replaced by the lymphatic spread of cancer. (Courtesy of Ralph Weissleder, MD, PhD, and Mukesh Harisinghani, Massachusetts General Hospital) (See Color Figures 9-1a and 9-1b in the insert.)*

*tumor segmentation*) using software that employs mathematical algorithms that distinguish between normal and abnormal tissue. In addition, a special MR imaging technique called *diffusion-tensor imaging* not only detects the presence of water but also tracks the direction of the flow of water along bundles of nerves. Knowing the direction of flow along neural pathways enables reconstruction of diffusion-tensor images that detail the location of important nerve bundles in relation to the tumor (Fig. 9-2). This advanced imaging guidance can inform the surgeon's approach to the tumor, allowing him or her to better preserve the patient's normal functioning. Intermittent imaging during the surgery or even future intraoperative imaging, using an MR-compatible operating room (OR), can inform the surgeon of how the landscape changes as he or she resects the abnormality. Advanced imaging-guided ORs like the AMIGO (Advanced Medical Imaging Operating Room), at the Brigham and Women's Hospital in Boston, will combine numerous computerized anatomical and functional imaging methods to direct improved surgical intervention (personal communication, Ferenc Jolesz, November 2008). In other words, these imaging tools will eventually provide surgeons live three-dimensional images of the surgical field to guide their activities.

Once the resection nears completion, another technology, earlier in its development, might enable a surgeon to determine if he or she has completely removed the cancerous tissue from the surgical site. Dubbed *tumor paint* by molecular researcher Ralph Weissleder at Massachusetts General Hospital, it is a biological agent with a high affinity for molecular receptors on the surface of tumor cells. Sprayed on the open surgical field and illuminated by a near infrared optical source, the agent will "light up" any tumor cells left behind by the surgeon, enabling more complete removal and reducing the likelihood of recurring illness.[6]

*MR-Guided Focused Ultrasound*    Advanced imaging visualization has important implications for making conventional neurosurgery safer and more effective. However, these techniques are essential to a novel noninvasive method of treating brain cancer now in limited clinical use. This innovation, known as *MR-guided*

FIGURE 9-2

Graphic three-dimensional representation of diffusion tensor MRI imaging of the brain. Major nerve tracks are shown in relation to a brain tumor (arrow) to help surgeons plan for as complete a removal of the tumor as possible while sparing important nerves in the region. (Courtesy of Ron Kikinis, PhD, Brigham and Women's Hospital) (See Color Figure 9-2 in the insert.)

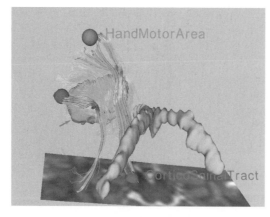

[6]  Personal communication, Ralph Weissleder, November 2008.

*focused ultrasound* (MRgFUS) ablation, uses an MRI scanner integrated with a device capable of emitting high-powered ultrasound waves to destroy tumors. Repetitive MRI imaging simultaneously informs the operators of what tissue has been destroyed, depicts the margins of the remaining tumor, and, via an MRI pulse sequence that elicits temperature information, indicates the level of heating (and hence, the risk of causing destruction) of surrounding normal neural pathways critical to the patient (Hynynen et al. 1997; Ram et al. 2006 ). As with other image-guided techniques, the goals are twofold: (1) destroy as much tumor tissue as possible and (2) injure as little of the surrounding normal tissue as possible to best preserve the patient's normal functioning postoperatively.

MRgFUS ablation has been shown to be effective in the treatment of uterine fibroids (Hindley et al. 2004). Researchers are testing the effectiveness of the device for other uses, like the treatment of breast (Fig. 9-3) and brain cancer, metastases from distant tumors, and conditions such as epilepsy, Alzheimer's disease, and Parkinson's disease (Bradley 2009). More than 70 MRgFUS devices have been placed in institutions around the world. Present constraints on the development of this technology involve the length of the sessions, the accuracy of targeting the focused ultrasound beam, diffusion of heat into surrounding tissues, and the costs and benefits versus those of established treatment modalities such as open surgery or targeted radiotherapy.

The Defense Advanced Research Projects Agency (DARPA), which helped fund miniaturization and hardening of ultrasound technology for use in combat situations, is now developing high-intensity focused ultrasound (HIFU) applications that do not rely upon MR guidance to enable a medic in the field to use ultrasound both to locate and seal off deep arterial bleeding, a leading cause of death for soldiers injured by roadside bombs or improvised explosive devices.[7] The technology has

FIGURE 9-3

*Sagittal contrast-enhanced MRI scans of the breast (a) prior to and (b) following MRgFUS ablation. Image (a) shows the enhancing breast cancer (arrow). Image (b) shows necrosis in the previous location of the tumor six days following the procedure. The treated area (arrows) is much larger than the tumor to be sure that cancer cells at the margin of the mass are destroyed. (Courtesy of Drs. N. McNannold, F. Jolesz, and C. Tempany, Brigham and Women's Hospital.)*

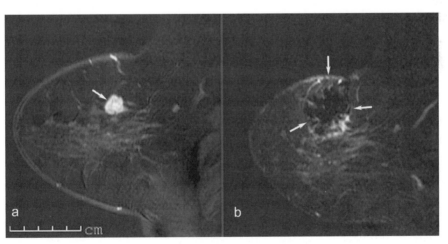

---

7  DARPA gave two contracts to device manufacturers in 2006 to develop such devices, as well as Doppler ultrasound tools to locate deep bleeding sites. See http://www.darpa.mil/dso/thrusts/bio/mainhuman/dbac/index.htm for a description of the Deep Bleeder Acoustical Coagulation program.

already proven effective in animal studies in quickly cauterizing deep arterial bleeding with minimal effect on surrounding tissues (Veazy and Zderic 2007)

*A Combination Technology to Treat Brain Metastases from Breast Cancer*    Cancer cells express a variety of proteins either not generated by normal tissue or expressed at much lower levels. These proteins create an environment conducive to the growth and spread of cancers. In breast cancer, one of these proteins is an enzyme called *epidermal growth factor* (EGF). An antibody has been developed as a drug (trastuzumab, marketed as Herceptin) that blocks the receptor on the cell that activates EGF. Trastuzumab is an effective targeted treatment for many patients with metastatic breast cancer whose cancer cells overexpress EGF, but it is ineffective for patients whose cells do not.

Unfortunately, brain metastases from breast cancer present a special problem with respect to trastuzumab treatment. The capillaries serving brain tissue are lined with cells (i.e., the *endothelium*) that are especially tightly bound to one another (i.e., the *blood–brain barrier*)—more so than in other tissues. As a result, few therapeutic molecules are small enough to escape the capillaries and penetrate into tumor tissue. Trastuzamab is a midsized molecule that normally does not cross the blood–brain barrier in sufficient concentration to be effective.

Researchers have found that gaps can be created temporarily between endothelial cells by applying low-frequency, high-power ultrasound energy to regions being perfused by an ultrasound contrast agent comprised of microscopic bubbles (naturally, known in the trade as *microbubbles*). Guidance by MRI (MRgFUS) makes it possible to focus the ultrasonic energy on the metastatic tumor masses and measure the effect of the treatment in allowing trastuzumab to pass into the targeted cancerous tissue (Kinoshita et al. 2006).

This creative technique might be extended to other brain conditions for which the blood–brain barrier poses a therapeutic constraint. The method is in preclinical testing.

*A PET Predictor of the Most Effective Treatment and Dose*    High-dose radiation is an effective treatment for many cancers. Radiation therapy is often employed when a tumor is too extensive for surgical resection, sometimes as an alternative treatment to surgery, or sometimes in addition to surgery. Imaging technologies like MR and CT have long been used to guide radiation therapy as a means of better focusing the destructive effect of radiation on the cancerous tissues while minimizing side effects by reducing the dose normal organs receive as much as possible.

Recent advances in understanding tumor physiology have shown that malignant tumors are heterogeneous. The tumor mass is comprised not only of cancerous tissue but also of hemorrhage (blood and blood products), necrosis (dead cancerous tissue that has outgrown its blood supply), and fibrosis (the body's reaction to inflammation). An emerging technology—*intensity-modulated radiation therapy* (IMRT)—addresses this inhomogeneity by "segmenting" the dose received according to what level of radiation is needed to be effective in different parts of the tumor.

Hypoxic tissue—living tissue that has lower levels of oxygen reaching the cells—is characteristic of some tumors, like cancer of the cervix, and is particularly resistant

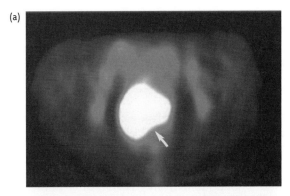

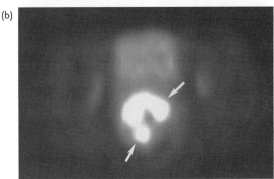

FIGURE 9-4

*Axial PET/CT scan through the lower pelvis. (a) The PET/CT image with 18-FDG shows a large, metabolically active mass (arrow) in the cervix representing cervical carcinoma. (b) The 64-CuATSM PET image reveals that the mass contains large areas of hypoxia (arrows) that may be resistant to a routine radiation treatment dose. (Courtesy of Mehdi Adineh, PhD, American College of Radiology) (See Color Figure 9-4 in the insert.)*

to the effects of radiation. Identification of hypoxic regions would inform radiation oncologists seeking to optimize their therapy. Until recently, there has been no practical, noninvasive way to accurately identify hypoxic regions of tumors. However, the development of a positron-emitting radionuclide, copper-64-ATSM ([64-CU]-diacetyl-bis($N$(4)-methylthiasemicarbazone), holds promise as a biomarker of hypoxia for treating tumors with hypoxic regions (Fig. 9-4) (Chao et al. 2001).

A principal problem with copper-64-ATSM is that the very short half-life of the radionuclide requires the presence of a very expensive-to-operate cyclotron virtually next door to the PET scanner. Copper-64-ATSM is undergoing early clinical trials (http://www.acrin.org).

*Hyperpolarized Noble Gases as Contrast Agents for MRI of the Lungs* Because there are few structures containing hydrogen atoms in the lungs, the depiction of pulmonary disorders has been a blind spot for MR imaging. Investigators at a number of sites, notably the University of Virginia, the University of Pennsylvania, and Duke University, have addressed this failing by employing an apparatus developed by Princeton University physicists. The device uses lasers to hyperpolarize the so-called noble or inert gases, like helium and xenon, making them susceptible to MR imaging in the same way we described for hydrogen in Chapter 1 (Salerno et al. 2001). The technique, which is being tested in human trials, has primarily been applied using helium to investigate ventilation disturbances like asthma, chronic obstructive pulmonary disease, and cystic fibrosis, where investigators believe hyperpolarized gas imaging could help guide and monitor treatment by defining the areas of most severely disordered air flow (Fig. 9-5). Increasingly, xenon is being used to evaluate the transfer of gases across the alveolar (air space) membrane—critical to blood oxygenation and diminished in many diseases causing inflammation and edema (Rupert et al. 2004).

### Software to Quantify Treatment-Related Changes in Cancer Patients

A great deal of clinical imaging deals with tracking the appearance of disease from one exam to the next to determine whether a condition is progressing or responding to treatment. For many aspects of modern imaging, the reporting of changes from one study to the next is done qualitatively based on often imprecise criteria. There is a need for more exacting measures, which are reflective of the disease status and ideally predictive of the prognosis, to guide treatment decisions.

Measures used in clinical trials to track treatment-related changes are increasingly employed in clinical practice. The current standard for evaluating the treatment of solid tumors is the so-called RECIST (Response Evaluation Criteria in Solid Tumors) measurement, a unidimensional length across the broadest diameter of the tumor mass. Changes in the RECIST measurement are translated (according to the percent change and an arcane set of rules) into one of several categories to determine whether a subject in a clinical trial is responding and/or is eligible to continue to receive treatment as part of the trial (major categories are stable disease, partial and complete disease regression, and disease progression) (Eisenhauer et al. 2009). This is an example of using imaging as a *surrogate endpoint*—an endpoint that reflects the true endpoints of disease, like life or death, but that is less time-consuming and expensive to employ.

Unfortunately, effective targeted treatments may not show a change in tumor size for months, long after the value of knowing whether a treatment is working has diminished. New, targeted molecular therapies may halt the growth of tumors without completely destroying them and may not show any size changes at all. The efficient development of new drugs and improved clinical care demand more accurate imaging approaches to quantify the effect of treatment.

FIGURE 9-5

*(a) Axial CT image of the midthorax and (b) corresponding axial MRI image using hyperpolarized helium gas as a contrast agent for the air spaces of the lungs (alveolae) in a patient with a left lung transplant. The MRI scan employs a special MR technique measuring the apparent diffusion coefficient (ADC), which reflects the size of the alveolae. The left lung (arrow) has a homogeneous low ADC, consistent with normal-size alveolae. The right lung is heterogeneous and depicts higher ADC consistent with the patient's known chronic obstructive lung disease, which has destroyed alveolae. The images of the experimental MRI correspond well with the CT scan. The CT scan shows a right lung that is hyperexpanded (the heart [H] is pushed to the left) and has fewer normal markings (appears blacker) than the normal left transplanted lung. (Courtesy of Talissa Altes, MD, PhD, the University of Virginia) (See Color Figure 9-5 in the insert.)*

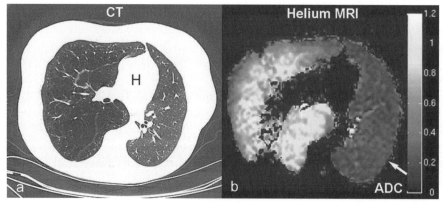

A host of new measurements are under study to determine if they depict the effects of drugs on cancer earlier and more accurately. They include refinements of anatomical measurement (e.g., the analysis of tumor volume) and new physiological approaches. New methods like dynamic contrast-enhanced (DCE) MRI (Fig. 9-6) and diffusion-weighted MRI to assess changes in tumor blood flow, magnetic resonance spectroscopy (MRS) to evaluate biochemical changes, and PET employing specialized radionuclides targeted to specific tumor markers (Fig. 9-7) may eventually replace RECIST as better markers of whether a drug is effective in treating cancer.

There is a burgeoning software application set to fulfill these needs. Products are being developed to perform key measurements for a host of conditions—cancer, autoimmune and inflammatory processes, and infection. These programs are already being employed in research and practice. New software programs are illuminating differences in pathology from one scan to the next or comparing the patient's scan against an atlas of normal individuals. Ultimately, new methods of viewing and quantifying the effects of treatment will be more automated, more accurate, and more representative of how disease and treatment are affecting patients. In other words imaging will serve as a noninvasive biomarker of treatment response.

*Data Mining to Improve Health Outcomes* The data generated by the preceding examples of future technologies are powerful in offering insights into how disease develops and into how to improve patient care. However, the value of imaging data is amplified when those data are stored in an integrated fashion with clinical,

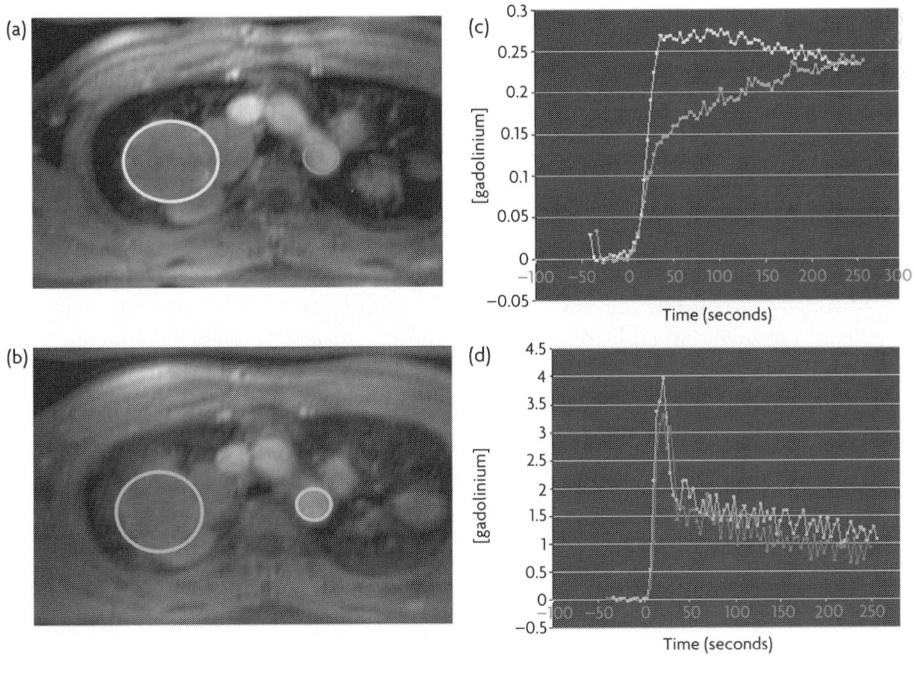

FIGURE 9-6

*Dynamic contrast-enhanced (DCE) MRI exam showing a change in the renal cell carcinoma (kidney cancer) enhancement prior to and 21 days following treatment with a therapeutic agent that interferes with blood vessel development in tumors (sorafinib). The yellow and green circled regions of interest mark the tumors (a) before and (b) after the treatment. In (c) the corresponding green line on the graph shows a slower and longer rise in the gadolinium contrast concentration (vertical axis) in the tumor following sorafinib therapy, indicating a reduction in tumor blood flow and/or leakiness of the blood vessels (permeability) relative to the pretreatment yellow line. (d) The red and blue lines reflect the passage of the gadolinium through the aorta on the pretreatment (a) and posttreatment (b) scans, respectively. They are virtually identical, confirming that the differences shown in (c) are not related to technical factors. (Courtesy of Mark Rosen, MD, PhD, the University of Pennsylvania) (Republished with the permission of Landes Bioscience. The image originally appeared as part of Figure 2 in: Flahery KT, Rosen MA, Heitjen DF, et al. Pilot study of DCE-MRI to predict progression-free survival with sorafinib therapy in renal cell carcinoma. Cancer Biology & Therapy. 2008;7:496–501.) (See Color Figure 9-6 in the insert.)*

FIGURE 9-7

*Axial CT (a) and corresponding PET scans (b) of the head in the axial, sagittal, and coronal planes. The PET scan employs a special 18-F compound that attaches to abnormal myelin (arrows) (substance covering the surface of neural tissue), associated with Alzheimer's disease. (Courtesy of Mehdi Adineh, PhD, American College of Radiology) (See Color Figure 9-7 in the insert.)*

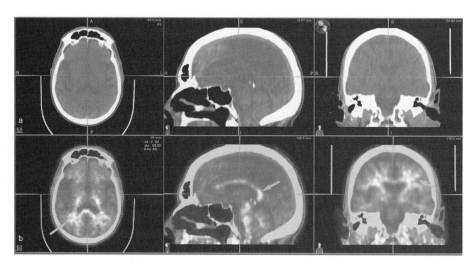

demographic, histological,[8] genomic, and proteonomic[9] data. Integrated databases will allow clinicians and epidemiologists to investigate the relationships among the data. The associations they unearth will be invaluable in helping researchers to better understand disease mechanisms and pathways. Such relationships would better inform health care providers and policymakers about what imaging practices provide greater value to patients, and when and under what circumstances to use them.

The development of such integrated databases is occurring just in time. Part of the 2009 federal economic stimulus legislation provided $1.1 billion to fund *comparative effectiveness research* (CER). The principal goal of CER is to identify which health practices are most effective in controlling or eliminating disease.[10] Imaging practices are amply represented in the "top 100" problems to be addressed.[11] The CER projects ask questions like: Which is better: colonoscopy or CTC to identify colonic polyps? Ultrasonography or MRI to diagnose fetal abnormalities? Computed tomography or MRI to determine whether a liver metastasis is resectable or whether a liver can be transplanted?

Prior to health reform and the acute concern over health cost growth, such questions were considered too mundane to bother with. As a consequence, CER has historically been underfunded. If considered at all, these issues were addressed by clinical trials or by modeling disease pathways using existing data to support decision analyses. However, in addition to supporting traditional NIH-style clinical trials, CER will also attempt to tap into the real world of clinical practice on a large scale. Mining large national databases, reflecting the diagnostic and therapeutic inputs of millions of episodes of patient care and their related health outcomes, has the potential to help achieve the goals of CER. A number of professional organizations have

---

[8]  The results of examining the cells of diseased tissues.

[9]  The proteins produced by cells, as directed by the genome.

[10]  http://www.hhs.gov/recovery/programs/cer/index.html.

[11]  http://www.iom.edu/cerpriorities.

begun to develop databases that ultimately will support CER data mining, like the ACR's National Radiology Data Registry (NRDR).[12]

*Computer-Aided Diagnosis (CAD) of Imaging Studies*    Computer-aided detection (CAD) software programs are in active development to help radiologists be more accurate in finding difficult-to-see abnormalities. These programs already act as a "second reader" to identify areas of concern that radiologists might otherwise miss on mammograms, lung and liver CT scans, and CTC studies (Fig. 9-8). Experimental smart systems compare a patient's brain scans to a computerized atlas of normal images and depict regions that deviate from the normal range, indicative of degenerative conditions like Alzheimer's disease.[13] It is not farfetched to imagine that future improvements in software might enable automated imaging detection. Systems that assist physicians with much of their workload already exist in other specialties. PAP smears undergo automated processing, with only suspicious cases viewed by pathologists. Similarly, the output of electrocardiograms and 24-hour Holter monitors are analyzed by software that spits out diagnoses, most of which are cursorily reviewed by cardiologists.

As refinements of high-technology imaging produce scans with many more hundreds or thousands of images, CAD might help focus radiologists' analysis by flagging specific images for detailed review, improving radiologists' productivity. Eventually, smart systems might be able to completely supplant radiologists for specific proven indications by providing detailed differential diagnoses, listing each possible cause for the constellation of CAD-detected imaging findings and an associated probability to guide further diagnosis and treatment.

The events of 9/11 have promoted this trend. Companies originally focused on using smart systems to identify potential threats to public security—particularly air travel screening technologies—are now translating their inventions into the early detection of human disorders using imaging.

FIGURE 9-8

*Three-dimensional reconstruction of a CTC exam showing a broad-based (sessile) polyp (arrow) projecting from the colon wall. (a) Without computer-aided detection (CAD); (b) the CAD software "paints" a blue tone on suspicious areas, in this case correctly detecting the polyp. (Courtesy of Jeff Hoffmeister, MD, iCAD Medical Systems) (See Color Figures 9-8a and 9-8b in the insert.)*

(a)
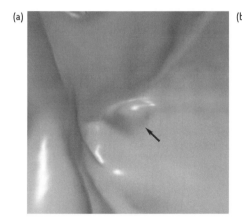

(b)
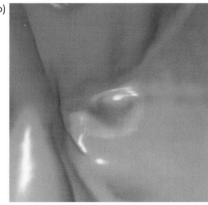

[12] http://www.acr.org/SecondaryMainMenuCategories/quality_safety/NRDR.aspx.
[13] Personal communication, R. Nick Bryan, May 2009.

## Between the Science and Helping Patients, Numerous Hurdles

The time and cost of developing new imaging technologies are potent barriers to the translation of promising applications into clinical practice. In addition, there is the undefinable risk that promising technologies may not make it through the regulatory approval system discussed in Chapter 5. At the end of the lengthy and expensive development and approval process, there must be a reasonable chance that the large investment will be rewarded or companies will not invest in commercializing new ideas.

The next section will discuss the research path to commercialization and its relationship to regulatory approval to market the product. It will then explore the financial implications of developing technologies to address the demands of personalized medicine. Finally, it will consider how the general and medical economies might promote or retard future imaging innovation.

*Research and Regulation*   In Chapter 5, the transition of a new imaging technology from discovery to clinical practice was likened to a salmon climbing a series of fish ladders.[14] This section provides a more in-depth understanding of the research required before a product is approved for commercial use.

All novel drugs and medical devices start with an idea that the originator deems to be a potential enhancement to health. Good ideas for medical innovations derive from diverse sources: random individuals working in their garages or laboratories, faculty members of academic centers, practicing clinicians, electrical engineers, software developers and researchers employed by the largest device and pharmaceutical companies, to name just a few.

Ideas are inexpensive (indeed, sometimes free!). In contrast, research on creative ideas in medicine can be quite expensive. Research gets more costly the further an idea progresses through the developmental stages of preclinical, translational, and clinical research (Hillman and Gatsonis 2008). From the societal perspective, the goals of the research are to learn if and how the technology works, to be sure it is safe, and to determine for which organ systems and diseases the technology might be used. For the inventor or manufacturer, however, the ultimate objective is to obtain regulatory approval by the FDA to market and sell a new technology. Until this occurs, all activity is expense. There is no offsetting revenue.

The iterative development and testing of new imaging devices is well described in an evaluation hierarchy (Table 9-1) portraying a "pilgrim's progress" over a number of hurdles. Initially, physicists and physicians collaborate in making explicit how a technology works and refining its capacity to detect and diagnose disease (the technical factors in Table 9-1). Typically, new devices or new applications for existing devices initially undergo testing of key parameters like spatial and contrast resolution

---

[14] We cannot do full justice to the process here. For an excellent review of the hurdles to acceptance see Raab GG, Parr DH. From medical invention to clinical practice: the reimbursement challenge facing new device procedures and technology—Part I: issues in medical device assessment. *J Am Coll Radiol.* 2006;3:694–702; Part II-3:772–777; Part III-3:842–850.

TABLE 9-1  *Hierarchy of Diagnostic Technology Assessment*

| Level of the Hierarchy | What Is Evaluated? | Stage of Development |
| --- | --- | --- |
| Technical factors | Imaging mechanism; spatial, contrast, and temporal resolution | Early |
| Observational studies (case reports and larger case series) | Potential applications; performance in best-case scenarios | Early |
| Diagnostic accuracy | Ability to discriminate between abnormal and normal structures | Middevelopment |
| Diagnostic impact | Effect of the imaging result on physicians' diagnostic considerations | Later |
| Therapeutic impact | Effect of the imaging result on physicians' therapeutic considerations | Later |
| Health outcomes | Effect of using the technology on patient's health | Mature technology |
| Cost | Costs of using the technology and imaging and nonimaging costs incurred as a result | Mature technology |
| Societal impact | Estimation of value—the cost of deriving a specific level of benefit | Mature technology |

on phantoms.[15] Technical testing answers questions like: What physical properties are actually being imaged? How quickly can an image be exposed? What are the smallest objects the device can resolve? How sensitive is the technology to contrast differences (on a scale from white to black) between types of tissues? Clearly, if the new technology cannot surpass the performance of existing ones in this highly idealized setting, or in some way display unique and important information of potential clinical value, there is no future for the technology.[16]

Successful preclinical devices are candidates for *first-in-man* or *translational* evaluation (case reports and case series). This is a major decision point, because evaluation in humans ups the financial ante considerably. The principal goals of early human evaluation are to learn of any unexpected harms (referred to in clinical trials lingo as *adverse events*) and to get some insight into how the new technology might be used in practice. Since manufacturers don't own clinical venues, they must form alliances with clinical facilities like teaching hospitals or multispecialty clinics to perform these early evaluations.

---

[15] A phantom is a nonbiological representation of the intended use of an application. As an example, a chest X-ray phantom might be made of a plastic that has X-ray absorption capabilities similar to those of the soft tissues of the thorax, with a hollow space in the middle to represent the air-containing lungs. In a more advanced version, objects could be placed in the phantom to simulate lung diseases.

[16] There are mathematical approaches to determining what level of effectiveness a new technology must achieve to surpass existing technologies.

Historically, companies developed research agreements with academic medical centers. More recently, community-based medical practices and teleradiology corporations also have begun to participate in clinical research with industry as a hedge against declining practice revenues. The products of translational imaging research tend to be case reports and case series. These scientific communications provide insights into potential clinical applications, but they usually are heavily biased in favor of the technology.[17] Imaging companies have learned that positive early reports from the field often generate interest in a new technology that can carry over into eventual adoption. These relationships are changing because of increasing scrutiny of how industry sponsorship potentially influences the outcomes of clinical trials (Lewin 2009).

Later evaluations might involve several clinical centers collecting data on the more promising clinical applications of the technology. The goal of this early *clinical* phase of development is to accrue more rigorous data that will justify corporate decisions to either terminate development or initiate an expensive *pivotal* clinical trial to fulfill the requirements for regulatory approval. Nearly always, the purpose of developmental research on new diagnostic devices is to determine the accuracy of a test (diagnostic accuracy) by answering such questions as: How rarely do radiologists interpreting an image miss an important abnormality? How often do they overcall abnormalities that don't exist?

While accuracy is the traditional endpoint for diagnostic technologies, some payers are questioning its relevance. A diagnostic test can be accurate without affecting a physician's diagnostic considerations (diagnostic impact), the therapy a patient receives (therapeutic impact), or the outcome of an episode of illness (health outcomes; see Figure 5-4 for a review of the role diagnostic tests play in these key processes). These latter endpoints, while more relevant, can be difficult to measure and, along with evaluation of the cost of using a new technology, tend to be of greater interest to academic researchers than to companies focused on gaining FDA approval. The FDA rarely requires their investigation.

The FDA treats drugs and biological agents (including imaging contrast agents and radiopharmaceuticals) in a manner similar to devices, but the path to approval generally requires more rigor and tends to be more expensive (Hoffman et al. 2007). With drugs, there usually is a prolonged laboratory phase during which repeated iterations of a compound are refined and tested for biological activity. Successful compounds are then tested on animal models of human disease[18] to determine whether the biological activity seen in the test tube holds up in a complex living system, gain some insight into the mechanism of action, and evaluate the compound for overt safety concerns. All of this activity is termed *preclinical*.

---

[17] A discussion of the biases of observational research, typical of translational evaluations, is beyond the scope of this book, but the principal biases uniformly work toward a more positive view of the innovation than would occur under more scientific research designs or a more positive view of the technology's actual performance in practice.

[18] Animal models exist for a broad range of diseases. Mouse models are particularly common. Models are based on either changing an animal's genetics or some surgical or pharmacological procedure.

As with devices, taking a successful preclinical compound into clinical testing means that the developer accepts much greater expense. There are four phases to clinical drug development and postapproval investigation: phases I and II focus on drug safety, determining the mechanism of action in humans, and getting an inkling of whether the drug will work effectively.

Companies must make a critical decision at the end of phase II. There is a saying in the pharmaceutical industry: "If a drug is going to fail, let it fail fast." While the expense of getting to this point is considerable, it pales in comparison to what must be spent in phase III for a large multicenter human trial (the *pivotal* trial) with sufficient sample size to convince the FDA of a drug's value. Even if the FDA approves the new drug, it may require a company to continue to collect phase IV data after an innovation is cleared for release into clinical practice to ensure that there are no long-term serious side effects when potentially millions of patients are exposed to the compound. In addition, a company may wish to pursue phase IV research to generate data for marketing purposes.

Future imaging technologies will present a number of new challenges to regulation. Incorporating *user fees* (e.g., charges to companies developing technologies) into the FDA's revenue stream in the 1990s reduced but did not eliminate the delays caused by chronic underfunding. The FDA will be challenged to handle the potential barrage created by P4 medicine. Many new imaging modalities will not fit neatly into the traditional pigeonholes of drug, device, or biological agent. They will be combination technologies (Fig. 9-9)—in the sense that they require both a device and an agent to operate, fuse multiple types of images into one, or simultaneously fulfill diagnostic and therapeutic missions.

Given its mission and the media frenzies that have accompanied past errors in drug and device approvals, the FDA operates in a cautious manner. In concert with

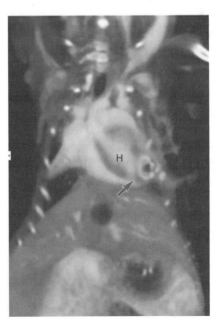

FIGURE 9-9

*Fusion image combining optical imaging using a fluorescent targeted agent (Prosense) and CT image showing a focal myocardial infarction (heart attack—arrow) in a mouse model (the arrow points to the region of infarction at the apex of the heart). Prosense is specifically designed to image a protease (an enzyme) that is present in large amounts in myocardial infarction. Prosense will progress to early clinical trials in 2010. (Courtesy of Ralph Weissleder, MD, PhD, and Matthias Nahrendorf, MD, PhD, Massachusetts General Hospital) (See Color Figure 9-9 in the insert.)*

insufficient funding, this caution has had a retarding effect on innovation. The time and expense of moving new agents and devices through the FDA approval process contributed to a twelve year decline in the number of approved new drugs.[19] The effect has been increasingly to move product research and development offshore.

The FDA recognizes that a problem exists. The agency has proposed several process innovations geared to increasing speed and reducing cost. One promising step forward is the exploratory Investigative New Drug (IND) application. An exploratory IND allows investigators to conduct preliminary human testing of a new agent on a small number of subjects for feasibility. The idea is to allow sponsors to either fail fast or gain better insight into the potential of a new agent at low expense. To some extent, the exploratory IND has been underutilized.

The other major innovation is what FDA calls the *Critical Path* to developing new pathways to approval. One aspect of this is to use validated imaging methods as surrogate endpoints for patient health outcomes to hasten the conclusion of trials and allow the use of smaller numbers of subjects to lead to conclusive results. An example of a surrogate endpoint using imaging is the RECIST measurement mentioned above. In some instances, a decrease in the diameter of a tumor is considered by the FDA to be equivalent to an improved clinical outcome. The RECIST measurement's poor correlation with health outcomes for many tumors and treatments means that new surrogate endpoints are needed. However, the Critical Path program has been underfunded and has not progressed significantly since its introduction in 2007.[20]

Finally, although the political barriers might be steep, there should be some consideration of furthering international reciprocity of device and drug approvals. The current approach of each country or region's regulatory authority evaluating the technologies of global companies is wasteful and inefficient. The current state of valuable innovations being available in one part of the world but not another is an anomaly in the context of most other economic sectors and ignores the growing phenomenon of medical tourism. Joining with other world regulatory bodies, such as the European Agency for the Evaluation of Medicinal Products (EMEA) and abiding universally by the resultant decisions would have the effect of pooling resources and expediting the adoption of valuable new imaging technologies into practice.

*The Economic Environment*    Attaining the right to market a new drug or device is a huge achievement for a company, but it is only the beginning. If insurers don't pay providers for the use of the new technology, the regulatory success may prove to be a hollow victory.

Chapter 5 described the fish ladders that a new product must clear to achieve Medicare coverage and payment. Briefly, once there is some use of the technology in practice, interested specialties and their advocates may clamor for a Category III billing code. Category III codes are flagged in practitioners' requests for Medicare payment for a procedure, but they themselves are not actually paid as are approved Category I codes. The purpose is to allow tracking of the diffusion and use of the innovation. Widespread use brings a new imaging device, contrast agent, or procedure

---

[19] http://www.fda.gov/oc/initiatives/criticalpath/whitepaper.html.
[20] http://www.fda.gov/oc/initiatives/criticalpath.

to consideration by the CPT (Common Procedural Terminology) Editorial Panel for Category I coding. However, even the assignment of a Category I code does not ensure Medicare payment. An application for payment and a proposal for the amount usually come to CMS from either the manufacturer or an interested professional organization on behalf of its clinician members.

This is an arcane and uncertain process. In principle, whether a technology is in common use and provides benefit to patients are supposed to be the key determinants of whether providers are paid for its use. The custom in the past was that CMS should not intrude on the practice of medicine, and the agency has not explicitly factored cost into its deliberations. Nonetheless, there is a persistent belief among companies and providers that cost considerations play a major role in determining coverage policy as moneys have grown tighter (Dhruva et al. 2009). Having to demonstrate that a product not only benefits patients but does so at a lower cost than existing products is, for most innovations, an impossible hurdle, particularly given the current state of methodological rigor in the field (Otero et al. 2008).

Given the current economic and political climate, achieving third-party payment is likely to become an even more difficult barrier to overcome in the future. As of this writing in 2010, the U.S. economy remains mired in a deep recession. While health care wasn't the primary cause of the economic meltdown, the declining economy has exposed the cost of health care to a previously unknown level of scrutiny. Health economists make straight-line extrapolations[21] of the present health cost trend and predict unsustainable spending levels in the future. There is increasing suspicion in the policy community that technical advances in medicine do not translate reliably into improvements in health, even as individual patients and their families demand access to them. While the health care reform legislation passed in 2010 did not explicitly change how health care is paid for, it urged experimentation with many new methods for restructuring payments to providers that might fundamentally affect the way new technologies are accepted into practice and paid for.

All of what is happening in the broader world of medicine and health care payment has important implications for the development of valuable imaging innovations. A principal engine for generating and exploring ideas has been the funding of independent investigators by the NIH. Funding of the NIH declined in real dollars for six consecutive years during the Bush administration. The trend finally reversed in 2009 with the economic stimulus program, which provided a significant ($10 billion) amount of new funding over a two-year period.[22] Hopefully, this was not merely a one-time surge of funding, but rather a rebasing of federal research support that will be sustained in an economic recovery.

The economic downturn has resulted in a shakeout of both academic imaging faculties and the small incubator companies that were major sources of innovation. During a late 2008 trip to Boston to research this book, the authors drove past block after block of nearly empty new buildings that had been built by Harvard and MIT specifically to house the research efforts of start-up companies based on their

---

[21] This is rarely a good idea. There is little in life that continues along an unaltered course for an extended time.

[22] Presentation by John Niederhuber to the NCI Clinical Trials and Translational Advisory Committee, March 2009.

faculties' intellectual property. The manufacturing giants in the imaging industry have undergone several rounds of layoffs. The downturn in imaging equipment sales has made them more cautious and pressured their budgets for new product development. While the most innovative and the best funded will likely survive, the effect has been a resetting of the developmental clock. Technologies that may have been 5 years from the marketplace may now be 8 or 10 years away. Some big-risk/big-reward technologies may have been killed for lack of corporate capacity to assume more risk.

Personalized imaging technologies face a particular problem: segmenting an already tight market. The financial success of technologies like CT, MRI, and 18F-fluorodesoxyglucose (FDG) PET has been related, in large part, to their applicability to numerous conditions and large numbers of patients. Broad applications mean large sales and profits for companies that have assumed the financial risks of developing them.

The problem with personalized medical technologies is that they are, by definition, designed for specific individuals and conditions. The more targeted a technology is to a specific use, the smaller the market and the harder it is to justify assuming the risk of product development. As one observer put it with respect to the continuing micro-reclassification of cancer, "Every tumor is going to be a rare tumor."[23] This truth explains much about why some targeted imaging discoveries—including some of those described above—have lingered so long in preclinical and translational stages without progressing to clinical practice.

Companies are struggling to find a financial rationale for targeted agents in a world in which molecular medicine is daily reclassifying major diseases into smaller markets of more accurately defined conditions. It is possible that, at least for new therapeutic drugs, new imaging agents can become part of the solution, as they have for some new "personalized" cancer drugs. That is, a specific test may be required to determine if the agent will actually have the desired therapeutic effect for a specific patient. Imaging and pharmaceutical companies might well join forces to provide paired diagnostic and therapeutic agents for major conditions like atherosclerotic cardiovascular disease and cancer that would be sold together.

An example of how authorities can help ease the introduction of more targeted, P4 imaging agents is the rule CMS is promulgating that allows payment for new PET and other nuclear medicine agents for a limited trial period immediately after FDA approval. Companies marketing new nuclear agents can apply for a two- to three-year *pass-through* payment that is based on the average sales price of the product. The program allows companies to recoup some of their development costs while CMS is considering its definitive payment decision.[24] The policy also applies to new therapeutic drugs and biological agents. A similar policy would greatly enhance incentives promoting device development.

Being able to short-circuit the path to payment, even if only for a short while, can really help a company struggling at the end of a long development process. Bringing a new diagnostic contrast agent to market can cost as much as $150 million

[23] Joel Tepper, meeting of the NCI Clinical Trials and Translational Advisory Committee, July 2009.
[24] http://www.asnc.org/content_8672.cfm.

(Nunn 2006). The cost of bringing a new therapeutic drug to market has risen 55% over the past decade (Mathieu 2002) and is now estimated to cost $1 billion or more over 10–17 years of development (Reichert 2003).[25]

The development of new diagnostic and therapeutic agents will benefit from programs like the FDA Critical Path or provisional reimbursement that could help reduce the arduousness of the fish ladders. Imaging could assist materially in this process. Imaging methods like PET, or optical imaging or other methods employing specifically targeted agents, might someday predict the specific clinical circumstances in which a therapy will be effective, indicate the most effective dose range, and reflect early and accurately the patient's health outcome. In turn, this would allow for more rapid and smaller trials and, consequently, less expensive drug development. Candidate imaging tests for these roles exist today. What is required is validation and acceptance of these tests by the FDA as surrogate endpoints for use in therapeutic clinical trials.

## Managing the Risks of Medical Innovation—a Parable

A striking example of how environmental factors can play out in real-world business decision making is found in the story of how General Electric Medical Systems (GEMS) came to pursue product development for MRI. In the early 1980s, MRI was just beginning to work its way into clinical practice. At that time, GEMS—the 800-pound gorilla of medical imaging—stood on the sidelines, uncertain of whether and how to pursue MRI, as smaller companies introduced their scanners and sold units to GEMS's traditional customers.

The company had delayed its decision because of the large required investment and the many uncertainties associated with MRI. Did MRI provide enough new information beyond what CT offered to warrant purchasers spending such a large amount of money?[26] How would selling MRI scanners affect the sales of GEMS's CT scanner, which dominated the market and was generating huge profits? Which of the several distinctly different MRI technologies[27] should they pursue? How would federal and state restrictions on providers' purchasing major medical equipment affect GEMS's ability to recoup its considerable development costs and make a profit?[28] Would insurers eventually pay for MRI exams?[29] Without insurance payment, patients would have to pay out of pocket, and sales of the technology would amount to little.

The initial decision made by GEMS was to develop and sell a premium version of a "me too" product—a 0.5 Tesla scanner similar to that of some of the other

[25] This amount includes the costs of all the *dry holes*—the unsuccessful drugs—that the company pursued, as well as R&D overhead, compliance costs, and so on spread over the agents that succeeded in receiving FDA approval.

[26] Magnetic resonance imaging and the modifications to buildings necessary to make it work safely and effectively made the outlays at least twice those of a CT scanner.

[27] Different manufacturers variously used permanent, resistive, and superconducting magnets as the basis for MRI. Each technology had both advantages and problems.

[28] We describe Certificate of Need regulations at length in Chapters 6 and 7.

[29] Medicare did not cover MRI exams, nor did private payers.

manufacturers. Walt Robb, GEMS's president, directed Roland Reddington's research group to downscale the 1.5 Tesla unit they had been using to investigate magnetic resonance spectroscopy (MRS) to 0.5 Tesla and focus on the development of a commercial MRI scanner. Reddington ignored the first directive but took the second to heart. He switched the focus of his group from spectroscopy to imaging. To the researchers' delight, images of the brain (like CT, the initial intended clinical use for MRI) at 1.5 Tesla were extraordinary, far superior to those that other manufacturers were generating at the lower magnetic field strength.

Now GEMS had a real basis for differentiating their product from the competition, but they confronted another problem. It would take longer to develop a high-field device than a 0.5 Tesla scanner. All the while, GEMS would be losing valuable market share. Therefore, GEMS needed to plant the idea in the minds of potential purchasers that it might be a mistake to buy a device before GEMS came out with their MRI scanner. As Reddington put it to his colleagues:

> "Blow smoke; develop as fast as you can; publish everything that you do; and keep people waiting for whatever it is that GE will do next, so that they don't spend their money on someone else's machine."[30]

The result was that GEMS received 50 orders, each for over $1 million, before the first device was shipped in the fall of 1984. It was an amazing start, but even as GEMS' strategy was beginning to bear fruit, the deteriorating economic environment threatened its long-term success. At least 25 companies were selling MRI devices; the worldwide health care economy was still recovering from the 1981–1982 recession; and changing Medicare payment methods[31] were causing hospitals (the primary sales target) to be more circumspect in their purchases of high-cost equipment. There still was very limited insurance payment for expensive MRI scans.

Still, GEMS persevered. Ultimately, as the environment grew more favorable and competition among providers drove MRI acquisition (Hillman et al. 1987a, 1987b), GEMS assumed a leadership position in a highly profitable new business.[32]

The story of GEMS and MRI is instructive from a number of viewpoints. New medical technologies take years to develop from an idea into a potentially useful clinical product. They take years more to achieve regulatory and reimbursement approval and still longer to work their way into broad acceptance in medical practice. As noted above, the time and expense of bringing an innovation through the entire process can be extraordinary. Managing the risks of medical innovation is a complex, big-stakes game.

---

[30] Managing innovation at GE Medical Systems. University of Virginia Darden School Foundation document 0000-1402-508C-000050FB. http://store.darden.virginia.edu.

[31] Bundling payments into diagnostic related groups (DRGs). The DRG method emphasizes lowering costs per admission and minimizing the use of diagnostic and therapeutic technologies as a means of improving hospital profitability.

[32] The preceding anecdote is synopsized from Managing innovation at GE Medical Systems. University of Virginia Darden School Foundation document 0000-1402-508C-000050FB. http://store.darden.virginia.edu.

## Challenges for the Future Practice of Radiology

The practice of radiology is changing. The development of new imaging technologies and new applications of existing ones are principally responsible, but so are advances in IT, the arrival of the boomer generation at late middle age, the advent of molecular medicine, and boundary disputes with other disciplines that use the same technologies. This section focuses on trends affecting radiologists and how they might respond to the public's need for medical imaging in the future.

*The Growth in Imaging Work*    Earlier, it was noted that medical imaging has been for most of the last fifteen years the fastest-growing physician-directed expenditure in all of health care. Imaging work has grown in two regards. One has been the rapidly increasing volume and cost of imaging procedures, which is a principal issue in this book. The other has been the mounting complexity of the exams that radiologists interpret. This greater complexity is largely a function of faster and higher-resolution scanners that are designed to image smaller abnormalities than previously. New, more complicated imaging protocols developed by radiologists to reduce misses are performed in seconds, a fraction of the time previously required. Computers rapidly reconstruct images into multiple planes or views. As a result, CT, MRI, and PET scans that used to consist of tens of images now often encompass 1000 or more. The radiologist must view each image before his or her interpretation is complete.

This would be an impossible task except for the transition during the past decade from film to digital imaging interpretation. Using advanced workstations and viewing images on high-resolution monitors, radiologists can review image sets more quickly than in the past by looking at them in *stacked* mode—in essence, a movie of sequential slices through the body. Advances in image viewing and interpretation technology have greatly improved radiologists' productivity, allowing them to read more and more complex examinations in the same amount of time as they expended previously.

More advanced technological solutions to increasing workloads are being developed. Engineers and their radiologist collaborators are introducing new three-dimensional viewing techniques that might further reduce the time per case needed to make accurate diagnoses. Computer-aided detection (CAD) algorithms scan images and can help radiologists focus on the detection of subtle abnormalities. Such software may eventually become sophisticated enough to manage some of radiologists' more mundane detection tasks, freeing up additional time for them to better address more complicated imaging interpretation.

However, technological solutions alone are unlikely to keep pace with the demand for imaging exams over the long term. Inevitably, radiologists and referring physicians must confront the fundamental problem that not all of the imaging being performed is necessary to the goal of medical care—improving patients' health. Indeed, the most direct approach to addressing future workforce shortages would be to eliminate marginal and unnecessary imaging studies. This is not as easy as it may seem. There is a relatively weak evidentiary basis for much of physician practice, and radiology is no exception.

In addition, the financial incentives to perform more imaging converge with the professional and patient biases described throughout this book: that more care means better care. Despite considerable evidence to the contrary, this bias underpins the aggressive use of medical imaging (Appleby 2008). The combination of better evidence for determining what imaging is best for patients, computerized systems that efficiently apply that knowledge to ordering needed tests, and elimination of aberrant financial incentives that induce unnecessary imaging would go a long way toward ameliorating a future shortage of imaging expertise while controlling imaging-related costs.

*Generalism versus Subspecialization*   The way radiology groups are organized and operate is changing to address the stresses of radiological practice. In particular, increasing demand for subspecialized radiology is disrupting the traditional general practice model discussed earlier in this book.

The value of generalism is being challenged by the physicians who refer patients to radiologists for their imaging procedures and those who pay for care. Some nonradiologist physicians who have chosen to incorporate high-technology imaging into their practices assert that, as dedicated organ system specialists, they can perform and interpret imaging examinations specific to their specialty better than general radiologists, whose practices cover all technologies and organ systems. They say that the traditional radiology practice model creates a knowledge mismatch between generalist radiologists and a client base of specialist physicians who have received some training in and grown more sophisticated about the specific imaging exams they employ in their specialties. In the business-speak of our times, these physicians are saying that there is no *value added* by consulting generalist radiologists.

Another force promoting the progression toward subspecialized image interpretations is the payment community. Their principal argument is that seeking a subspecialist's opinion initially produces a more definitive diagnosis. Doing it better the first time, they say, reduces the likelihood of clinicians ordering follow-up studies to reduce diagnostic uncertainty. Therefore, steering exams to subspecialists might save them money when viewed from the perspective of overall costs.

The rise of teleradiology has made large-scale interpretation by subspecialist radiologists practical, since teleradiology allows imaging examinations to be interpreted in an entirely different place from where the exams were performed. Health insurers and their RBM surrogates are beginning to steer their beneficiaries' exams across town or across the country to subspecialist radiologists with whom they have contracted in order to attain subspecialist expertise at affordable payment rates. This practice allows payers to purchase subspecialist interpretations at rates equal to or below those they might pay the facilities generating the exams while validating a claim for higher quality that they can market to health plans and employers.

An example of a business employing these practices is Premerus, owned by the RBM MedSolutions. Premerus is piloting in Phoenix, Arizona, the concept of subspecialty imaging interpretation as a cost-saving measure for its client, Aetna. While acknowledging that its data have not been accessible to outside scrutiny, the company claims that this approach has produced considerable downstream savings. While some of the cost reduction is related to fewer follow-up imaging exams, the greatest fraction of savings is attributable, they say, to more accurate treatment decisions.[33] On its Web site home page, MedSolutions advertises that Premerus saves payers a whopping $4.45 per member per month.[34]

Over the past few years, radiology has responded by moving toward greater subspecialization. As mentioned earlier, nearly all radiology residents now add one to three years of subspecialty fellowship training in an organ system or modality beyond their residency (Smith et al. 2009). An organ system fellowship might focus on imaging the gastrointestinal tract or kidneys, or possibly the central nervous or musculoskeletal systems; a modality fellowship would concentrate on a technology like ultrasound or MRI. The majority of community radiologists report that they now mostly practice in one or a small number of subspecialty areas (Smith et al. 2009).

In recognition of the need for greater imaging subspecialization, the ABR is redesigning its final certifying examination, which radiology residents must pass to become credentialed as radiologists. Beginning in 2011, the board will allow trainees to select a small number of subspecialty areas on which they will be examined rather than mandating, as it does now, broad but shallower competency in all aspects of the specialty. Radiology residency training programs are in the throes of redesigning their training requirements to synchronize with the new mandates. Interestingly, current residents are not necessarily happy with the turn of events. At the 2008 ACR annual meeting and Chapter Leadership Conference, the nearly 200 members of the ACR Residents and Fellows Section, representing trainees nationwide, overwhelmingly expressed a desire to utilize all aspects of their radiology training as general radiologists in their future practices.

General radiology doubtless will persist, either in its definitive form or in hybridized generalist/subspecialist practices. The generalist serves an important role in small hospitals and rural settings, as well as in public hospitals and care systems. Even in larger urban and suburban practices, general radiologists could interpret a large fraction of straightforward exams and triage difficult cases to subspecialists, making the workflow of their groups more efficient. Nonetheless, the demands of the imaging marketplace ensure that there will be a need for more subspecialized imaging in the future. Persistent resistance to subspecialization could create a mismatch between the desires of radiologists and their clients that could damage future radiology practice.

*The Reconfiguration of Imaging Practice*    In Chapter 7, the increasing involvement of nonradiologists in medical imaging was a major theme. The future is likely to witness a further breakdown of the traditional patterns of providing imaging care and, eventually, new imaging practice models.

The disruptive changes that will reshape imaging practice include the migration of imaging toward detailing cellular and subcellular processes; societal demand for more integrated and collaborative care; possible new payment models that pay providers per episode of illness rather than per visit, per hospitalization or per scan; the development of smaller, cheaper, and easier-to-use technologies by companies

---

[33] Personal communication, Gregg Allen, MD, December 2009.
[34] http://www.medsolutions.com.

seeking expanded markets; patients' wishes for more convenience and participation in their care; and teaching the educational content to the providers of future imaging care.

This last influence will prove particularly important. Much of the democratization of imaging technology will be shaped by changes in the education and training of young clinicians. As described in Chapter 1, the contemporary training of radiologists involves an extended apprenticeship focused mainly on learning to recognize patterns of gross disease. Functional and molecular imaging techniques are taught with highly variable intensity in the more than 200 radiology training programs across the United States. This is because there is presently little demand in the radiology job market for individuals who are expert in molecular techniques. Radiologists' traditional work is plentiful and has generated high incomes for practitioners. Hence, there is little incentive for academic programs or trainees to emphasize molecular imaging training. This is less true for medical subspecialists who work daily with the molecular pathways of their diseases and with treatments of interest that imaging might address.

At the same time, advanced imaging techniques are increasingly being integrated into the training of other specialists. As examples, the training of cardiologists involves extensive experience with modalities directly applicable to the heart and blood vessels, like conventional angiography, nuclear medicine, ultrasonography, and CT. Neurology and neurosurgery training depends heavily on CT and MRI scanning of the brain. Orthopedics trainees spend time reviewing radiographs and MRI exams of their patients' bones and joints. The practice of the surgical subspecialties increasingly depends on imaging guidance, motivating providers to adopt imaging modalities into their practices.

Technological innovation is supporting the trend. For instance, there is already a burgeoning business in single-purpose MRI scanners—instruments specifically designed to image only the organs of interest of a particular specialist, like a limb or the brain. These devices need little, if any, shielding, take up much less space than traditional scanners, and are much less expensive to purchase; in addition, insurers pay the same for an exam as one of higher quality performed on a much more expensive machine.

Another example, the wide dissemination of ultrasonography devices among primary care and emergency room physicians as tools for physical examination, would not have been possible without advances in portability and lower cost. This highly operator-dependent technology will require intensive training in residency rotations to be effectively used. Both the practice of ultrasonography by primary care physicians and the downstream referrals it will generate will inevitably alter established patterns of care. Indeed, ultrasonography may become so democratized and its use so routinely a part of a physical exam that the payment may be bundled into the fee for patient evaluation and management and only rarely paid separately.

Advances in image processing similarly may lower the barriers to entry into imaging. The PACS technology has had the effect of lessening radiologists' control of images by decentralizing where images are interpreted. Some specialized physicians who have focused organ system expertise may feel comfortable interpreting the parts of an imaging examination related to their specialty area (e.g., a gastroenterologist identifying polyps within the colon on a CTC study). However, they may feel less secure interpreting all of the other information on a set of images (a CTC exam also displays the genitourinary, cardiovascular, lymphatic, and other structures in the abdomen). Future enhancements to software like the CAD programs described earlier in this chapter have the potential to enable a broader array of providers to participate in image interpretation.

As one dramatic example of how advanced future software might help address this issue, consider this anecdote. Philips Medical Systems proposed to address the problem of incidental findings in CTA by using image processing to subtract everything from the image field but the intravenously injected contrast material in the blood vessels. The idea was to produce a CT scanner that would appeal to office-based cardiology and vascular surgery practices, enabling physicians to avoid interpreting, or even viewing, parts of the scan that made them uncomfortable. The concern that the product would generate the same amount of radiation as a conventional CT scan and cost as much, while providing much less information, caused the company to abandon the new system—at least for now.

*The Transition to Molecular Imaging*   Although some contemporary imaging techniques, like PET, address physiology, the bulk of radiological practice since the discovery of the Roentgen rays has focused on differentiating normal and abnormal anatomy. This remains true for most modern high-technology examinations. As discussed throughout the book, anatomical imaging has greatly improved patient care. Still, the surface of imaging capability has hardly been scratched. What is variously referred to as *molecular, functional,* or *mechanistic imaging* has extraordinary potential to address knotty problems in human health.

Molecular medicine researchers seek to improve care by identifying a host of elements—enzymes, proteins, and cell surface receptors, for example—that are active in promoting the pathophysiology of specific diseases. The goal is to identify disease in its earliest state, choose the most effective treatment the first time, predict and monitor the outcome of treatment, and, by doing all of this, reduce both illness and the cost of treatment. Imaging is expected to play an important role in addressing all of these objectives.

Molecular imaging is an example of a disruptive technology because it has the potential to change not only what imaging specialists do but also how medicine is organized and who ends up doing this new work (Hillman and Neiman 2002). Even today, with molecular imaging on the horizon, radiologists are almost entirely trained in anatomical imaging. Few radiologists participate in the research that is bringing molecular imaging to fruition, despite the fact that much of the research is conducted in academic radiology departments under the aegis of doctoral scientists. In the end, even new radiologists just beginning their careers are ill equipped to practice molecular imaging.

So, who will practice molecular imaging once it is sufficiently advanced to be a sizable fraction of all imaging? It might well be radiologists, who have mastered the imaging modalities like PET and MRI that currently use molecular probes. However, like other disruptive technologies, molecular imaging provides opportunities for other physician specialists to fill what is currently an underoccupied niche. This is particularly the case because molecular imaging offers the promise of consolidating both diagnostic and therapeutic elements on the same molecule or probe. The capacity both to identify an abnormal focus and treat it with the same agent, then evaluate the response of the abnormality over time, surely will prove attractive to therapeutic specialists with focused knowledge of the subcellular mechanisms of disease.

Indeed, molecular imaging potentially puts the two major diagnostic specialties, radiology and pathology, on converging pathways. Pathologists increasingly have moved their practices into the molecular realm. Their specialty involves a great deal of imaging, although usually of tissue samples displayed on slides rather than images of the insides of living humans. The past few decades already have seen some alignment of the two specialties. Anatomical imaging has grown sophisticated enough that it often provides a more accurate diagnosis than biopsy specimens.[35] A recent publication detailed the accuracy of CT and MRI in performing what the authors called the "minimally invasive autopsy" (Weustink et al. 2009). It is possible that, eventually, important parts of radiology and pathology will merge into a single new specialty of *molecular diagnostics*, with expertise that spans the continua from anatomical to functional and from tissue specimens to living humans.

A partial consolidation of radiology and pathology might lead to the development of an entirely new training regimen that would embrace the best of both specialties and discard what has become vestigial. The risk to radiology is disaggregation, with some components of current practice remaining radiology and others falling to molecular diagnosis. However, a new department of molecular diagnosis might benefit society by putting at patients' service more focused expertise and providing greater efficiencies for the health care system.

## Summary

This chapter has focused on the forces that will shape the future of imaging. It is incontestable that the current state of imaging science could once again spawn new technologies that might surpass the imaging revolution of the past 40 years. However, it is clear that the path to innovation will be encumbered by restraining influences in both the medical and economic environments. The societal demand for greater value for health care expenditures and the promise of more effective, less harmful personalized diagnosis and treatment will help determine the direction of technological innovation.

Scientific and societal imperatives likewise will drive changes in the financial models of imaging technology development. Changes in regulatory requirements must recognize that emerging molecular imaging technologies do not fit the current regulatory pigeonholes. New regulatory approaches should recognize the unique needs of combination products that rely on the interaction of multiple components. Companies will have to develop original business models to support product development that will serve the needs of 4P medicine and still return a profit.

All of this is a tall order. Since the introduction of MRI in the early 1980s, advances in imaging have been mostly incremental in nature. What has been described in this chapter is quite different—the potential for another giant leap in the contributions of imaging to patient care. To illustrate how profoundly another revolution in imaging

---

[35] A biopsy is a sample of the tissue in the abnormal region. Since most disease is heterogeneous, specimens may not accurately represent the condition causing the problem.

might improve care, we invented a mythical device, the Omniscient, which in a single painless visit could assess an individual's risk for serious disease, detect whether the condition was present, evaluate the likelihood that the abnormality would ultimately affect a patient's health or life span, and treat the finding with little harm to the patient's normal tissues. If the imaging community can respond to the challenges of the environment, the invention of a real set of imaging technologies mimicking the qualities of the Omniscient may eventually emerge. The barriers to such inventions are daunting. The risks to innovators are significant. But as Zerhouni has said, "The greatest risk in science is to stop taking risks."[36]

# References

Appleby J. The case of CT angiography: how Americans view and embrace new technology. *Health Aff.* 2008;27:1515–1521.

Bradley WG. MR-guided focused ultrasound: a potentially disruptive technology. *J Am Coll Radiol.* 2009;6:510–513.

Chao KS, Bosch WR, Mutic S, et al. A novel approach to overcome hypoxic tumor resistance: Cu-ATSM-guided intensity-modulated radiation therapy. *Int J Radiat Oncol Biol Phys.* 2001;49:1171–1182.

Dhruva SS, Phurrough SE, Salive ME, et al. CMS's landmark decision on CT colonography— examining the relevant data. *N Engl J Med.* 2009;360:2699–2701.

Eisenhauer EA, Therasse P, Bogaerts J, et al. New response evaluation criteria in solid tumors: revised RECIST guideline (version 1.1). *Eur J Cancer.* 2009;45:228–247.

Harrisinghani MG, Barentsz J, Hahn PF, et al. Noninvasive detection of clinically occult lymph-node metastases in prostate cancer. *N Engl J Med.* 2003;348:2491–2499.

Hillman BJ, Gatsonis C. When is the right time to conduct a clinical trial of a diagnostic imaging technology? *Radiology.* 2008; 248:12–15.

Hillman BJ, Neiman HL. Translating molecular imaging research into radiological practice—Proceedings of the American College of Radiology Colloquium. *Radiology.* 2002;222:19–24.

Hillman BJ, Neu CR, Winkler JD, et al. The diffusion of magnetic resonance imaging scanners in a changing U.S. health care environment. I. Acquirers' considerations and actions. *J Technol Assess Health Care.* 1987a;3:545–554.

Hillman BJ, Neu CR, Winkler JD, et al. The diffusion of magnetic resonance imaging scanners in a changing U.S. health care environment. II. How experiences with X-ray computed tomography influenced providers' plans for magnetic resonance imaging scanners. *J Technol Assess Health Care.* 1987b;3:554–559.

Hindley J, Gedroyc WM, Regan L, et al. MRI guidance of focused ultrasound therapy of uterine fibroids: early results. *AJR Am J Roentgenol.* 2004;183:1713–1719.

Hoffman JM, Gambhir SS, Kelloff GJ. Regulatory and reimbursement challenges for molecular imaging. *Radiology.* 2007;245:645–660.

Hricak H, Gatsonis CG, Coakley F. Early invasive cervical cancer: tumor delineation by magnetic resonance imaging, computed tomography, and clinical examination, verified by pathologic results, in the ACRIN-6651/COG-183 intergroup study. *J Clin Oncol.* 2006;24:5687–5694.

Hynynen K, Vykhodtseva NI, Chung JH, et al. Thermal effects of ultrasound on the brain: determination with MR imaging. *Radiology.* 1997;204:247–253.

---

[36] Elias Zerhouni, Moorefield Lecture to the ACR annual meeting and Chapter Leadership Conference, May 2009.

Islam T, Josephson L. Current state and future applications of active targeting in malignancies using superparamagnetic iron oxide nanoparticles. *Cancer Biomark.* 2009;5:99–107.

Kinoshita M, McDannold N, Jolesz FA, et al. Non-invasive localized delivery of Herceptin to the mouse brain by MRI-guided focused ultrasound-induced blood-brain barrier disruption. *Proc Natl Acad Sci USA.* 2006;103:11719–11723.

Lewin JS. Industrial-academic relationships: departmental collaborations. *Radiology.* 2009;250:23–27.

Mathieu MP, ed. *PAREXEL's Pharmaceutical R&D Statistical Sourcebook 2002/2003.* Waltham MA: Parexel International, 2002.

Nunn AD. The cost of developing imaging agents for routine clinical use. *Invest Radiol.* 2006;41:206–212.

Otero HJ, Rybicki FJ, Greenberg D, et al. Twenty years of cost-effectiveness analysis in medical imaging. Are we improving? *Radiology.* 2008;249:917–924.

Ram Z, Cohen ZR, Harnoff S, et al. Magnetic resonance imaging-guided, high-intensity focused ultrasound for brain tumor therapy. *Neurosurgery.* 2006;59:946–959.

Reichert JM. Trends in development and approval times for new therapeutics in the United States. *Nat Rev Drug Discov.* 2003;2:695–702.

Rupert K, Mata JF, Brookman JR, et al. Exploring lung function with hyperpolarized 129-Xe magnetic resonance. *Magn Reson Med.* 2004;51:676–687.

Salerno M, Altes TA, Brookman JR, et al. Dynamic spiral MRI of pulmonary gas flow using hyperpolarized He: preliminary studies in healthy and diseased lungs. *Magn Reson Med.* 2001;46:667–677.

Schwartz LM, Woloshin S, Floyd FJ, et al. Enthusiasm for screening in the United States. *JAMA.* 2004;291:71–78.

Smith GS, Thrall JH, Pentecost MJ, et al. Subspecialization in radiology and radiation oncology. *JACR.* 2009;6:147–159.

Veazy S, Zderic V. Hemorrhage control using high intensity focused ultrasound. *Int J Hypertherm.* 2007;23:203–211.

Weustink AC, Hunink MGM, Van Dyke CF, et al. Minimally invasive autopsy: alternative to conventional autopsy? *Radiology.* 2009;250:897–904.

Zerhouni EA. Major trends in the imaging sciences: 2007 Eugene P. Pendergrass New Horizons Lecture. *Radiology.* 2008;249:403–409.

# 10

# Making the Best Use of Imaging's Expansive Toolbox

This book has explored a remarkable dual success story: the emergence of medical imaging's remarkable technology and the rise of the clinical specialty of radiology, the discipline that helped develop medical imaging into what it is today.

The annealing of the "intellectual DNA" of several disciplines has made radiology—a medical specialty of gearheads and restless tinkerers—the rivals of software engineers as the most successful contemporary knowledge discipline. For generations, radiologists have collaborated with physicists, engineers, and computer scientists—across industry, academia, and community-based practice—and borrowed liberally from them to refine and extend the capabilities of mature technologies to the point where they have become even more useful. As such, radiologists are a superb example of *hybrid vigor*[1] applied to a knowledge industry.

New knowledge of the radiofrequency spectrum, co-opted both from pure science and military and commercial applications, found uses in medical imaging with remarkable speed. Since the early 1970s, imaging also has leveraged Moore's Law. As computing power has continuously increased, so have the reach and refinement of computerized imaging methods. Today, radiologists and imaging scientists are pushing the envelope of scientific innovation in systems biology and molecular medicine.

Based on diagnostic advances, radiology leapt the fence to invasive, curative medicine. Innovations in interventional radiology techniques have provided ways of curing human illness that are less costly per intervention and less risky than previous methods. The success of interventional radiology has disrupted the traditional division of labor among specialists. Radiologists also anticipated a flattened,

---

[1] Hybrid vigor is a proposition in genetics whereby parents with differing traits combine their genomes to produce offspring with characteristics superior to those of either parent.

networked world and created the technical infrastructure to utilize broadband Internet years before it was available to them. The universal availability of images anytime, anywhere threatens further disruption in the traditional organization and processes for delivering medical care.

Advances in imaging have fundamentally transformed medicine by providing ways of visualizing human pathology more accurately and definitively than the naked human eye. However, all of this progress has come at a price. The disruption caused by many of radiology's most valuable innovations has disturbed the practices of other specialists, spawning economic and professional conflicts. These conflicts remain unresolved and have the potential to unnerve patients and damage medicine's public image. Just as significantly, imaging is now squarely in the gun sights of those seeking to contain the growth in health care costs. Along with pharmaceutical spending (now in a decade-long deceleration), imaging spending has been identified by the policy community as a prime contributor to an unsustainable rate of growth in health care spending in the United States.

Through 2006, imaging spending grew at more than double the rate of health care spending in the United States as a whole. There was a marked leveling off of imaging cost growth (as there was for all of health care expenditures) during 2007–2008. It is too soon to tell how much of this cooling was a product of the deep recession and how much was due to the concerted efforts of payers, particularly Medicare, to reduce the growth of imaging costs.

While advances in technology and the aging of the population explain some of the growth in imaging spending, other contributors, discussed at length in Chapter 5, are causes for concern. Most importantly, it is certain that a substantial fraction of imaging utilization is unnecessary. A sketchy evidentiary basis for many imaging studies, as well as disordered and overly thorough diagnostic practices—learned in medical education and carried over into clinical practice—bear some of the responsibility. There is compelling evidence of economically motivated imaging that does not improve quality and adds to cost. Though efforts have been made since the early 1990s to contain moral hazard–driven imaging (discussed in Chapter 7), policymakers have not yet succeeded in finding the right balance between the economic interests of practitioners and the interests of patients and society. Fear of malpractice liability drives some unknown but probably sizable fraction of examinations that return little patient benefit.

Since the inappropriate use of imaging is a multifactorial problem, there is no single answer to how to improve the current situation. A variety of policy changes will be required for the United States to derive greater value from the use of advanced imaging technology. This chapter examines some important policy considerations and suggests opportunities for improvement, with the goal of improving care for patients and ensuring access to future valuable imaging innovations.

## What Do We Want as Patients?

Learning how to use imaging's powerful capabilities more intelligently and thoughtfully is a vital objective for a sustainable health care system. Properly employed and paid for, imaging advances will continue making health care safer and more effective. Achieving that goal requires the cooperation of patients. A major reason imaging volumes and costs have grown as rapidly as they have is that patients have demanded and received imaging examinations even when imaging has had little to offer.

Understanding how this situation has come about requires answering the question "What do patients really want?" In our view, patients want accurate, thoughtful, and dispassionate assessments of their clinical condition by clinicians who are both well trained and appropriately equipped to provide those assessments. Patients want physicians to provide safe, timely, and appropriate care. Patients want physicians to act in their interests, as free from economic conflicts and motivations as possible.

These patient goals are best addressed by practitioners who work as a team with patients and their families—each serving the role for which they are best trained—in a purposeful collaboration to find the best solution to the patient's medical problems. For this to occur, the way physicians are paid must be altered from the current incentives that reward the provision of more imaging care. Any new payment method affecting imaging should provide incentives for multidisciplinary teams to develop and employ processes that encourage the best outcomes.

How to do this is more complex than it may seem, because a more thoughtful and cautious payment policy for imaging cannot be created in an economic vacuum. Much of the progress in imaging has been made possible not only by societal investments in basic sciences like mathematics, physics, biology, and defense technology, but also by research and development investment by private industry. There is a need for accelerated and sustained government investment in basic and applied research in both the physical and biological sciences that will ultimately fuel further innovations in imaging technology. These investments tend to come in spurts, interspersed with lengthy periods of negative real growth, rather than as a steady, predictable government commitment.

Ultimately, though, innovation will be powered by how, and how much, private and public insurers will pay for imaging services. Capital flows into imaging from capital markets and other sources that cater to industry. Payment policies that promote more conservative and thoughtful use of imaging services must be pursued with the awareness that they will affect the pace and scope of future technological progress. Corporations that cannot anticipate a return on their investments in imaging technology will direct their capital elsewhere. Regulation that increases the costs of research and development will also have a chilling effect on the diffusion of innovations into clinical practice. Thus, any change in regulatory policies affecting imaging must consider whether patients will ultimately suffer for lack of access to important new discoveries.

Having said, this, some middle course must be taken that encourages innovation while discouraging the non-beneficial use of imaging drugs, contrast agents, and devices.

## Addressing the Causes of Unnecessary Utilization

It is important to reiterate that much of the growth in imaging services has been entirely appropriate and valuable to patients. Remarkable advances in medical imaging continue unabated even as this book is being written. Improvements in CT, MRI, PET, and image-guided treatment technologies are producing new clinical applications that make diagnosis and treatment safer and better than ever before.

Nonetheless, a number of powerful influences promote non-beneficial, inappropriate utilization. The root problem is with the practice cultures of physicians. The prevailing mindset is to do whatever it takes to achieve diagnostic certainty—often pursuing this goal to unrealistic levels. This culturally ingrained approach is termed *flat of the curve* medicine because expenditures continue to climb even though the application of another test does little to improve the care patients receive.

Flat of the curve medicine begins with education and training. Physicians are educated and predominantly serve their training years in academic medical centers (AMCs). Physicians working in AMCs tend to care for the sickest of the sick. In these environs, physicians-in-training are encouraged by their chiefs and teachers to leave no stone unturned. When they go out into community practice (as the great majority do), many perpetuate the high-technology approach to clinical care they learned in the AMCs despite the change in their practice environment and (for many) the lesser complexity of their patients' clinical problems. Young physicians' training to test aggressively converges with patients' desire to receive more care and with powerful financial incentives to adopt and employ profitable diagnostic technologies. The result can be disastrous overuse with little positive effect on patients' health.

The most effective solution to the non-beneficial use of imaging will take a long time to achieve. Clinical faculties in medical schools and teaching hospitals must become more conscious of the aspects of academic culture that breed inefficiencies in their own clinical practices. This means returning to a past epoch in which the goal was to make an efficient, *elegant* diagnosis. An elegant diagnosis is one that asks the right questions, takes stock of the probabilities, and employs only those tools that can reasonably address the patient's complaints. Rather than learning blindly to fire expensive and showy diagnostic shotgun blasts, young physicians need to be taught how to combine assessments of the probability of disease and the performance of imaging tests into a coherent testing plan. The appropriate diagnostic course would avoid testing when testing is of limited value and employ only the most appropriate imaging when it was indicated. This approach would heed the well-worn medical adage: "When you hear hoof beats, think horses, not zebras."

Radiologists could play a much more important role in guiding a return to more rational, resource-efficient use of imaging than they have to date. Radiology medical school curricula have focused too much on the instruction of the rudiments of imaging interpretation and too little on how imaging could be employed more effectively in patient care. A greater emphasis on how nascent physicians should access consultation with radiologists on whether imaging might be beneficial for a given case or which imaging exam would be most appropriate would better serve society.

More generally, the broad electronic availability of images and radiologists' interpretations has greatly reduced consultation between radiologists and referring clinicians. Radiologists too often acquiesce to marginal or unnecessary exams for fear of alienating referring clinicians or perhaps because an unnecessary exam generates the same payment as an appropriate one. The *orders* radiologists receive for imaging examinations are actually requests for consultation and should more often treated as such. Each consultation is a *teachable moment*. The accumulation of teachable moments over time might have a potent effect on changing the culture of imaging practice for the better.

Ultimately, however, for medical practice to return to elegant diagnosis requires society and our political system to address the principal barriers to more thoughtful, more rational practice: a legal tort system that promotes the practice of defensive medicine in order to minimize legal liability; aberrant financial incentives to overuse imaging technologies; and the thin evidentiary basis for defining the best imaging care for many clinical indications.

## Reforming Our Tort Liability System

The role that tort liability plays in encouraging inappropriate or marginally unnecessary imaging examinations has been discussed in several chapters. While it is not the root cause of the growth in imaging spending, it plays a very important supporting role by amplifying the expensive search for medical certainty, which is the main culprit.

To think about this constructively, it is important to recognize that medicine is still as much art as science. Mistakes will inevitably occur in what is, at its best, an imperfect and fundamentally human process. Good communication between the clinical team and patients and their families when things go wrong is an important beginning point. Frank acknowledgment of mistakes by the clinical team and aggressive efforts to mitigate the damage caused will go some way toward reducing the incidence of tort liability claims and, eventually, their cost.

Chapter 1 briefly explored an important imbalance in our legal system that all physicians face: doctors are much more likely to be sued if they fail to employ diagnostic testing than if they test too much. The significant financial risk of a malpractice action reinforces the tendency to conduct overly thorough diagnostic workups. The possibility of a million-dollar (or more) malpractice judgment powerfully reinforces the tendency learned during medical education and training to "throw the kitchen sink" at a clinical problem. As a result, the many physicians who are sensitive to medical-legal risk tend to order exams that are not strictly necessary for high-quality care. Similarly, risk-averse radiologists are likely to overcall findings and suggest additional imaging exams to cover themselves, further aggravating the problem.

In dealing with physicians' concerns over medical liability, the simplistic notion of restricting punitive or noneconomic damages (known as *malpractice caps*) does not effectively address the perceived risk in performing diagnostic work. More innovative solutions are essential to reduce the referral and interpretation of unnecessary exams.

Collaborative mechanisms that encourage honest discussion of what went wrong in diagnostic miscalls, such as mediation and arbitration, could play an important role in controlling malpractice expenses. Another idea is to implement and extend beyond hospital practice settings both credentialing and skills-based restrictions on who performs and interprets imaging examinations. At a minimum, this might reduce the incidence of malpractice and, eventually, malpractice insurance premiums. Another interesting possibility would be to design special *health courts* that take the process out of the traditional tort liability/jury trial track but keep actions in the judicial system (Barringer 2005). It is also possible that adaptations of the *no-fault* compensation models that have helped stabilize the liability costs in vaccine development may have a role to play in managing the consequences of missed diagnoses. All these strategies are worth pursuing.

More robust and widely disseminated appropriateness guidelines, integrated into order entry software (discussed in Chapter 5) to help physicians request the most appropriate examination for their patients, would enable clinicians to be less wasteful in their ordering patterns while providing some cover against capricious legal actions. Physicians using guideline-directed order entry systems should receive discounts on their malpractice premiums because they will be practicing safer and more conservative medicine. Scientifically validated standards of appropriateness are the right substitute for ad hoc application of *community standards* to govern when and how imaging should be used. A legal determination of whether a physician relied on scientific standards to order imaging examinations would be a vast improvement upon the too often arbitrary decisions of emotionally charged lay juries.

A more definitive solution to the defensive medicine problem would be to outlaw the practice of contingency fees and to institute a formula whereby the loser pays court costs. Just as argued above with regard to moral hazard–driven imaging, the current contingency fee approach of most plaintiffs' attorneys presents a moral hazard of its own. A lawyer's perception that there is too little money in a case can disenfranchise a patient with a legitimate complaint; alternatively, the smell of big money can provoke a frivolous lawsuit. Putting medical liability lawyers on a fee schedule similar to the physicians' RBRVS, with a prescribed compensation schedule for different kinds of injuries, would correct the current aberrant incentives, ensure that injured patients receive a higher percentage of the compensation awarded for the real injuries they suffer, and diminish the impact of defensive medicine on systemic costs. Unfortunately, it is lawyers who mostly make the laws in Congress and state legislatures and, simultaneously, powerfully influence them through campaign contributions and the political process. As a result, this perfectly logical approach is likely to be a nonstarter.

## More and Better Studies of Appropriateness and Clinical Effectiveness

It is neither naive nor idealistic to expect a better evidentiary basis for deciding when to order imaging studies and what test works best for a given clinical indication. Coverage and payment policy should be fact-based. To make it so will require an enhanced and sustained investment in clinical outcomes and comparative effectiveness research (CER). Despite the complexities of CER (discussed in Chapter 5), better and more complete information on what imaging studies are appropriate, and in what circumstances, is achievable.

Better evidence and the use of practice guidelines and decision trees[2] based on that evidence, along with incentives to adopt best practices, comprise the optimal solution to the current problem of duplicative testing—using multiple technologies that do the same thing. Less accurate technologies would be used less frequently, and there would be a reduced tendency to employ multiple overlapping, tests if there were better evidence-based guidelines to help clinicians decide what to order and when.

The problem of how to encourage evidence accumulation interacts with the decisions regarding insurance coverage (particularly Medicare coverage) and payment levels for new technologies. Setting the evidence bar too high too early carries the risk that promising emerging tools—such as various molecular imaging methods—will be prematurely discarded before there is sufficient clinical experience to determine

---

[2] Decision trees chart sequential tests and treatments based on the results of earlier testing. They are necessary for situations where a single test is usually insufficient to diagnose the patient's problem.

whether full-scale scientific evaluation of its comparative effectiveness and cost/ benefit information is worthwhile. It would also reduce the incentives for manufacturers to invest in developing or building out the tools in the first place.

To address this problem, both Medicare and private insurers should support the notion of *coverage with evidence development* (CED). This method should apply to selected high-impact technologies that may most significantly affect health or societal costs. Already, CED has seen considerable use. The CMS promulgated guidelines in 2005 to encourage prospective research on promising devices and pharmaceutical innovations when, in the agency's view, there was an insufficient evidentiary basis to justify a national coverage determination for Medicare payment. Since then, CED has been applied to such diverse technologies as implantable defibrillators, lung reduction surgery for chronic obstructive pulmonary disease, and FDG-PET scanning for the evaluation of Alzheimer's disease and oncology (Tunis and Pearson 2006).

Currently, under CED, provisional Medicare coverage and payment are granted to providers who contribute data to the evaluation of the benefit derived from employing the technology. Only providers supplying data to *deemed research* studies (i.e., registries and clinical trials approved by CMS) are eligible for payment.

An alternative approach would be to pay all providers a provisional payment rate during the period of the CED ruling. This method has the advantage of generating broader clinical experience than might be accrued through deemed studies alone. Providers who submitted data to the deemed studies would receive a bonus for their trouble. To help steer patients to the physicians submitting data, patients would be required to pay a higher copayment to nonparticipating physicians to help offset the cost of the bonus. This copayment might also serve as a modest brake on the moral hazard–driven use that has plagued new diagnostic and therapeutic imaging tools.

The accelerated development of a more rigorous factual basis for health care decisions (including prominent mention of imaging) received a boost in the 2009 economic stimulus legislation. The American Relief and Recovery Act (ARRA) allocated more than $1 billion to increase funding for CER. Several members of the Obama administration, notably Budget Director Peter Orszag, are strong proponents of this type of research, suggesting that additional federal funding for CER will be forthcoming in future years.

An increased federal government commitment to CER research and implementation of the results in determinations of what actually gets paid for by public and private insurers would help reduce duplicative imaging expenditures. This could be encouraged by a three- to four-year stepwise phase-out of insurers' payments for performing outmoded procedures. Older, less effective technologies should pass more rapidly out of usage rather than lingering in practice, as they do today.

Few providers or payers would dispute that a better evidence basis would lead to more beneficial, less costly care. The argument has centered on who should pay for the research to generate the information that would underlie better medical decision making. On the government side, NIH funding of clinical trials generates data to support advancing clinical practice and remains a bulwark underlying CER. One would think that private insurers also would contribute to the advancement of better clinical knowledge. It would be hard for any disinterested observer to conclude that insurers have no "skin in the game."

However, insurers have argued in the past that providers are the ultimate beneficiaries and have generally refused to participate to any real extent in funding outcomes or cost-effectiveness research. For payers, it has been a classic "problem of the commons" concern. Research done by any one of them benefits all. This position has become outmoded. Given the need for better clinical knowledge to support coverage decision making, it will be difficult for payers to rationalize remaining on the sidelines in the future. The Patient Protection and Affordable Care Act, enacted in March, 2010, created a non-profit Patient-Centered Outcomes Research Institute to identify and conduct research on improving the effectiveness of medical treatment.

## Paying the Right Price for Imaging Procedures

It is not just coverage policy that should be evidence-based but payment policy as well. Present Medicare policy is grounded in the premise that payments to physicians should be reasonably related to their costs. However, there has been much carping among specialties about whether practice costs are fairly calculated. The ability to track and accurately assign practice expenses to the relative value of a procedure has been hampered by the methods employed and the tendency of the usually small number of physicians who participate in the surveys to game the activity in favor of their specialty. As a result, the evidence on which to base alterations of the current RBRVS fee payments for imaging under Medicare has been sketchy. The thinness of the data has led to what many practitioners consider arbitrary policy decisions (e.g., reduced fees for scanning adjacent body parts and recent changes in utilization factors for MR and CT scanners), raising questions about CMS's commitment to evidence-based policymaking.

In the absence of better data, coverage and payment decisions are politically fraught and subject to congressional input, which in turn is responsive to pressure from the medical professions, patient groups, and manufacturers (who sometimes work in remarkably tight linkage). Former Senate Majority Leader Tom Daschle and others have recommended that decisions about coverage and payment for new and existing technologies be depoliticized to the maximum extent possible and placed in the hands of an independent Federal Reserve–like agency for health care (Daschle et al. 2008). A provision to create an Independent Payment Advisory Board for the Medicare program in the 2010 health reform legislation will likely shape Medicare payment policy in the future.

This initiative may prove effective but, as with most things, the devil is in the details. How would such a panel be constituted? Which constituencies might be represented and which not? How will a sustainable and appropriate flow of funding be assured to create the evidentiary basis for policy decisions? Is it realistic to believe that we can completely depoliticize a process in which so much money is at stake?

## Rightsizing the Relationship between Cognitive and Technical Payments

One anomaly of the U.S. health care payment system is that it financially values procedures, particularly those that involve the use of high-technology tools, more than the fundamental exercise of human judgment. Practitioners who invest time in listening to patients and understanding their problems are compensated at rates far below those of practitioners who perform diagnostic or therapeutic procedures. As an application of this anomaly specifically to imaging, the technical component of imaging payment dwarfs the professional component, which compensates radiologists for exercising their educated diagnostic judgment (what is referred to in the trade as their *cognitive* work). This imbalance needs to be redressed to reduce the aberrant incentives that drive the financially motivated self-referral of advanced imaging procedures.

Because income from *evaluation and management* (E&M) services has lagged far behind the growth in physicians' expenses, many practitioners have turned to self-referral for laboratory and imaging services to fill the income gap. In the Marcus Welby era, this took the form of setting up small laboratories and X-ray suites in physicians' offices. In the modern high-technology era, advanced imaging such as CT, MRI and PET scanning has metastasized from hospitals and full-service imaging centers into individual physicians' offices.

Paying physicians more generously for exercising their clinical judgment will not necessarily halt the practice of self-referral overnight, but rightsizing the relationship between payments for cognitive services and the use of technology would be a start. To bolster the effect of fairer payment, federal rules governing the appropriateness of physicians' referral to clinical services in which they have an ownership interest need to be reexamined and modernized. However, to do so without solving the underlying problem that helped foster these developments in the first place would be unjust and counterproductive.

## Markedly Restricting Self-Referral for Imaging

As discussed in Chapter 7, principal-agent (physician) moral hazard has reared its ugly head in the imaging industry and made a major contribution to generating unnecessary costs. It has also undermined the legitimacy of the medical profession, which is honor-bound to put patients' needs before the economic interests of the practitioner. Federal law (the Stark II law) forbids practitioners from referring Medicare patients to free-standing services in which they or immediate family members have an ownership interest or billing Medicare for those services. Another set of Medicare regulations, the so-called anti-kickback provisions, forbids physicians from accepting payments in consideration of their referrals of Medicare patients for services.

While these laws have been sufficiently demanding to alter the ownership structure of freestanding imaging centers, they have left a gaping loophole—the in-office ancillary services (IOASE) exception—large enough to drive a Brinks truck through. The IOASE allows physicians to refer patients for imaging devices they place in their offices or in the same building in which they provide their primary patient care services. The IOASE was originally intended to protect practitioners' use of simple in-office laboratory tests (like those from desktop analyzers or dry chemistry tests like dipsticks) and office X-ray and ultrasound machines. It now protects individual practitioners' and medical groups' use of million-dollar MR, CT, and PET imaging equipment, technologies that were never intended to be sheltered when the law was passed in the early 1990s.

It is time to narrow this window of economic abuse dramatically. One intriguing thought is simply to restrict the IOASE to imaging services provided on the same day as the patient's visit to the physician. Such a restriction would recognize the value to the patient of convenient one-stop care. This approach would be easy to administer. If the imaging were billed for any day other than the day of the original visit, the physician would not receive payment for the imaging exam.

A more rigorous approach would be to prohibit self-referral for high-technology imaging in all physician office settings with very narrow *safe-harbor* corridors. Entities exempted from this prohibition might include academic practices that conduct clinical research requiring the equipment, multispecialty group practices where physicians are salaried and do not receive compensation based on the volume of services they or their colleagues order, or groups of radiologists or other practitioners in which the referring physician does not have the capacity to self-refer.

There could also be a safe harbor for groups that do not meet the above criteria but that have a definable and significant percentage of their group income derived from fixed, per capita (e.g., capitation) payments from health plans or where the group is large enough that the financial incentive for referral is diminishingly small. These and the restrictions proposed above could be phased in over five years to avoid creating economic havoc for physicians or physician groups who entered into ownership or leasing arrangements when such activities were legal.

Despite the claims of those who might be adversely affected, neither the same-day-only approach nor terminating the IOASE with narrow safe harbors would inhibit access to needed imaging studies. Rather, it would channel orders for imaging studies to those who have trained and specialized in imaging practice and are less affected by moral hazard—specifically, those providers who do not have the capacity to benefit financially by referring their patients to their own imaging operations.

The alternative policy approach is much less appealing. The GAO recently proposed amending the Medicare law to require prior authorization by a third-party reviewer, such as an RBM firm, to confirm the medical necessity of advanced imaging procedures. As earlier argued, this is a 1970s solution to a twenty-first-century problem. Patients are inconvenienced by delays and cancellations. The criteria by which they approve or disapprove examinations are proprietary, hence opaque and suspect. Prior authorization increases overall administrative expenses, with which the medical system already is overburdened. Using RBMs adds to practice and institutional overhead for every practitioner who orders an imaging study, implicating the entire community of users in what could be managed more directly. Intelligent decision support radiology order entry software would do a less costly, more effective job of screening out inappropriate studies, especially if its recommendations were backstopped by auditable enforcement of its protocols.

Finally, and apropos of earlier comments on evidence-based decision making, it would be helpful to further study the appropriateness of the ordering patterns of self-referring and radiologist-referring physicians. Such evaluation would help to establish a baseline for appropriate use. Evaluations of appropriateness should include a generalizable assessment of both self-referral and *auto-referral* (the latter being the effect of radiologists suggesting follow-on studies to the referring physician; see Chapter 7) to ensure that ownership incentives do not result in inappropriate radiologist-directed utilization patterns. There should not be an automatic presumption of virtue concerning the appropriateness of ordering follow-on exams merely because the radiologist does not initiate the diagnostic sequence.

## Accreditation of Practitioners and Facilities

Patients and their families should have access to imaging care performed by properly trained and equipped personnel, using safe, accurate, and well-maintained equipment, practicing within the orbit of appropriate professional preparation and experience. While tightening Stark II by closing the IOASE would help matters, it will be insufficient by itself to create a safer and more effective imaging environment.

The radiology community, led by the ACR, pioneered the approach of improving quality via the accreditation of facilities providing mammography services. This successful, initially voluntary, program specified detailed quality criteria for facilities providing mammography services. The approach was eventually codified into federal statute by the Mammography Quality Standards Act (MQSA) of 1994, which empowered the FDA to require accreditation of facilities providing this vital women's health service. The expense of adhering to MQSA chased out marginal-quality mammography providers. The success in improving quality standards in mammography is a recommendation of this approach for broader adoption in high-technology imaging.

Late in 2005, United Healthcare became the first private health plan to put providers on notice that they would require accreditation of facilities that perform high-technology imaging studies as a condition of paying for their services. This accreditation program was to have been implemented in 2009 but has been delayed indefinitely. CMS indicates that they will require credentialing of high-technology imaging by a deemed (by CMS) accrediting organization under new legal authority provided by the Medicare Improvement for Patients and Providers Act of 2008 (MIPPA). In late 2009, CMS deemed several quality of care organizations, including the ACR and the Joint Commission on Accreditation for Healthcare Organizations (JCAHO), to institute facility accreditation beginning 2012.

Quality improvement standards for the nonhospital outpatient sector[3] are long past due. It is anomalous that hospital imaging has been elaborately regulated by CMS to assess both professional and institutional qualifications but that no parallel process has existed for imaging practitioners and facilities, even if they perform invasive curative procedures. The MIPPA changes that situation and will require competency-based certification as a condition of receiving technical component payments under Medicare. Linking both the qualifications of practitioners and the technical capabilities of facilities to payment is the method most likely to ensure that patients get the quality of imaging services they deserve. It will help screen out marginal facilities that should probably not be providing imaging services, as well as raise the bar for the entire industry.

## Promoting Team-Based Imaging Services

Chapters 7 and 9 discussed how emerging imaging technologies and organizational changes are altering the traditional boundaries among medical disciplines. Imaging innovations are opening the door to broader adoption by multiple professional disciplines of tools that were initially developed in radiology. Indeed,

---

[3] Quality accreditation for hospital outpatient and inpatient services is the purview of the Joint Commission on Accreditation for Healthcare Organizations (JCAHO).

some components of what is presently radiology may end up being housed in entirely new disciplines — like interventional medicine or molecular diagnosis and therapy.

Inevitably, the reorganization of medical disciplines involves professional conflict and may raise questions in patients' minds about where they can receive the best care. The best care is provided when practitioners with overlapping knowledge work in teams that harness the best of what each physician offers to arrive at the appropriate diagnosis and course of treatment.

Cancer care is the best example of complementary multidiscipinary care in contemporary medicine. In the best cancer centers — like M.D. Anderson and Memorial Sloan Kettering cancer centers — patient care is provided by multidisciplinary teams. Medical oncologists, surgical oncologists, diagnostic and interventional radiologists, surgeons, radiation therapists, and allied health personnel work in seamless coordination based on agreed-upon clinical protocols. Cutting-edge cancer care requires that all the actors involved in diagnosis and treatment work from the same script and that the results can be accurately evaluated. Economic conflict is minimized at many of these centers by paying physicians salaries based on nationally established competitive norms for their specialties.

Radiologists are increasingly subspecializing, furthering their participation in this type of multidisciplinary care. The trend toward subspecialization is an irresistible product of broadening and deepening scientific knowledge about disease. The trend toward subspecialization in radiology recognizes that no individual, no matter how dedicated or intelligent, can master the vast amount of knowledge required to be an expert in all organ systems and all fields of medical imaging. Subspecialization will inevitably result in more intensive fellowship training of future radiologists in organ-specific anatomy, physiology, and biochemistry at both the gross and molecular levels.

Subspecialization should lead to closer collaboration with professional disciplines that have viewed radiology as a competitive threat — and vice versa. The challenge to radiology will be to resist its ingrained combative reflex in the name of defending its historical economic franchise. Patients are unnerved by intraprofessional disputes. They expect the clinical team to work together to resolve their problems. Failure to collaborate will eventually damage medicine's legitimacy in the eyes of those it serves and make it easier for populist politicians to impose regulatory schemes that damage patient care.

Unfortunately, the contemporary fee-for-service payment system reinforces fragmented practice models that inhibit team medicine. The fee-for-service model pays each practitioner separately and separates professional fees from facility charges (technical fees). The oddities of the traditional fee-based payment model have fostered economic competition among disciplines and, by doing so, have encouraged fragmented care.

Some in the policy community have proposed that the fee-for-service system be replaced by a system that would bundle (e.g., make a single unified) payment to a facility and all practitioners involved in an episode of illness as the means of fostering more collaborative care. Under a bundled payment system, all those participating in an episode of illness (from diagnosis through treatment and recovery or rehabilitation) would draw from a fixed, shared pool of funding. Under this system, physicians involved in an episode of care would be compelled to develop a script defining precisely the role of each clinical contributor, as well as a payment logic for compensating each of them. This script and payment logic would be created through inevitably contentious and difficult negotiation within and among hospital systems, physician groups, or community-based health plans.

This idea is worth exploring. However, it could take a decade or more of experimentation and evaluation research to see if bundled payments actually encourage cooperation in the delivery of care, improve clinical outcomes, make providers' compensation any more rational, and save money before the idea is ready for prime time.

In the meantime, it is possible that greater transparency and public disclosure could lead to patient convergence on diagnostic and therapeutic centers that encourage multidisciplinary care. If patients with cardiac issues, for example, better understood the potential benefit to them, they might freely choose a cardiac *center of excellence* where cardiologists, radiologists, and cardiac surgeons work closely together as a team rather than a closed cardiology practice or a freestanding imaging center. Health insurers could encourage this migration by forgiving the deductible for patients who consult insurer-certified centers of this type. Insurers could also elect to pay higher fees to practitioners who agree to participate in these coordinated activities.

Beyond team care, new payment approaches that encourage more convenient, less expensive single-session care might save money on unnecessary testing and hospitalization. As a part of a system of *value-based payments*, such care—which combined diagnosis and intervention in a single session—could receive added compensation in recognition of its contributions to safety and convenience and its reduction of total care expenditures. As illustrated by the hypothetical Omniscient technology described in Chapter 9, if new technologies emerge that reduce overall health care expenditures and provide greater convenience for patients, they should receive higher fees to encourage their future development and incorporation into practice.

Imagine if it were possible to diagnose and solve a threatening clinical problem, like a tumor or an unstable and threatening coronary plaque or bleeding in the abdominal cavity, in a single session without the use of anesthesia, invasive surgery, postoperative recovery, or a hospital stay. Wouldn't it be worth it to patients and society to pay a single, more generous global fee for the clinical team and facility than a group of separate fees for multiple sessions?

Similarly, there are single-session opportunities in acute care that fall uncomfortably in the gray zone between an outpatient procedure and inpatient hospitalization. Patients who arrive in the emergency room with unexplained abdominal pain, for example, will not only receive high-technology scanning but also may be treated with either image-guided interventional techniques or immediate surgical intervention in the same suite in which the diagnosis takes place. This type of acute intervention is actually a new type of medical service—not inpatient yet not strictly outpatient—importantly facilitated by imaging. The MR or CT scan is the pivotal event in determining the diagnosis and, in many circumstances, provides guidance for the treatment procedure.

A prominent contemporary example now under multicenter clinical investigation, as well as being offered as a clinical service in many emergency rooms, is the *triple rule-out CTA* for patients presenting with chest pain. If CTA can determine, less expensively and more effectively than the current multi-test and observation approach, that the source of the chest pain is a life-threatening heart attack, dissecting aneurysm, or pulmonary embolus (blood clot in the arteries to the lung), then it should be paid for more generously.

Even with bundled payments, there is still the moral hazard issue of inappropriate overuse leading to unnecessary downstream testing and treatment. Using the triple rule-out CTA example, more patients might get referred for the imaging exam than really need it because of the incentive proffered by the higher payment. In the parlance of health policy, there might be *indication creep*—patients who wouldn't normally qualify might begin to receive the procedure. Ultimately, we may be driven to accept that moral hazard is an inescapable fact of medical practice and focus our efforts on containing its worst abuses by using some of the other strategies— certification, tightened fraud and abuse provisions, and so on—discussed above.

## The Sorcerer's Apprentice Revisited

In the "Sorcerer's Apprentice" segment of the Disney film *Fantasia,* the wizard sternly reprimanded his assistant for playing with serious magic and sent him back to his chambers to clean up. Over the past three decades, advanced imaging has presented a classic example of how near-magical technologies have overmatched the ability of health care organizations and the payment system to use them as efficiently as the times demand. Our societal apprenticeship in learning to make responsible use of modern imaging technology has clearly not been completed.

Imaging and the professionals who employ it have made great contributions to the improvement of our health. Imaging science has enormous future potential to save both lives and money. Innumerable advances in imaging that could improve patient care are queued up in the development pipeline. To enjoy the fruits of imaging innovation in the future, it is essential to figure out how more efficiently to translate into medical practice the most valuable technologies and shelve the ones that are duplicative and wasteful.

How to use these powerful tools more thoughtfully and pay for them in a way that fosters continued technical and care delivery innovation is one of the most difficult challenges facing medicine over the next two decades. If caregivers and policymakers can remain optimistic and work together, they'll ultimately get it right.

## References

Barringer F. Health courts: a better approach to malpractice reform. *BNA Health Law Reporter,* 2005. http://commongood.org/healthcare-reading-cgpubs-opeds-43.html. Accessed December 17, 2009.

Daschle T, Lambrew JM, Greenberger SS. *Critical: What We Can Do about the Health-Care Crisis.* New York: Thomas Dunne Books, 2008.

Tunis SR, Pearson SD. Coverage options for promising technologies: Medicare's "coverage with evidence development." *Health Aff.* 2006;25:1218–1230.

# Index

Note: Page numbers followed by "*f*" and "*t*" denote figures and tables, respectively. Number following an "*n*" denotes the note number on the corresponding page.